While it is true Christopher Columbus might never have discovered the "New World" if he'd had a guidebook, it's also true that few of us have the gumption or wherewithal to spend two years wondering where it is we are wandering. Thankfully, Marcus Woolf has done more than enough wandering for all of us and the result is a wonderfully engaging guidebook that ensures your explorations of Atlanta's many wild and less wild trails are well planned and memorable for the right reasons.

—Michael Hodgson,
President of SNEWS, the premier trade website and magazine for the outdoor industry

If you have spirit and gumption to hit the trails, but maybe not the time to spend all day looking for them, this book is for you. Woolf's comprehensive guide will not only get you on some of the finest trails in the Southeast but will also prime you for deeper forays into the vast wilderness just beyond your Atlanta doorstep.

As an outdoor photographer, I have often asked Woolf for tips on this or that hiking area, since I know he has been to all of them. As a rock climber, I can also appreciate the inclusion of some great cliffs and boulderfields in this book—areas that can add diversity and adventure to the Atlanta hiker's experience.

—Andrew Kornylak,
outdoor photographer, climber, and Atlanta resident

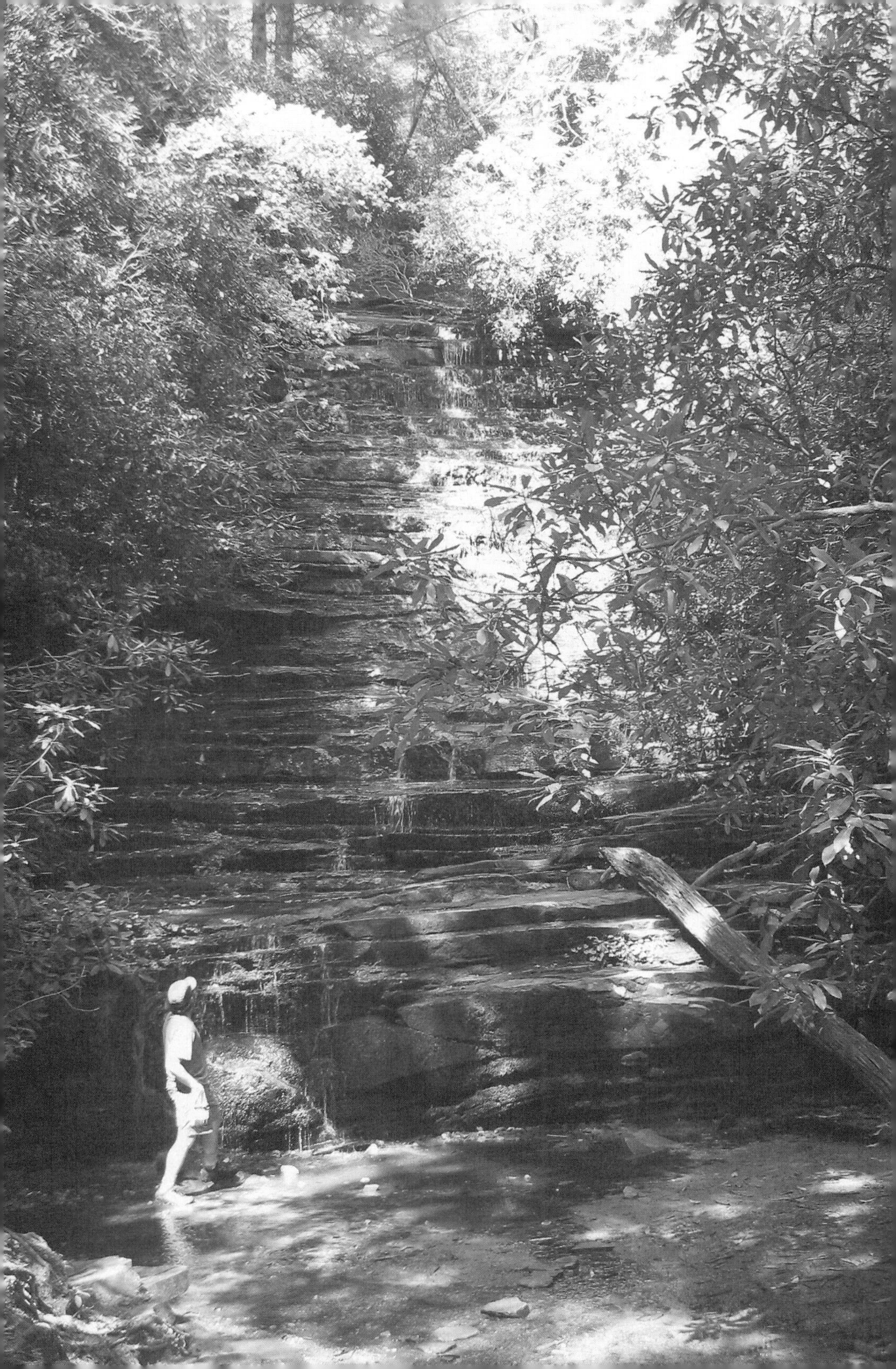

Afoot & Afield

Atlanta

A comprehensive hiking guide

Marcus Woolf

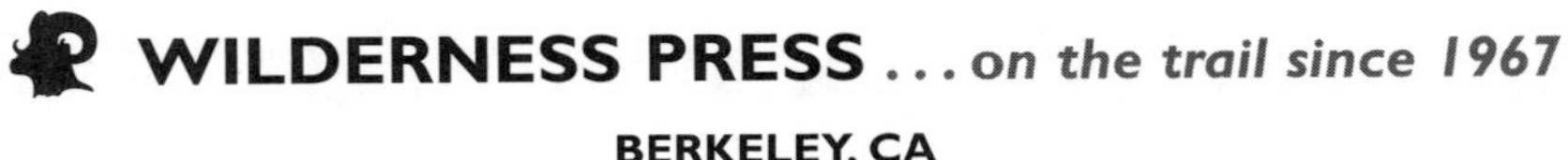

WILDERNESS PRESS . . . on the trail since 1967

BERKELEY, CA

Afoot & Afield Atlanta: A Comprehensive Hiking Guide

1st EDITION 2009

Front cover photo copyright © 2009 by Pat and Chuck Blackley
Interior photos, except where noted: Marcus Woolf
Maps: Bart Wright, Lohnes + Wright
Cover design: Andreas Schueller and Larry B. Van Dyke
Book design and layout: Andreas Schueller and Larry B. Van Dyke
Book editor: Laura Shauger

ISBN 978-0-89997-415-6

Manufactured in the United States of America

Published by: **Wilderness Press**
1345 8th Street
Berkeley, CA 94710
(800) 443-7227; FAX (510) 558-1696
info@wildernesspress.com
www.wildernesspress.com

Visit our website for a complete listing of our books and for ordering information.

Cover photo: A hiker at the junction of West Rim and Overlook trails in Cloudland Canyon State Park (Chapter 1: Trip 7)
Frontispiece: Panther Falls, Rabun Beach Recreation Area (Chapter 3: Trip 28)

SAFETY NOTICE: Although Wilderness Press and the author have made every attempt to ensure that the information in this book is accurate at press time, they are not responsible for any loss, damage, injury, or inconvenience that may occur to anyone while using this book. You are responsible for your own safety and health while in the wilderness. The fact that a trail is described in this book does not mean that it will be safe for you. Be aware that trail conditions can change from day to day. Always check local conditions, know your own limitations, and consult a map.

For Evan

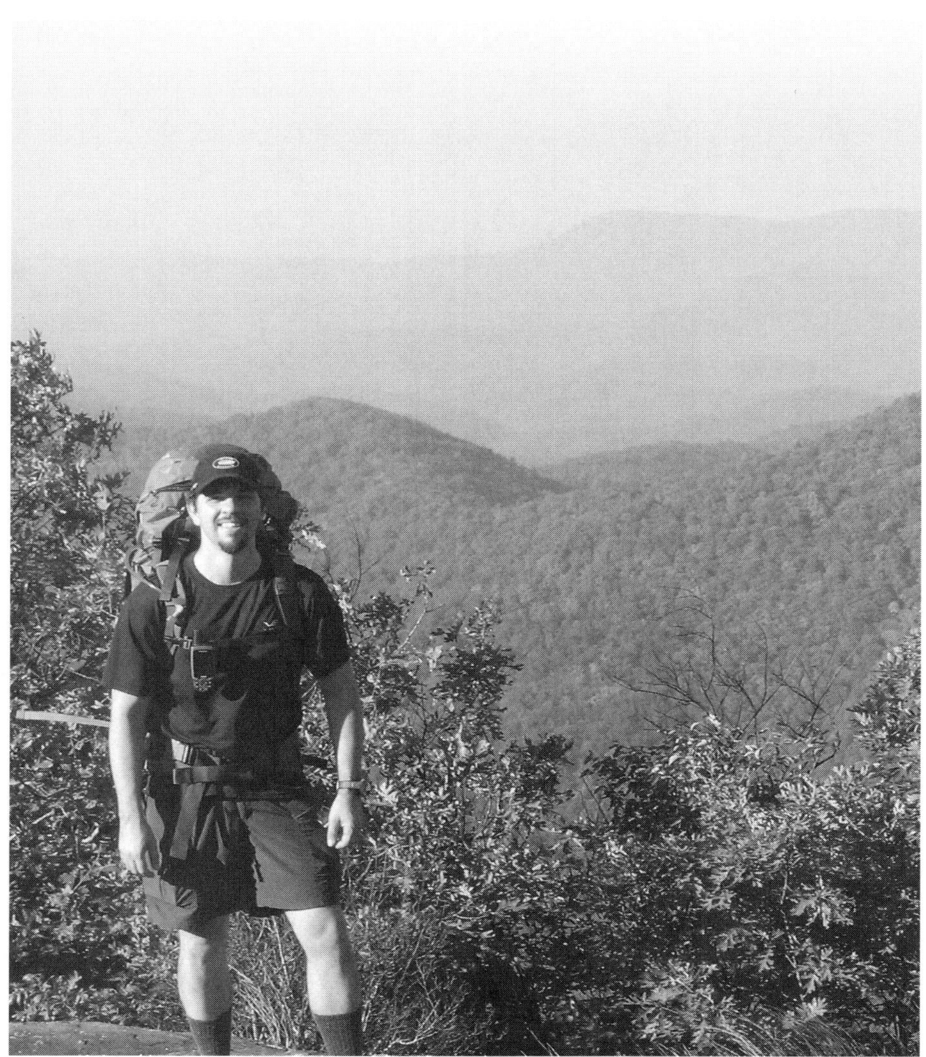

Author backpacking on the Appalachian Trail (Chapter 3: Trip 2)

Acknowledgments

The generosity and kindness of many people made this book possible. I would first like to thank my parents, brother, and grandfather whose love and support was the greatest thing I carried on each hike. Big thanks to Tom, Joe, Andy, and Karen who accompanied me on trails and pushed that measuring wheel. Much gratitude goes to Michael Hodgson, who has guided me in my journey to be an outdoor writer, as well as to Wendy Geister whose support is invaluable. Thanks Rob and Tigree for sharing your home.

Personnel with Georgia State Parks, the U.S. Forest Service, National Park Service, Georgia Department of Natural Resources, and other organizations provided critical information for the book. Special thanks to Forest Service members David Kirkindall, Larry Luckett, and Larry Thomas. There is probably no greater source of information concerning Chattahoochee River history than National Park Service Ranger Jerry Hightower. And I thank Chris Hughes of the Chattahoochee River National Recreation Area for supplying me with its Historic Resource Study.

Researching Georgia battlefields was a highlight of working on this project, and two great sources of knowledge were Interpretive Park Ranger Rebecca Karcher and Park Ranger Jim Staub of Chickamauga Battlefield.

Also, a big round of applause to all the people working to educate the public about Georgia's natural resources, such as Sandy Straw, naturalist with the Len Foote Hike Inn. And another round to organizations such as the Georgia Appalachian Trail Club and its volunteers who put in all the hard hours to maintain trails and ensure that we can have quality experiences outdoors.

Thanks to Kris Wagner of *Backpacker* magazine and to James Dziezynski and Brian Beffort for showing me the ropes on documenting trails. Also, thanks to Giff Beaton for contributing his birding expertise.

And thanks to Roslyn, Laura, and the team at Wilderness Press for giving me this opportunity and showing great patience.

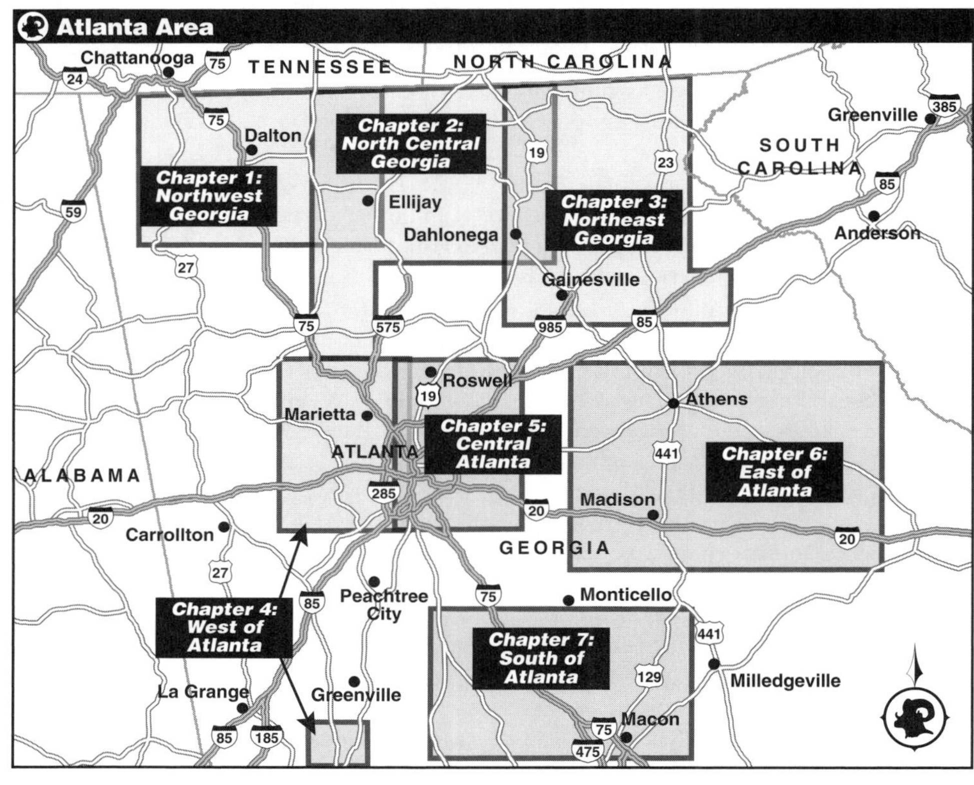
Atlanta Area
Chattanooga
TENNESSEE
NORTH CAROLINA
Dalton
Chapter 1: Northwest Georgia
Chapter 2: North Central Georgia
Ellijay
Dahlonega
Chapter 3: Northeast Georgia
Greenville
SOUTH CAROLINA
Anderson
Gainesville
Roswell
Marietta
ATLANTA
Chapter 5: Central Atlanta
Athens
Chapter 6: East of Atlanta
ALABAMA
Madison
Carrollton
GEORGIA
Peachtree City
Monticello
Chapter 4: West of Atlanta
Chapter 7: South of Atlanta
Milledgeville
La Grange
Greenville
Macon
24
75
59
27
575
985
85
19
23
385
441
285
20
129
185
475

Contents

Preface

"You better eat your Wheaties." I will never forget that park ranger's warning, spoken so many years ago. He was trying to warn my high school buddies and me that the trail we were about to attempt was pretty difficult. Of course, we paid no attention to him—hey, we were teenagers—and carrying little knowledge of what lay ahead, we stormed up the path. Hours later, several exhausted 16-year-olds lay strewn about a campsite, too whipped to whip up dinner. Our disregard for the ranger, and our failure to educate ourselves about the trail, led to much misery. These days we laugh about it, but nobody was laughing at the end of that hard day.

That experience really taught me the value of using guidebooks and other sources to actually *plan* a trip. A major motivation for writing this book was to help others avoid such trouble and truly enjoy their time while exploring trails surrounding Atlanta. My involvement in the project resulted from my experience serving as a GPS mapping correspondent for *Backpacker* magazine. Through this work, I not only learned the finer points of documenting a trail but I also encountered a great number of people from Atlanta who were new to hiking. Curious as to why I was scribbling in a notebook on the trail, they would often approach me and strike up conversations. And mostly, folks just wanted clear and concise information on good places where they could hike. This book is an extension of those conversations. My hope was to point people toward the places that I love to visit, and provide them with good information—but not overwhelm them—to help them easily plan an outdoor excursion and be prepared to travel safely.

I have included the majority of the available trails within a couple hours' drive of Atlanta, but in deciding what to leave in and what to omit, I focused on including those that are most enjoyable. I eliminated some areas where trails have become overgrown and very difficult to navigate. Some chapters, such as those concerning the Cohutta Wilderness and the Appalachian Trail, serve as a primer, offering details on selected hikes that will familiarize you with the area. Although the Georgia Pinhoti Trail is not included in this first edition, it will likely be covered in a future edition.

Occasionally I have flavored trip descriptions with my experiences while hiking, but be aware that you could have a very different experience, depending on weather and other variables. One of the best things you can carry on the trail is a flexible frame of mind—that and basic knowledge of the terrain and environment. It always helps to know if you need to eat your Wheaties.

All of these trail descriptions come with one important caveat: You'll probably have a better time if you avoid hiking during peak travel days. The population of the Atlanta metro area has exploded in the past 20 years, so on a warm spring Saturday, popular trails resemble Interstate 285 at rush hour. Granted, work and other responsibilities relegate most hiking to the weekends, but if you can arrange to hike on a weekday, you will be rewarded. That campsite you love so much will probably be unoccupied, and you could have that swimming hole with the waterfall to yourself for a little while.

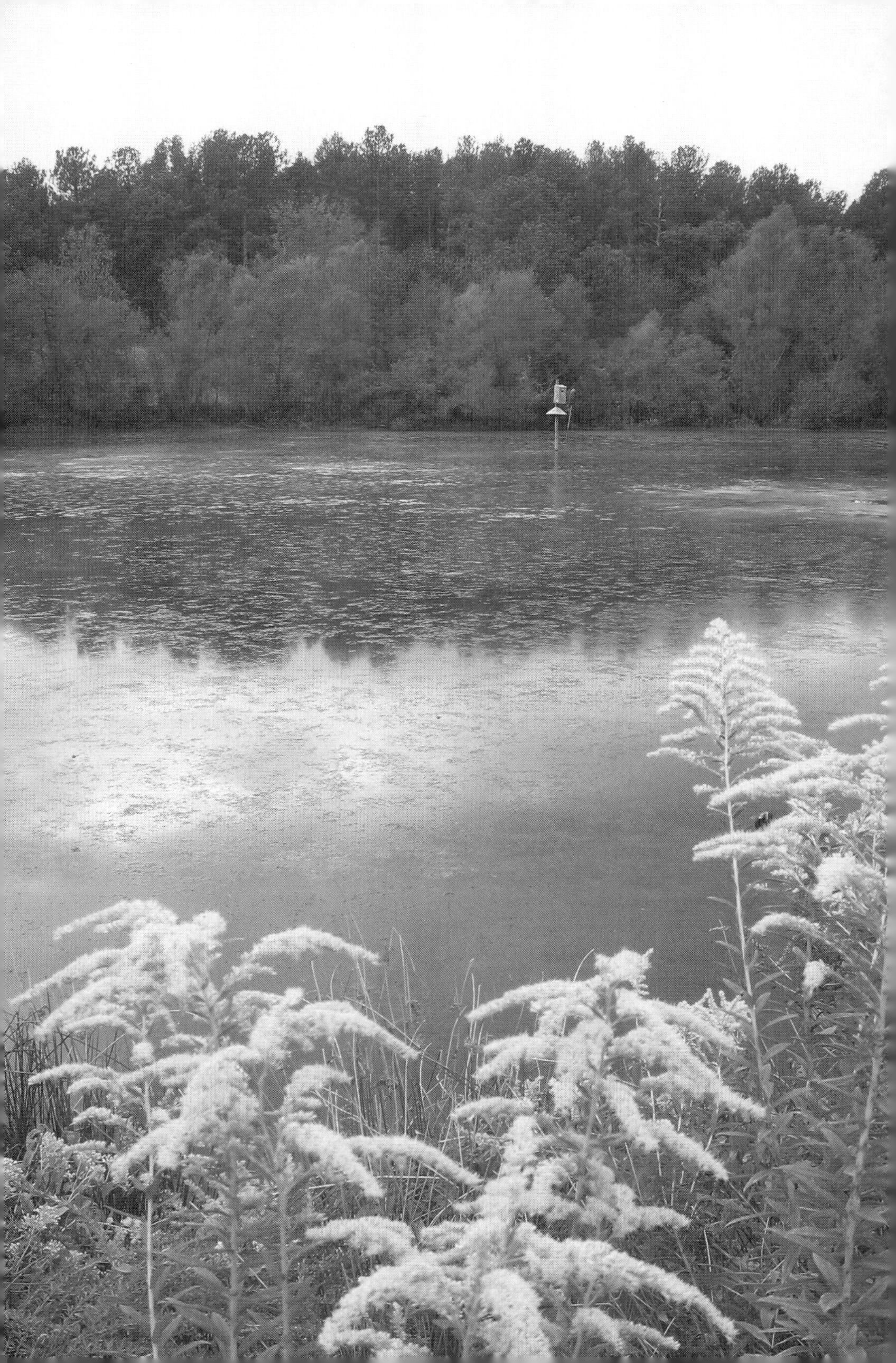

Introducing the Atlanta Area

Since the year 2000, Atlanta's metro area population has skyrocketed to include more than 5 million residents, and the 2007 U.S. Census Bureau declared that Atlanta was the fastest-growing city in the country. This explosive population growth and accompanying urban sprawl have obviously affected the number of natural areas where Atlanta residents can escape the congested world of concrete to walk in peaceful, green corridors. Each day, 55 acres of land are developed in the Atlanta area, according to the latest Georgia Statewide Comprehensive Outdoor Recreation Plan (2008–2013), but city and state officials have recognized that the lack of recreation land poses a serious risk not only to the health of the environment but also to the well-being of Atlantans.

Within the last 10 years parks and recreation departments for cities and counties have shifted their focus from constructing "high infrastructure" sites, such as ballparks, to creating green space and preserving wetlands. Georgia Governor Sonny Perdue has called for the state to create its first comprehensive land conservation plan where the state, private sector, and local governments and institutions would work to conserve natural spaces. This plan would help protect animal populations and habitats, preserve water sources, and create places for people to exercise, relax, and escape from the pressures of the city. The City of Atlanta is investigating one especially ambitious proposal, the BeltLine project, which would convert (over 25 years) a 22-mile rail corridor around the city into a continuous system of greenways. Should the project succeed it would relieve some pressure from one of Atlanta's most popular destination, the Chattahoochee River National Recreation Area.

Each year, about 3.5 million people visit the Chattahoochee River NRA's 13 park units that include 4500 acres along the Chattahoochee River. It includes 50 miles of trails that run through pine and hardwood forest and follow the banks of a 48-mile stretch of the river. A major destination for hikers, birders, anglers, kayakers and folks out for a midday walk, the river corridor supports a wide range of wildlife, such as foxes and deer, and you have a good chance of seeing a great blue heron soaring over the Chattahoochee.

As the greenways near Atlanta become crowded, more hikers are venturing beyond the metro area to explore Georgia trails. There's an abundance of forestland, parks, and other quiet woods within a two-hour drive of Atlanta. An amazing thing about Georgia is the sheer variety of landscapes that can be explored—within a

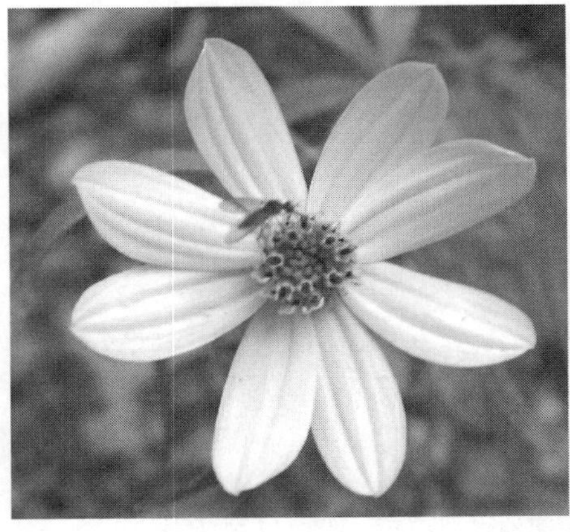

Arrowhead Wildlife Interpretive Trail (Chapter 1: Trip 14)

morning's drive, there are at least a dozen state parks that boast vast lakes, wetlands, forests of wildflowers, and high peaks with inspiring views. Also within reach of Atlanta are fascinating geologic formations, such as the vast granite outcrop at Panola Mountain State Park southeast of the city. As if you are stepping back in time, you can kneel down on the rocky slab to spy tiny plants that represent the earliest stage of forest life.

While the granite slabs at Panola hold almost hidden treasures, you can find grand displays of nature in the mountains of north Georgia. Spanning nearly the entire northern portion of the state, the Chattahoochee National Forest covers 750,000 acres with lofty peaks, deep river ravines, and broad, green valleys. Within the national forest, there are wildlife management areas devoted to conserving habitat, as well as parks that preserve the state's most impressive features, such as 2-mile-long and thousand-foot-deep Tallulah Gorge. Of the hundreds of miles of trails in north Georgia, there's a hike to suit every desire. You can take a brief walk through exotic forest of rhododendron and mountain laurel to a roaring waterfall or shoulder a daypack for a vigorous trek to Georgia's highest point at 4784 feet. If you're new to backpacking, places such as Vogel State Park provide easy access to backcountry trails that are perfect for an overnight trip. The Appalachian Trail (AT) in Georgia has several access points, allowing you to hike a section in a weekend, while experienced hikers can string together a multiday journey along the AT, or hike other long trails such as the Benton MacKaye.

A jewel of the Chattahoochee National Forest lies in the northwest section of the state. With 36,977 acres of mountainous terrain, the Cohutta Wilderness is a top choice if you wish to delve more deeply into remote forest. From high ridges of hardwoods and pines, you can descend into shaded groves of great hemlocks and deep cuts where wild rivers cut through the rugged landscape.

Georgia is blessed with great tracts of land where Atlantans can enjoy respite from the things of man. But equally intriguing are the paths that trace Georgia's human history. The Kennesaw

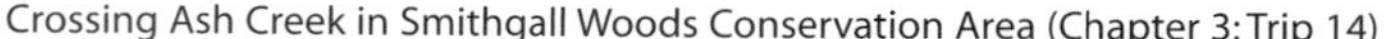

Crossing Ash Creek in Smithgall Woods Conservation Area (Chapter 3: Trip 14)

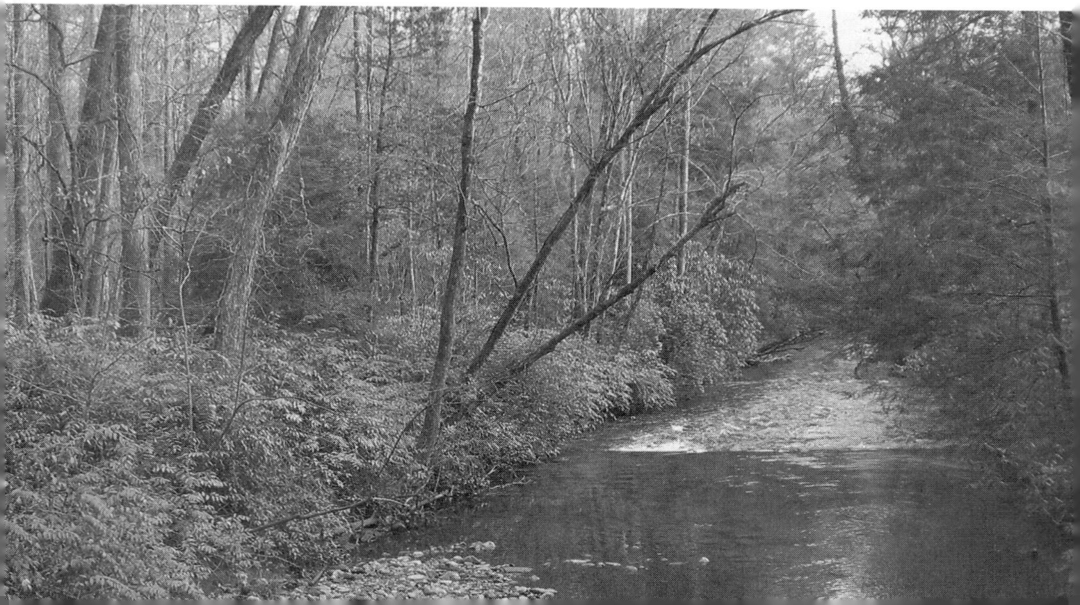

Mountain National Battlefield Park west of Atlanta has well-maintained trails with interpretive signs explaining one of the heaviest battles pitched during the Atlanta Campaign of the Civil War. A little farther west, the rolling woods of Pickett's Mill Battlefield have been preserved almost as they were when Union and Confederate troops clashed in a rare night battle. While there are no historical plaques or markers dotting the battlefield, the undulating terrain and dense woodlands are natural monuments and reminders of how Georgia's landscape made fighting extremely difficult. You'll have a very different experience walking the Chickamauga Battlefield near the border with Tennessee. One of the Civil War's deadliest battles was fought in the low fields and woodlands of Chickamauga, and the battlefield is replete with all manner of historical markers, from tablets to large, elaborate stone monuments. Documenting the action in remarkable detail, some markers note the specific hours that troops held certain plots of ground.

Another important aspect of Georgia's history is the effort to harness rivers to operate mills and generate power. In the early 1800s, settlers as well as Cherokee set up gristmills and sawmills along Georgia rivers and creeks. You can learn more about mill history by hiking Sweetwater Creek State Park southwest of Atlanta. Built in 1849, this mill—like so many others in Georgia—was burned by Union troops during the Civil War. In the late 1880s and early 1900s, work began to convert mills to generate power and meet the state's growing demand for electricity. One of the more high-profile projects was construction of the Morgan Falls Dam on the Chattahoochee River to feed a hydroelectric plant. And the Vickery Creek trails near Roswell explore this area where the Roswell Manufacturing Company operated one of the South's most important plants. But the industrial revolution was not confined to the Atlanta area. Watson Mill Bridge State Park east of Athens has trails that lead to the ruins of a hydroelectric plant that began operating near the South Fork River in 1905.

In the grand scheme of things, this is also recent history, as people have occupied Georgia for 10,000 years. To understand the full breadth of human history in Georgia, drive south to the Ocmulgee National Monument near Macon and stroll among the remains of a village where Native Americans constructed great earth mounds. You can view a meeting room in the reconstructed Earthlodge and climb to the summit of the Great Temple Mound to look over neighboring wetlands. Visitors should take time to visit Ocmulgee Monument's excellent museum, which chronicles human habitation on the site, from the Clovis people of the most recent ice age to settlers who established a trading post in the 1600s to exchange goods with the Creek Indians.

From Native American settlements to Civil War battlefields, lush riverbanks and wild and remote wilderness, Georgia trails traverse a great variety of landscapes and environments. Atlanta residents are truly blessed to have within reach such a broad spectrum of natural places to explore. As the Atlanta population continues to boom, people are learning to value green spaces where they can enjoy peaceful moments, reflect on the past, or simply clear their minds of city noise. The word *recreation* implies that this is a way to re-create yourself. A hike can bring calmness and clarity to your life, improve your physical and mental health, and open your eyes to a better understanding of the world around you.

Climate

The north and central regions of Georgia experience four true seasons, with mid- to late spring and fall being the optimum times to explore the outdoors. Early spring is the wettest season, and the northern mountains see temperature highs in the 60s and lows in the 30s and 40s. Early spring in the central region brings highs in the upper 60s and lower 70s and lows in the 40s and lower 50s. In mid- and late spring, north Georgia enjoys highs in the 70s and lows in the 50s, perfect for hiking and camping. During this period, temperatures in central Georgia can reach into the 80s while lows hover in the 60s.

Another prime hiking time is October, usually the driest month. In northern Georgia, fall temperatures climb to highs of 70s and 80s and drop into the 40s and 50s at night. For the central part of the state, highs in the fall range from upper 60s to upper 70s, while lows range from the low 40s to low 50s.

January tends to be the coldest month for north and central Georgia, with the mountains experiencing an average high of 49°F and an average low of 26°F. From January to March, the highs in central Georgia can range from the low 50s to the mid- and upper 60s, and sunny, winter days make for great hiking. Occasionally, a polar air mass will swing through, and the northern mountains will get hit with snowfall plus temperatures well below freezing. Still, a traveler can experience relatively mild days in winter, and the lack of foliage allows views of surrounding landscape that you simply won't get in spring, summer, and fall.

Throughout the northern and central regions, summers in Georgia are hot and humid, with highs in the 90s and lows in the 70s. The mountains can be 8 to 10 degrees cooler than lower regions in summer, but the humidity is still a factor. You'll find fewer travelers along the trails in July and August, when it's nice to hike next to a river, stream, or lake where you can swim to cool down.

Georgia receives moderate to heavy precipitation, about 40 to 50 inches per year, with the amount of rainfall generally even throughout the year. Rainfall amounts are higher in the upper elevations, and the mountains in the northeast can get 75 inches of precipitation in a year. In 2007, Georgia suffered severe drought with Atlanta receiving only 31.85 inches and Athens a mere 31.51 inches. Towns such as Helen and Hiawassee in north Georgia fared better, getting 45 to 50 inches of rain. As of September 2008, Atlanta had received 30.17 inches of rain, about 5 inches less than normally received by then. Many trails in this book were hiked during 2007 and 2008, when backcountry travel required careful thought and planning as stream flows were unpredictable. You will likely not have to be as careful, but you should still carry an ample water supply at all times.

A final climate consideration for outdoor travel is severe weather, especially tornadoes. In north and central Georgia, a tornado can strike anytime, but the greatest activity occurs from April to June.

Geology

The area of Georgia covered in this book includes four geologic zones: Valley and Ridge in northwest Georgia, the Blue Ridge in the northeast, Piedmont in the central area of the state, and the Fall Line separating the Piedmont from the Coastal Plain.

VALLEY AND RIDGE

As its name suggests, the Valley and Ridge area in northwest Georgia is comprised of a series of ridges and valleys that generally run from northeast to southwest. In the Paleozoic Era, this land was the bed of a shallow sea, and the landscape is comprised of limestone, sandstone, shale, and coal. Near the end of the Paleozoic Era, two tectonic plates collided, and metamorphic rock was pushed up and over sedimentary stone in northwest Georgia. This process bent the land into large folds, and a ripple effect to the northeast formed the Appalachian Mountains. Over time, erosion created what we see today—long ridges covered mostly with pine and oak forest and valleys between that serve as pastureland and farm fields.

BLUE RIDGE

The north-central and northeast regions of Georgia lie within the southern boundary of the Blue Ridge zone, which extends to Virginia. Millions of years ago, sheets of the earth's crust were compressed, thrust upward, and stacked to form the dramatic mountains ranging from 2000 feet to nearly 5000 feet in elevation. Here is Georgia's high point, Brasstown Bald, and towering peaks such as Yonah Mountain. The land in the eastern portion of Georgia's Blue Ridge is primarily comprised of igneous and metamorphic rock, such as granite and quartzite. Geologic activity in this region also formed deposits of marble, as well as the Gold Belt, which runs from the Alabama border to Lumpkin and White counties in northeast Georgia.

PIEDMONT PLATEAU

Atlanta, Athens, and the majority of Georgia's population lie within the Piedmont zone, which runs across the belly of the state, between the Valley and Ridge and Blue Ridge zones to the north and the Coastal Plain to the south. This region is mostly comprised of rolling hills, though faults in the southwestern Piedmont created Pine Mountain, which rises dramatically amid the surrounding lowlands. The rocks in the Piedmont zone are primarily igneous and metamorphic, which have weathered to form the red clay that is known so well in the state. This region also includes igneous granite, which makes up Stone Mountain and Panola Mountain near Atlanta. Important natural resources in the Piedmont include the Chattahoochee River, which follows the ancient Brevard Fault Zone that runs from Alabama to North Carolina. The Piedmont area was once a region of thriving oak and hickory forest, but the removal of timber and farming of cotton and tobacco have left the area largely covered in pines.

FALL LINE

This geologic boundary stretching from Columbus to Augusta separates Georgia's Piedmont and Upper Coastal Plain. It is dubbed the Fall Line because, as you move inland from the Coastal

Winding among the Rocktown boulders (Chapter 1: Trip 11)

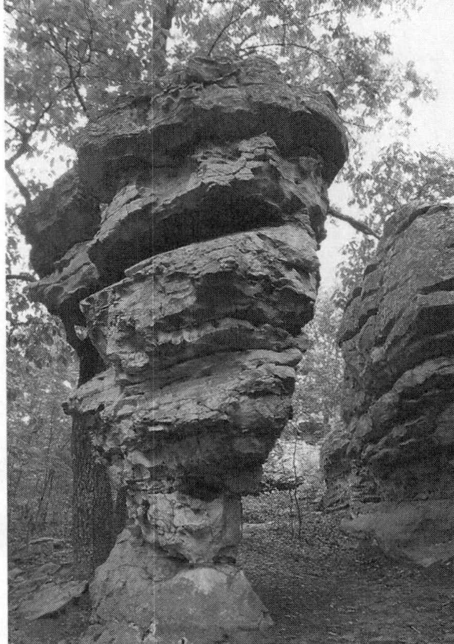

Plain, this is the first place you meet river rapids and waterfalls. Here, waterways such as the Ocmulgee River in Macon drop from the upland areas of metamorphic rock and clay soil into the lower landscape of the Coastal Plain, which is made up of sedimentary rock and sandy soil. In Georgia's early days, the Fall Line created a natural barrier for river navigation, and goods transported on rivers in the Coastal Plain had to be off-loaded at the Fall Line and transferred to other transports to be carried upstate. This exchange led to the development of cities, such as Columbus, Macon, and Augusta, on the Fall Line.

Forests

With more than 24 million acres of forestland, Georgia has the largest area of forest of any southern state. About half of the state's forests are primarily pine, while a third of the forestland is covered with hardwoods and the rest is a mix of pines and hardwoods.

OAK-HICKORY FOREST

The north Georgia mountains fall into the oak-hickory forest classification. Here you will find a wide variety of oaks such as white, chestnut, red, scarlet, and black. Some of the hickory species include shagbark, bitternut, and pignut. North Georgia's mountain slopes and stream basins are also home to hemlocks, which can grow to be 100 feet tall with trunks 4 feet in diameter. You'll see sweet birch as well in the hardwood coves of the mountains. Moist mountain areas support black cherry as well as butternut trees, which produce a fruit with a hairy yellow-green hull. Red maples grow on the slopes and in the valleys of the mountain region (and are also common in the Piedmont). One prominent tree in the region is the sourwood, with trunks that sometimes bend at great angles. Older sourwood trees have bark that resembles alligator skin with deep furrows.

Whether you're hiking in the Valley and Ridge, Blue Ridge, or Piedmont

A clear view through the hardwoods on the Miller Trek Trail, Brasstown Valley Resort (Chapter 3: Trip 8)

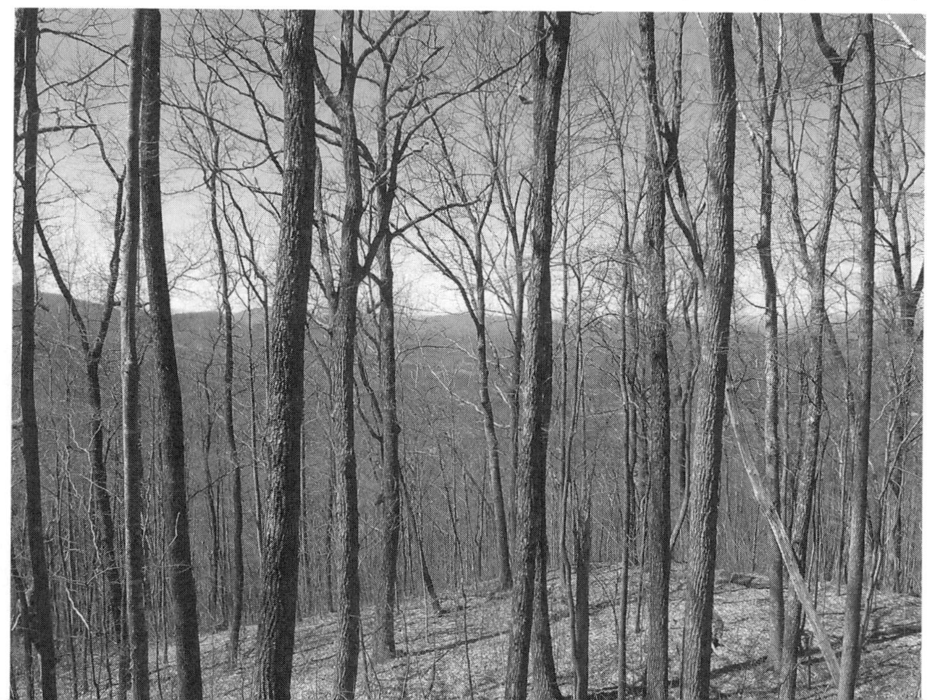

regions, you will notice a change in tree types in moist coves and along streambanks. River birch is common along streams and is identified by bark that peels off in curls. This is also the habitat for blue beech (20–30 feet high), as well as the much taller and often-seen American beech. This tree can be 80 feet high and has easily recognizable smooth, gray bark. Areas with moist soil in these parts of the state give life to Fraser magnolias, which have smooth, gray-brown bark and long, broad leaves that are green and glossy. In such regions, yellow poplars are common and grow to more than 100 feet in height. Yellow poplars have smooth bark that appears gray on older trees. In bottomlands and along streambanks, American sycamores can also be found.

PINES

A variety of pines also live throughout the state's northern and central regions. One type, the eastern white pine, tends to thrive in valleys and coves and has needles in clusters of five ranging from 3 to 5 inches long. In the upper reaches of the state, as well as the Piedmont, shortleaf pines can grow to be 100 feet tall. The yellow-green needles of the shortleaf pine are 3 to 5 inches long and grow in clusters of three. Living mostly on the high, dry ridges of northeast Georgia are pitch pines. They usually grow to about 50 feet in height, and in the early days of Georgia's settlement they were used to produce turpentine and charcoal.

The mountains and upper Piedmont support Virginia pines, which usually only reach about 40 feet high and are shorter than other pines. Their trunks appear orange-brown and often do not grow as straight as trunks of other pine species. Throughout the Piedmont loblolly pines, also known as southern yellow pines, are prominent. Loblolly pines have bark with deep furrows, and their needles are 6 to 9 inches long and appear in clusters of three.

PINE-HARDWOOD MIX

In the Piedmont, forests have a more even mix of pine and oak than in the upper mountains. Here, hardwoods such as black and red oak live among the various pine species, while water oak, often used for lumber, grows along streams in this region as well as the Coastal Plain.

The moist soil in the Piedmont's lowlands support the American elm as well. On trails in the Piedmont you'll likely see black walnut, which can be 100 feet high and produce a dark brown knot that grows within a yellow-green hull. Also common are sweetgum, which produces a spiked, round fruit that you'll see scattered along the trail. Residing in most parts of Georgia is the popular dogwood, which blooms in brilliant white or pink.

Plants & Wildflowers

The trails surrounding Atlanta are rich in plant life, with thousands of species too numerous to list here, but you will encounter several plants frequently that are worthy of mention. Some of the most beautiful forest areas in the northern mountains have thick groves of rhododendron, which bloom pink and white in late spring. Another member of the

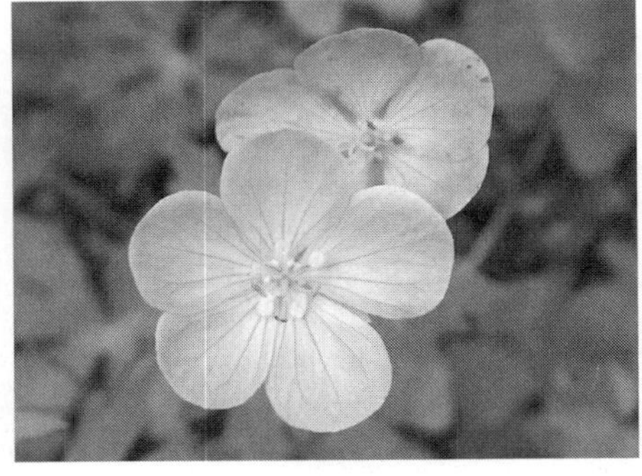

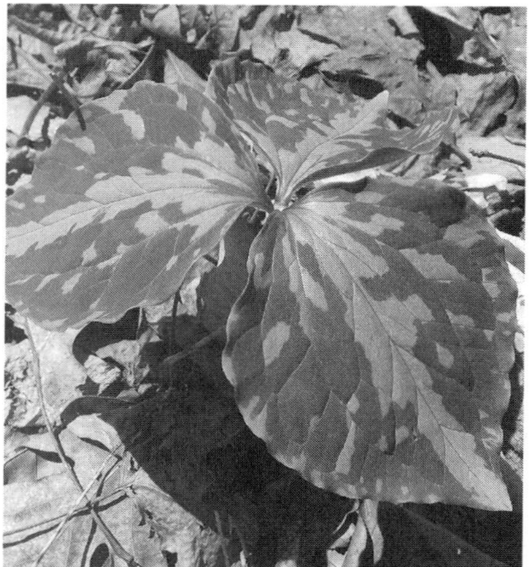
Trillium

rhododendron genus, flame azalea, is easily spotted in higher elevations, with its fiery orange blooms. Along the mountain slopes you will also encounter thickets of mountain laurel whose star-shaped flowers bloom pink and white from May to June. As you hike in Georgia's higher elevations you may encounter a strong, mucky odor; look to the sides of the trail to pick out heart-shaped galax, whose leaves turn red in winter. This plant was once harvested for holiday decorations. Other wildflower species of the Valley and Ridge and Blue Ridge areas include bloodroot, pink lady's slipper, trillium, May apple, and dwarf iris.

The woodlands of north Georgia are also rich in fern species. In areas with moist soil you can find rattlesnake ferns and large beds of New York ferns. Christmas ferns, which require drainage, tend to populate the mountain slopes.

Cinnamon ferns grow along streams and in swampy areas throughout Georgia, including the Piedmont region. Riverside trails in the Piedmont, such as those along the Chattahoochee River, are alive with violets, trillium, bloodroot, and Solomon's-seal.

A very different kind of Piedmont plant life can be found on the granite outcrops of Stone Mountain and Panola Mountain State Park. On the exposed slabs of rock, tiny diamorpha plants and other species grow in solution pits (small plots of shallow sand and soil). Some of these plants are nearly invisible without close inspection, and they represent the earliest stage of plant succession, whereby one plant community replaces another until the area reaches a climax, such as becoming a mature forest.

Animals

If you've never spooked a flock of wild turkey, you'd be surprised by the noise, as they explode from the trees like a gun blast. And if you have never watched deer grazing in an open field, you would be humbled by the peacefulness of that moment. Georgia trails provide excellent opportunities to observe birds, large mammals, reptiles, and other wildlife, whether you're exploring remote mountain trails or shepherding a child down a nature trail.

MAMMALS

At 2 AM one September night in the Cohutta Wilderness, I heard a gruff snort outside my tent. With the flick of a lantern switch, I could see the head and shoulders of a black bear on the other side of the mesh. Fortunately, my early morning visitor merely shuffled off. It was a heart-pounding moment to be sure, but also one of my favorite—nothing gets your head buzzing and heart racing like seeing a mammal in the wilderness. The forests of Georgia are the stomping grounds not only of black bears but also white-tailed deer, several species of bats, squirrels, mice, tiny shrews, raccoons, skunks, red foxes, and coyotes. I once saw an armadillo slip into a hole at the base of a tree while I was hiking a bottomland trail on Pine Mountain. And I faced the charge of an opossum while walking a path in northeast Georgia. (I took its hissing as a warning to not poach its dinner—a dead snake it had just dropped at the edge of the trail.) While an encounter with a large mammal (or short, stocky opossum) gets the adrenaline going, remember that you should view them with caution, but not necessarily as a threat. In my encounters with black bears I've found that if I call out to warn them of my presence and stand still for a few minutes, they will simply move on.

BIRDS

The state of Georgia is home to more than 300 species of birds, and several spots are considered good birding areas, such as F. D. Roosevelt State Park southwest of Atlanta, Kennesaw Mountain slightly northwest of the city, the Chattahoochee River National Recreation Area, and the state's northeast mountains.

The mountains in northeast Georgia are especially interesting as this is the southern terminus for some birds typically seen in more northern areas and not found elsewhere in Georgia. Georgia birding expert Giff Beaton identifies the trail up to the summit of Brasstown Bald as a great place to look for some of Georgia's highest-elevation breeders. "Here you might see veery and rose-breasted grosbeak, along with the more typical mountain species," he says. "Watch and listen above for the croaking of common ravens, which have a nest near here, and always watch above for hawks as well, since broad-winged hawks nest here too."

President F. D. Roosevelt was a birding enthusiast all his life, so it's fitting that the National Audubon Society has declared Pine Mountain (the location of F. D. Roosevelt State Park) a place of importance for birding. Beaton suspects that this high mountain range might also have northern species like scarlet tanager and ovenbird. Hardwood forests have other interesting species, such as summer tanager, wood thrush, great crested flycatcher, yellow-throated warbler, black-and-white warbler, plus red-eyed and yellow-throated vireo.

While hiking trails along the Chattahoochee River, look for migrants such as common yellowthroat, as well as wood ducks, great blue herons, and red-headed woodpeckers. In the Gold Branch unit

"Browse enclosure" along Non-Game Interpretive Trail, Moccasin Creek State Park (Chapter 3: Trip 23)

BROWSE EXCLOSURE
This wire cage is designed to demonstrate the grazing pressure exerted on this food plot by deer, turkeys, bears, rabbits, groundhogs and other wildlife. Large differences in forage height and plant composition inside and outside the cages indicate heavy use. Depending on the species of plant, the weather and alternate food sources, use is generally greatest in winter and early spring when native forage is dormant.

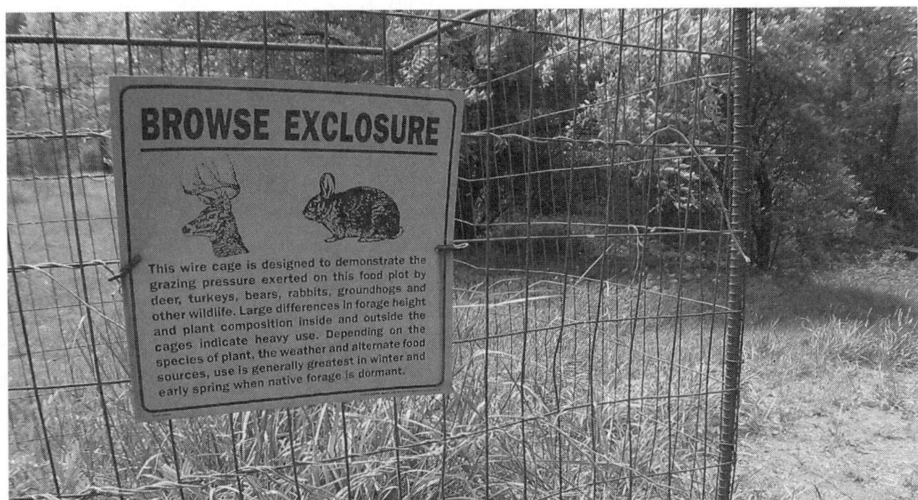

you might also see swans cruising across a river inlet.

Falcons and hawks can be seen soaring over the Kennesaw Mountain National Battlefield Park. And this is a prime spot to look for some 20 species of warblers.

Many hiking areas in the Piedmont region feature marshes and beaver ponds. In pretty much any pond habitat look year-round for waterbirds, breeding wood ducks, green herons, and red-winged blackbirds. In summer you might see swallows feeding on insects over the water.

AMPHIBIANS & REPTILES

There are about 30 species of frogs in Georgia, 12 of which inhabit the small ponds in Smithgall Woods near Cleveland. These include bellowing bullfrogs, the green "banjo" frog that makes a plucking sounds and the wood frog that sort of cackles. The American toad also inhabits Smithgall's wetlands. As you hike along the Chattahoochee River and other waterways in the Piedmont, look for the upland chorus frog, which is between ¾ and 1³/₈ inches long and has a brown or gray body. All across Georgia you can see the eastern box turtle. I have encountered them many places, from streamside trails at Pine Mountain to an elevation of 4000 feet on the Wagon Trail leading to the state's high point at Brasstown Bald.

Salamanders are another type of amphibian seen in Georgia wetlands. In northern areas, such as Moccasin Creek State Park near Clayton, look for the spotted salamander, which has a blue-black body with yellow spots and orange stripes on its back.

Dozens of reptile species live in the woodlands of north and central Georgia, including lizards, snakes, and turtles. A group of large snapping turtles inhabit the Big Pond in the Reynolds Nature Preserve south of Atlanta. They can grow to be more than a foot in length, and adult snapping turtles in the wild can weigh 10 to 30 pounds.

Georgia's various habitats support more than 40 species of venomous and nonvenomous snakes. The venomous copperhead has a stout body colored a dull brown and wrapped with bands the shape of an hourglass. Timber rattlesnakes make their home both on rocky slopes and swampy areas and have a gray or tan body with dark bands. The venomous cottonmouth, or water moccasin, lives in the wetlands and river habitats of Georgia's Piedmont. It has a thick body of brown, yellow, or almost black and dark bands. Cottonmouths can reach four feet in length and have a big, triangular head.

One of the most common species in Georgia is the nonvenomous rat snake. There are black, yellow, and gray varieties, and adults can be more than five feet long. (While working on this book, I encountered an impressive black rat snake some six feet long in the Chicopee Woods near Gainesville.) These snakes are constrictors and feed on squirrels, birds, mice, and lizards. Other common, nonvenomous species you might see are the brown snake, eastern kingsnake, and the black racer.

Comfort, Safety, & Etiquette

The trails within reach of Atlanta afford a wide range of hiking experiences. You can take a brief afternoon stroll on a flat, easy path or travel for days in rugged backcountry. Some journeys require much more planning than others, but a hike of any type and duration will be more enjoyable if you take a bit of time to consider things such as your route, the environment you will explore, and things you need to carry. Some knowledge and planning can go a long way in making you safer and more comfortable in the outdoors.

Weather & the Environment

Before hitting the trail, consider the weather you will face, and dress appropriately for the full spectrum of weather you might experience. Fall daytime temperatures in the Georgia mountains can reach the 70s, while afternoons can be quite cool. Dress in layers so that you can shed or add clothing to regulate your body temperature. Because weather is not totally predictable, it's also a good idea to pack a waterproof shell when traveling in fall or winter to not only keep you dry in rain but also to shield you from chilly winds.

Spring is a great time to enjoy blooming wildflowers along the trail, but it's also the season for severe thunderstorms and tornadoes. If you are in the backcountry, avoid hiking and camping on exposed ridges when lightning is present.

Strong rains can also affect river levels, and some paths, such as the Jacks River Trail in the Cohutta Wilderness, may include several stream crossings. Before your trip, you can call the appropriate agency to check on water levels. You should take extreme caution when crossing swift streams, and it's a good idea to use trekking poles to improve your balance.

Summers in Georgia are hot and humid, and the key thing to remember is to drink plenty of water. In the backcountry, stream levels are inconsistent, and drought conditions can leave a creek bone dry. On multiday trips, try to carry as much water as possible, and consult the appropriate agency to learn about current stream conditions. If you take water from streams, be sure to treat it by using a filter or by boiling it to avoid getting sick from waterborne bacteria.

Insects such as mosquitoes can be heavy along the trails in summer, so be sure to pack whatever repellent you prefer. An insect repellent with at least 30% DEET or 20% Picaridin will also ward off ticks, which are a concern during the spring. It's recommended that you wear long pants during tick season. You should also check your body from time to time to see if ticks have hitched a ride. They tend to latch on to warm moist areas, and frequently hide out where the top seams of your socks meet your skin.

One thing a lot of people don't think about is sun exposure. Many of Georgia's trails are shaded by forest, but you can still catch quite a few rays during a day of hiking, so pack (and apply) a high-SPF sunscreen, preferably something that is waterproof to hold up during heavy sweating.

Preparation

Many people, especially those new to hiking, have a difficult time knowing just how far they can walk in a day without wearing themselves out—especially when loaded down with a 40-pound backpack. Take an honest assessment of your physical abilities, particularly when you are considering a long hike over difficult terrain. And remember that heat, cold, rain, and the terrain can limit the number of miles you can hike. Before you set out, try to examine a topographic map of the area to see just how much climbing and descending will be involved. This book includes an estimate of the total elevation gain and loss for each trip—the higher the numbers, the more difficult the hike.

Examine maps to become familiar with the area you will visit. A little studying will come in handy should you get confused and take a trail that is not part of your planned route. Also if you are planning an overnight hike, consult maps or the appropriate agency to identify available campsites, and prepare a plan B. If you wind up traveling much slower than expected, you may have to bed down somewhere other than your top campsite choice. If you are planning to use water from streams, be sure to examine the map and other information sources for reliable water sources.

Clothing

Another important step in the planning process is determining the clothing and gear you need. And there may be no more important piece of equipment than your footwear. An ill-fitting pair of shoes or boots can quickly ruin a day in the woods. Whether you choose to wear a lightweight pair of low-cut hiking shoes, a midweight pair of boots, or heavy, all-leather boots, get your footwear well in advance of your hike and test it before hitting the trail. You don't want to find out halfway through a long day's journey that your shoes don't fit. For cold, wet conditions, people often seek out a shoe or boot with a waterproof membrane such as Gore-Tex or Event. That's a good idea, but keep in mind that, in the South, high levels of humidity limit the ability of waterproof footwear to breathe. Some people prefer to buy a synthetic or leather shoe without a membrane and then add topical waterproofing agents.

It's also a good idea to invest in a lightweight jacket, or shell, with a waterproof membrane. As with footwear, these products will not breathe as well in the South as they would in a less-humid western environment, but it's better than having something than doesn't breathe at all.

For your other lathers of clothing, opt for things made with synthetic fabrics, rather than cotton. Synthetic fabrics will have a better chance of drying, and in cold weather they will not suck warmth away from your body as much as cotton would. To prevent blisters, try a synthetic sock, which will pull moisture away from your feet. Merino wool socks (which do not itch like traditional wool) are preferable to cotton.

The key to staying comfortable on the trail is to regulate your body temperature so that you are not too cold nor too hot for long periods. The trick is to dress in layers. For the fall and winter seasons, or even early spring, pack a thin top and bottom, a light or midweight layer to wear over that, and an insulated jacket to top it off. The final piece is your waterproof shell.

We lose much of our heat from our extremities, such as our head and hands. One of the quickest ways to warm up (especially if you're cold at night) is to put on gloves and a synthetic fleece or wool hat.

Equipment

If you're headed out for a morning trail run, you may not need to carry more than a bottle of water and a light snack or energy gel. But, if you plan to spend a full day or multiple days on the trail, consider packing the following:

WATER & FOOD

When dayhiking, plan to carry all the water you will need for the entire day—typically one to two quarts, depending on the weather (you may need more on a hot, humid summer day), and the difficulty of the trail. Do not count on drawing water from streams and springs unless you have confirmed that they are flowing. And be sure to filter or treat all water taken from natural sources.

When hiking in cold weather, keep in mind that you should bring a stove or other heat source to make a warm drink in case you get wet and chilled. It's also a good idea to carry energy bars that can deliver quick fuel to increase your energy level.

MAP & COMPASS

Even experienced hikers can become disoriented in the outdoors, especially at the end of a long, tiring hike. And in some places, such as designated wilderness areas, trails may not be marked with signs. Whenever possible you should carry a map to aid in your navigation. Before you set out on your trip, learn the basics of reading a map and matching contour lines and other map features to your surroundings while traveling in the environment. You can give yourself some peace of mind by learning to use a compass and to properly orient your map.

Agencies responsible for trails in an area can generally provide you with the most accurate map available. USGS 7.5-minute maps also offer good detail, but you should be aware that you might need several maps to cover the entire area of a route.

Outdoor gear shops also provide excellent maps for particular trails, such as the Appalachian Trail. These sometimes include helpful features such as elevation profiles that give you an idea of the type of terrain you'll encounter along the way. Many newer maps also have waterproof coatings, which can extend the life of your map in wet weather.

Another good source is the National Geographic TOPO! series of maps on CD, which were used to help create the maps in this book. This program allows you to create a seamless topographic map of your entire route, and you can zoom in or out to make a map of the general area, as well as a close-up of the trail. You can look at the elevation change, build an elevation profile, calculate distance, and identify waypoints that have been provided in this book.

Global Positioning System (GPS) receivers have become increasingly popular because they make land navigation easier. But, like any tool, a GPS receiver is only helpful if you take time to learn how to use it and realize its limitations. First, remember that batteries can fail, so you should not rely solely on a GPS receiver—always carry a map and compass. Also, some Georgia trails venture into deep ravines and heavy foliage where it can be difficult for the receiver to get a good signal with the satellite system, so you should get a GPS receiver with a strong antenna.

FIRST-AID KIT

You can put together your own first-aid kit or purchase one from a gear store. Modern kits come in a wide range of sizes to accommodate different types of trips and various group sizes. No matter what type of kit you carry, be sure to understand how to use its components, and always carry any manual provided with a kit. It's tough to take a crash course in an emergency situation.

For low-risk hikes lasting a day or less, a basic kit is fine. A basic kit should include:

- Manual
- Bandages, including gauze and medical tape. Moleskin is very handy for treating hot spots and even preventing blisters. Tincture of benzoin will help moleskin adhere to skin better.
- Antiseptic to clean wounds
- Drugs, including something to reduce fever (like acetaminophen), something to reduce inflammation (like ibuprofen), electrolyte tablets to overcome dehydration, and antacid tablets
- Prescription medicines
- Cutting tools, like scissors or a razor
- Hydrocortisone cream for skin irritations
- Tweezers
- Duct tape

The amount of bandages and drugs will depend on the size of the group. Many preassembled kits indicate the number of people a kit will serve over a certain amount of time. Note that these numbers may be inflated, meaning the kits include twice as much stuff as you'd actually need. But some buffer is built in so you will have enough supplies to handle the unexpected.

For longer trips that go well out of range of medical attention, a more sophisticated kit is needed. The big question is whether the kit can deal with at least one major injury or laceration. An advanced kit should include:

- Large bandages to stop bleeding
- Extra bandages
- Drugs to treat burns and skin irritations and possibly prescription drugs for serious pain
- Tools to immobilize limbs, such as a splint and sling

INSECT REPELLENT

The most effective insect repellents include DEET, though you can choose products with higher or lower levels depending on your skin sensitivity. You might also consider repellents containing Picaridin. Natural alternatives, such as repellents with certain plant oils, can also work, but you might need to apply them more often.

SOURCE OF FIRE

In an emergency situation, a fire can provide warmth, serve as a signal to rescuers, and improve your state of mind. Carry waterproof matches or some other fire source, plus small candles, to help ignite kindling.

KNIFE OR MULTI-TOOL

Whether you need to construct a shelter or repair a piece of gear, a knife or multi-tool can be a critical piece of gear. You probably don't need a massive tool with everything except the kitchen sink, but a locking blade, screwdriver, and tweezers (if there isn't already a pair in your first-aid kit) are good implements to have.

WHISTLE

Should you become injured or separated from your hiking partners, a whistle is a great help in attracting attention. Its sound will generally be much louder and travel farther than the sound of your voice. There are many lightweight, durable plastic emergency whistles on the market, and first-aid kits often include one. Plus, many backpacks now have small whistles integrated into the sternum strap.

TREKKING POLES

Over the course of a long journey, trekking poles help to distribute your weight and reduce the accumulated pressure and weight put on your legs and knees. They are especially helpful in reducing fatigue on steep descents. Also, trekking poles stabilize your body during stream crossings. If you use them, be sure to adjust and use them while maintaining good posture.

GAITERS

Southern trails can get pretty muddy after a good, hard rain, and a pair of low-profile gaiters can help keep moisture, mud, and trail debris from sneaking into your shoes or boots.

SANDALS OR WATER SHOES

Slip on some sandals or water shoes for stream crossings to keep your hiking shoes or boots dry. They are also good to wear around camp as they will allow swollen feet to breathe and recover.

CELL PHONE

People often debate whether cell phones belong on the trail. Some people believe that they are a crutch or offer a false sense of security, but some people have used them to be rescued in emergency situations. If you carry one, consider it a last resort, not something to rely on. On many trails you won't be able to get a signal anyway. And, unless you need to use it in an emergency, please keep it turned off and avoid using it to call someone just to chat. A ringing cell phone is a real bummer for those trying to escape the noises of civilization.

Safety Measures

There are many precautions you can take to stay safe when traveling in the backcountry. One of the most important is to let someone know where you are going, particularly if you'll be hiking alone or plan to be gone for more than just a few hours. Provide a friend or relative your itinerary, including the day you plan to return. Provide that person a phone number for the appropriate agency responsible for the area where you will be hiking. Notify rangers or other authorities of your itinerary. (You can do this when getting required permits.) Put a copy of your itinerary on your dashboard.

Do not leave valuables in your vehicle. Trailhead break-ins are not frequent in most areas, but they happen. If you are in bear territory, do not leave food in your vehicle. You would be amazed at the things bears have done to rear windows and even car doors while trying to get to food.

Hike in a group if possible. This not only adds security but you will feel safer if you are not alone if you get lost. Plus, in an emergency situation it's best if someone can remain with an injured person while someone else goes for help.

The key to staying found is to be aware of your surroundings. It's easy to miss a trail junction or accidentally take the wrong path. If your map indicates you should be ascending, and you find yourself on a long descent, stop to examine your map and the terrain around you. If you get lost, find a comfortable spot with shelter (or construct a shelter) and stay put. A rescue team can find you more easily if you are not wandering.

Campfires can liven up a camping trip, but take extreme caution around them. During times of drought, or when there are posted warnings of high fire danger, avoid building one. Always use available or designated fire rings or pits, and only use dead, downed wood. Never leave a campfire unattended, and always thoroughly smother and extinguish any campfires before going to sleep.

Trail Etiquette

The good news is that more and more people in the Atlanta area are getting out and enjoying the many beautiful trails. The bad news is that some popular and easily accessible trails are suffering from overuse and neglect. Some camping spots have been highly eroded, trees have been chopped down for fires and you might even see toilet paper littering the ground beneath bushes. When you hike, be considerate of those who will follow you. They deserve the same high-quality experience you are seeking. To minimize your impact on the environment, follow these guidelines created by the Leave No Trace Center for Outdoor Ethics:

- **Plan ahead and prepare.** Know the regulations and special concerns for the area you'll visit. Schedule your trip to avoid high times of use, and visit in small groups when possible.
- **Travel and camp on durable surfaces,** such as established trails and campsites, rock, gravel, dry grasses, or snow. Camp at least 200 feet from lakes and streams when possible. Avoid altering a campsite, and try to use existing trails and campsites.
- **Dispose of waste properly.** If you pack it in, pack it out. Inspect your campsite before you leave for spilled foods. Pack out all trash, leftover food, and litter. Deposit solid human waste in catholes dug 6 to 8 inches deep at least 200 feet from water, camp, and trails. Cover and disguise the cathole when finished. Pack out toilet paper and hygiene products.
- **Leave what you find.** Examine but do not touch cultural or historic artifacts. Leave rocks, plants, and other natural objects as you find them. Do not build structures or makeshift furniture or dig trenches.
- **Minimize campfire impacts.** Consider using a lightweight stove for cooking and a candle lantern or battery-powered headlamp for light. (A candle lantern can double as a source of heat and light in an emergency.) Where fires are permitted, use established fire rings. Keep fires small, and use dead and downed wood. Put fires out completely.
- **Respect wildlife.** Observe wildlife from a distance, and do not follow or approach any animals. Never feed wildlife—feeding damages their health, alters natural behaviors, and exposes them to predators and other dangers. Protect wildlife and your food by storing rations and trash securely.
- **Respect other visitors and protect the quality of their experience.** Be courteous and yield to others on the trail. Take breaks and camp away from trails and other visitors. Let nature's sounds prevail. Avoid loud voices and noises.

Using This Book

The book is arranged into seven regional chapters: northwest Georgia, north central Georgia, northeast Georgia, west of Atlanta, central Atlanta, east of Atlanta, and south of Atlanta. Each chapter includes trips arranged roughly from west to east. Each trip is a very specific hike on a trail or series of connected trails. Some areas have numerous paths that can be walked in different sequences and directions, but I have tried to simplify things by making each trip an exact journey. Each trip consists of capsulized summaries, highlights, driving directions, facility information, and the actual hike directions.

Capsulized Summaries

Each trip begins with a capsulized summary that includes the following information: distance and trip type, hiking time, difficulty level, total elevation gain and/or loss, trail uses, best times to hike, agency, and recommended maps.

DISTANCE & TRIP TYPE

The first figure listed in this section is an estimate of the total hiking distance for each loop or out-and-back hike, including outbound and return journey. The trail mileage for most trips was calculated using a measuring wheel and GPS receiver, but keep in mind that mileages in this book may differ from what you see on trail signs or certain maps. All these different sources can often conflict because they've been calculated by different people using different methods over time.

The other listing in this section is the trip type, which consists of a loop, semiloop, out-and-back trip, or point-to-point (or shuttle) hike.

HIKING TIME

This is an estimate of the walking time for the average person for each trip. Estimates are based on walking 2 miles per hour on easy to moderate terrain, and 1.5 miles per hour on strenuous terrain. Hiking times do not include rest stops; your actual time on the trail will vary depending on how often and how long you stop.

DIFFICULTY LEVEL

Although it's somewhat subjective, the difficulty rating for each trip is based on distance, total elevation gain, and the type of terrain. The ratings are as follows:

Easy: A relatively short trip with little elevation gain and loss.

Moderate: A trip that requires several hours of walking and/or includes a few climbs and descents but does not cover a great change in elevation.

Strenuous: A long trip covering many miles and requiring several hours. This trip might include steep ascents and descents and great gains and losses in elevation.

ELEVATION GAIN/LOSS

The elevation gain and loss figures are a sum of all the uphill and downhill segments of the hike, including the outbound and return portions of the trip.

TRAIL USES

While all of the trails are suitable for hiking, some are also good for mountain biking, horseback riding, backpacking, or bringing along your canine companion. The trail use section lists the appropriate uses for each of the hikes. Of the trails that allow dogs, most require that they be on a leash no longer than 6 feet. Trips that measure 3 miles or less, and cover easy to moderate terrain may be marked as being "good for kids."

Mountain biking is allowed on a few of the trails in this book. It's good idea to be alert when hiking these trails, and yield to riders. Some multiuse trails in this book are also used by horseback riders.

Trails labeled for backpacking are good for overnight or multiday trips and have areas along the trail suitable for camping. In most areas other than those classified as wilderness, there are designated campsites. Check with the agency responsible for the area for information about required permits and advance registration.

BEST TIMES

Most trails in this book are suitable for hiking during any season of the year. Fall is a prime season due to favorable weather and attractive foliage. Spring is also popular due to mild temperatures and blooming wildflowers. Keep in mind that some trails in higher elevations will have better views in winter due to the reduced foliage, but you should take extra caution to be prepared for cold temperatures. Summer can be extremely hot and humid, so be sure to carry plenty of water to avoid dehydration.

AGENCY

This section lists the government agencies or administrators responsible for the land through which the trails run. They can provide you with information on maps, fees, special guided hikes, educational programs, campsites, facilities, and much more to aid your planning. If you want to contact them or visit their website, see Appendix 3 for their mailing address, location, phone number, and website (if available).

RECOMMENDED MAPS

Some areas, particularly Georgia State Parks, the National Park Service, and U.S. Forest Service, provide good trail maps, some of which are available at park offices and some online. Most agencies will also mail a map to you if you write or call them. Good commercial maps are also available from National Geographic Maps, particularly their Trails Illustrated line. Another option is to use USGS 7.5-minute quadrangle maps with a 1:24,000 scale (2.64 inches on the maps equals 1 mile). Try to get the most up-to-date map possible, as trails are sometimes rerouted. The maps provided in this book were created using a GPS receiver and serve as a general guide.

Highlights, Driving Directions, & Facilities

Just after the summary information in each trip, a highlights section mentions interesting historical details about the area or notable natural features. Each trip includes driving directions from the central metro area of Atlanta and beginning on major roads, such as Interstates 85, 75, and 285. Each trip also includes a mention of the facilities, such as restrooms, water sources, and campgrounds available in the trailhead area.

GPS Waypoints

The maps in this book include numbered waypoints that indicate trailheads, important trail junctions, notable natural features, and backcountry campsites. On maps that show multiple trips, the waypoint number is preceded by the trip number. For each waypoint you will find corresponding UTM (Universal Transverse Mercator) coordinates. The UTM coordinate system is basically a grid that specifies locations on the Earth's surface. Each UTM coordinate includes the

UTM zone plus easting and northing coordinates. For example, if the waypoint coordinate is 17S 237034E 3863796N, the UTM zone is 17S, easting is 237034, and northing is 3863796.

The UTM coordinates for each trip are listed at the end of the trip description for easy reference. Before you go on your trip you can enter these coordinates into a GPS receiver to create waypoints. You can use these waypoints to create a route. As you hike, the GPS receiver will display your location, and also steer you toward each waypoint along the route.

Remember that a GPS receiver should never be used as your sole navigation device. As with any electronic equipment, batteries can fail, making the receiver useless. Carry at least a map (preferably a topographic map) and a compass. Before traveling, take time to learn how to use your GPS receiver properly. You should also learn how to read a topographic map and use it in conjunction with a compass.

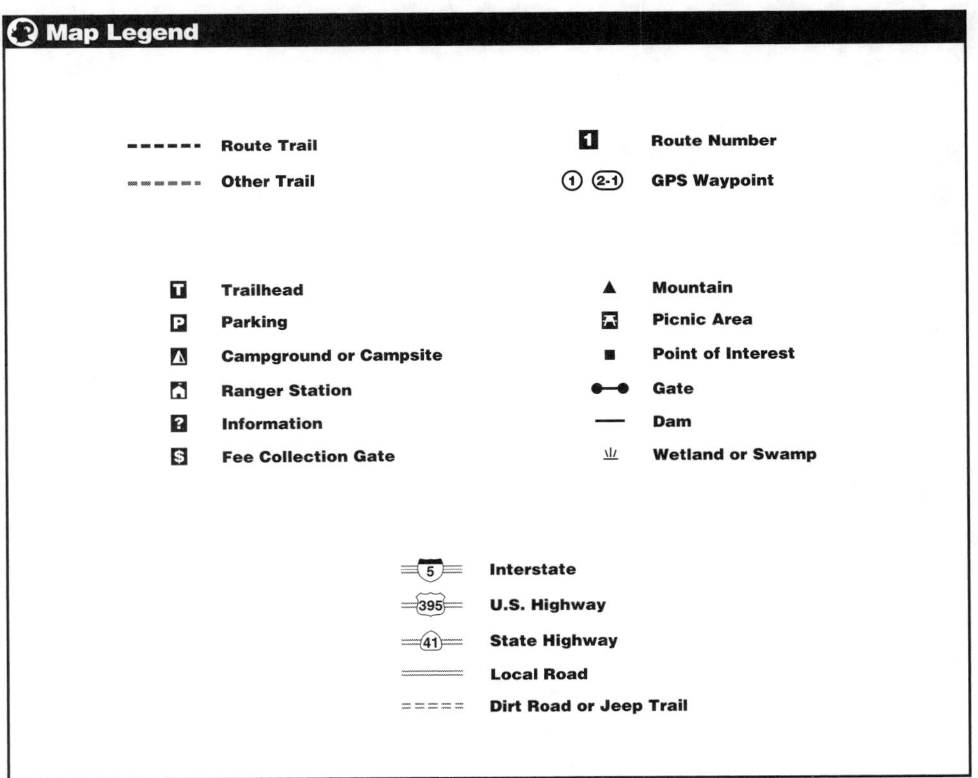

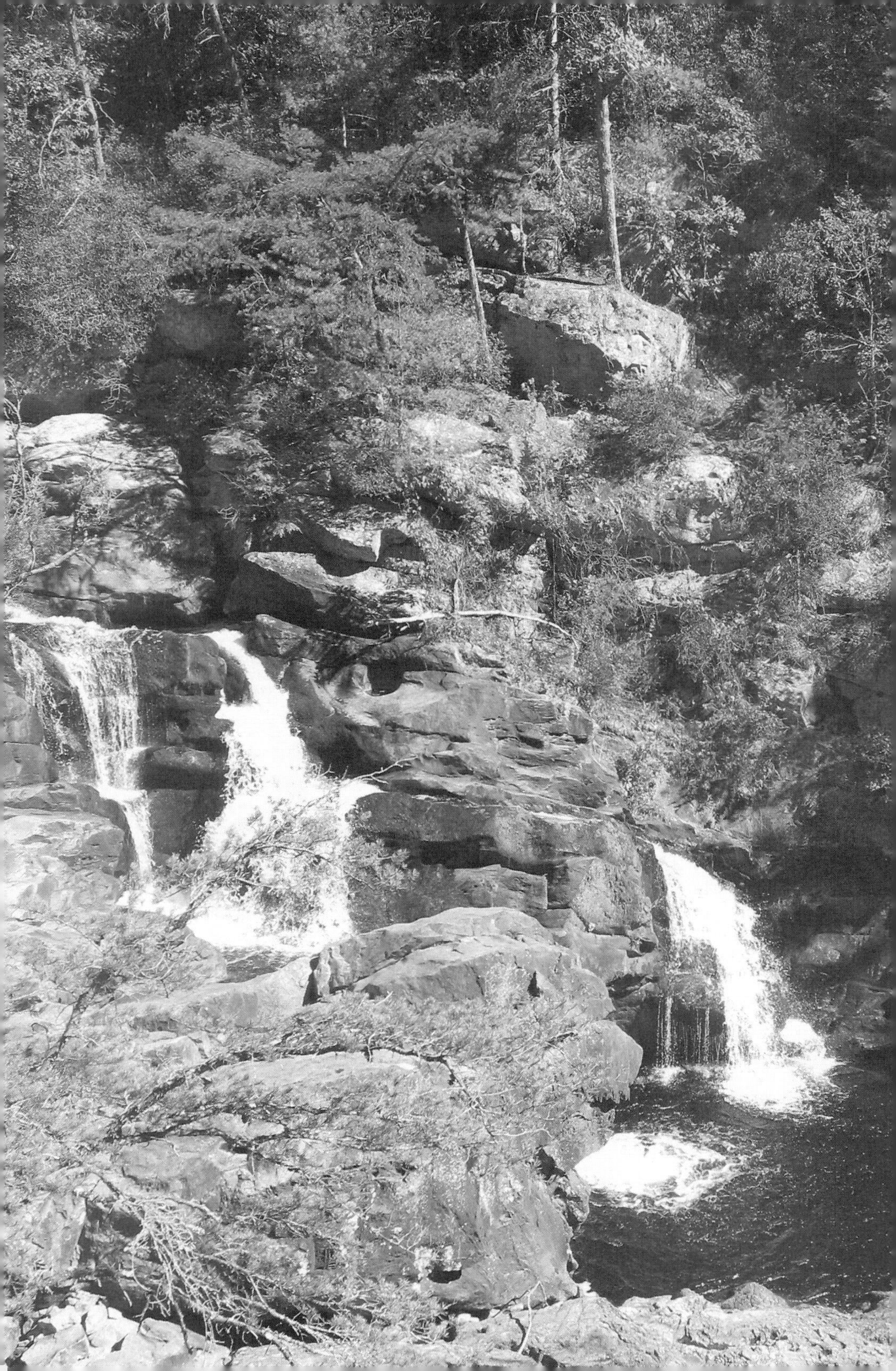

Chapter 1
Northwest Georgia

From the towering cliffs and waterfalls of Cloudland Canyon to the curious boulders atop Pigeon Mountain, northwest Georgia includes some of the state's most fascinating and dramatic natural features. Hikers will also find a great diversity of trips, from multiday backcountry treks deep within the Cohutta Wilderness to day trips strolling down wildlife interpretive trails. This region is also notable for a number of historic sites where those curious about state history can walk among a Cherokee settlement and traverse the rugged battlegrounds of the Civil War. From the lush ravine that hides the Chickamauga Creek Trail to the stirring memorials that dot the Chickamauga Battlefield, the trails in this region explore the natural and human history of Georgia.

Cohutta Wilderness

Quiet. Solitude. The middle of nowhere. These things become more elusive as civilization creeps up on the Georgia's green spaces. But the ridgebacks and river bottoms of the Cohutta Wilderness can carry you far away from the city rumble. Spanning 36,977 acres, the Cohutta is one of the largest wilderness areas in the Southeast. From 1915 to 1930, the Conasauga River Lumber Company extracted timber from about 70 percent of the area, but the U.S. Forest Service purchased most of the land between 1934 and 1935. The forest started its slow recovery, and then in 1975 the Cohutta became Georgia's first designated wilderness area. With this high level of protection, the forest is preserved in as natural a state as possible, prohibiting timber harvesting, human-made structures, and the use of motorized vehicles on the trails. The Cohutta Wilderness has more than 92 miles of hiking trails, and the adjoining 8082-acre Big Frog Wilderness has another 33 miles, making this one

Jacks River Trail (Trip 5)

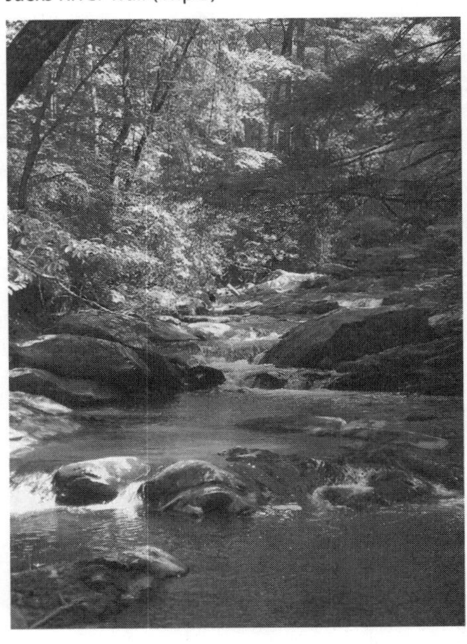

Jacks River Falls (Trip 2)

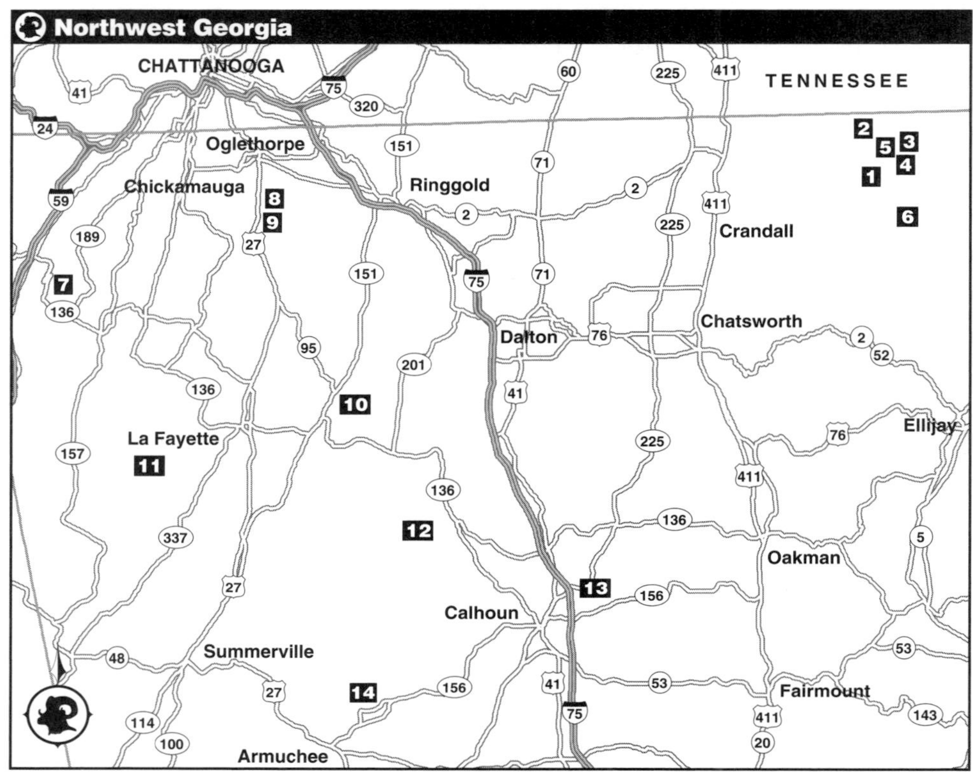

of the most massive tracts of contiguous forest in the eastern U.S. The five overnight hikes and dayhikes included in this chapter are a good sampling of the area's diverse terrain.

Beyond the five trips described in this chapter in this wilderness area, you might consider consulting a map of the area and checking out several others: The 1.8-mile, moderate Chestnut Lead Trail descends to Conasauga River and intersects with the Conasauga River Trail. The 13.1-mile, moderate Conasauga River Trail begins at the southeastern edge of the Cohutta Wilderness at Betty Gap and follows the attractive Conasauga River to a parking area off of Forest Service Road 17-B in the northwest section of the wilderness. Easy-to-moderate Hickory Creek Trail, 8.6 miles, runs south from the western side of the wilderness near Forest Service Road 51 to cross the Conasauga River and end at its intersection with the Conasauga River Trail. The 3.4-mile, strenuous but popular Panther Creek Trail runs between the Conasauga River Trail and the East Cowpen Trail, passing the lengthy cascades of Panther Creek Falls. The 3.9-mile moderate Rice Camp Trail begins at the western side of the wilderness at Forest Service Road 51 and crosses several streams before rising to cross a ridge and drop to end at its intersection with the Jacks River Trail. The 3.4-mile Tearbritches Trail begins at the southwestern edge of the wilderness at Forest Service Road 68 with a strenuous climb over Bald Mountain, but becomes easier as it descend to its junction with the Conasauga River Trail.

Chickamauga Battlefield

Civil War historian Shelby Foote wrote that among Civil War battles, Chickamauga was "not only the greatest battle of the West, but would also be, for the numbers engaged, the bloodiest of the war." The wounded and killed included an estimated 16,170 Union soldiers and 18,454 Confederate soldiers. Despite their losses, the Rebels prevailed, though this would be their final major victory in the war.

This battle was part of the Union offensive in southern Tennessee and northwest Georgia to capture Chattanooga. As a railroad hub and important manufacturing center, Chattanooga was seen as a vital objective for the Federal forces.

In September 1863, the Union Army of the Cumberland, led by Maj. Gen. William Rosecrans, moved toward Chattanooga, while the Confederate Army of Tennessee, led by Gen. Braxton Bragg, set up on the bank of Chickamauga Creek and prepared to block the Union advance.

The battle began on September 19 and raged into the next day, with the Confederates and Union soldiers launching a series of attacks and counterattacks in dense forest that was occasionally broken by farm fields. It was a chaotic scene as the tangled woods limited the visibility of the fighting men, causing great confusion.

The Confederates made several unsuccessful attempts to break the Union lines. Then, on September 20, Union Gen. William Rosecrans inadvertently created a gap in his line of men, and forces under Confederate Gen. James Longstreet took advantage by plowing through the hole and driving a large portion of the Union Army out of the area. That evening, the entire Union Army withdrew to positions near Chattanooga.

Union Army headquarters site at Chickamauga Battlefield (Trip 8)

FIELD HEADQUARTERS.
ARMY OF THE CUMBERLAND.
MAJ. GEN. W. S. ROSECRANS.
SEPT. 20, 1863. 10 A.M. TO 11.15 A.M.

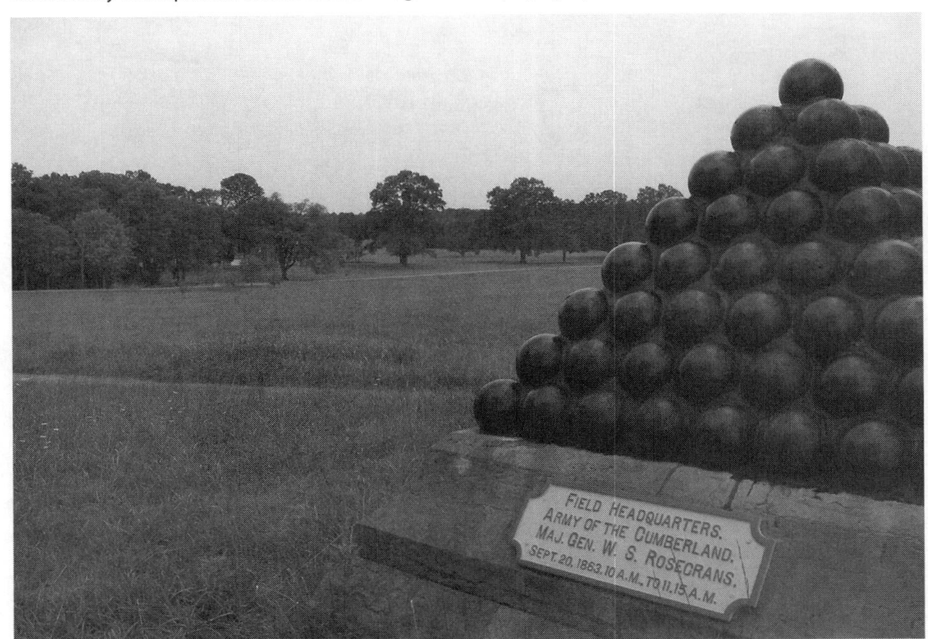

Benton MacKaye Trail

Named for the man who first proposed the construction of the Appalachian Trail (AT), the Benton MacKaye Trail (BMT) stretches 300 miles from the top of Springer Mountain in Georgia to Davenport Gap on the northern fringe of Great Smoky Mountains National Park. MacKaye not only envisioned what is now the AT, but he also hoped that a series of side trails would link the AT to other green spaces along the route, including a path along the Blue Ridge in the southern Appalachian mountains. The surge in backpacking in the 1970s increased traffic on the AT, and the U.S. Forest Service worked with trail clubs to construct a series of alternate trails that would be less developed and have no established campsites or shelters. Employees of the Georgia Department of Natural Resources pushed the idea forward, working with the Forest Service and trail clubs. Formed in 1980, the Benton MacKaye Trail Association began plotting the course for this new trail system, and by 1989 the 80 miles of the BMT that run through Georgia were completed. Work continued to construct the BMT's northern course, and on July 16, 2005, the plan was completed and the entire trail was officially opened.

For the purposes of this book, I have included selected hikes on the Georgia portion of the Benton MacKaye Trail. If you wish to explore it further, I encourage you to visit the Benton MacKaye Trail Association website at www.bmta.org. The association does an excellent job maintaining the trail through the work of volunteers, and it is a prime resource for detailed information. Another great resource is Tim Homan's *Hiking the Benton MacKaye Trail.*

Hiking the Benton MacKaye Trail between Dyer and Watson gaps (Trip 6)

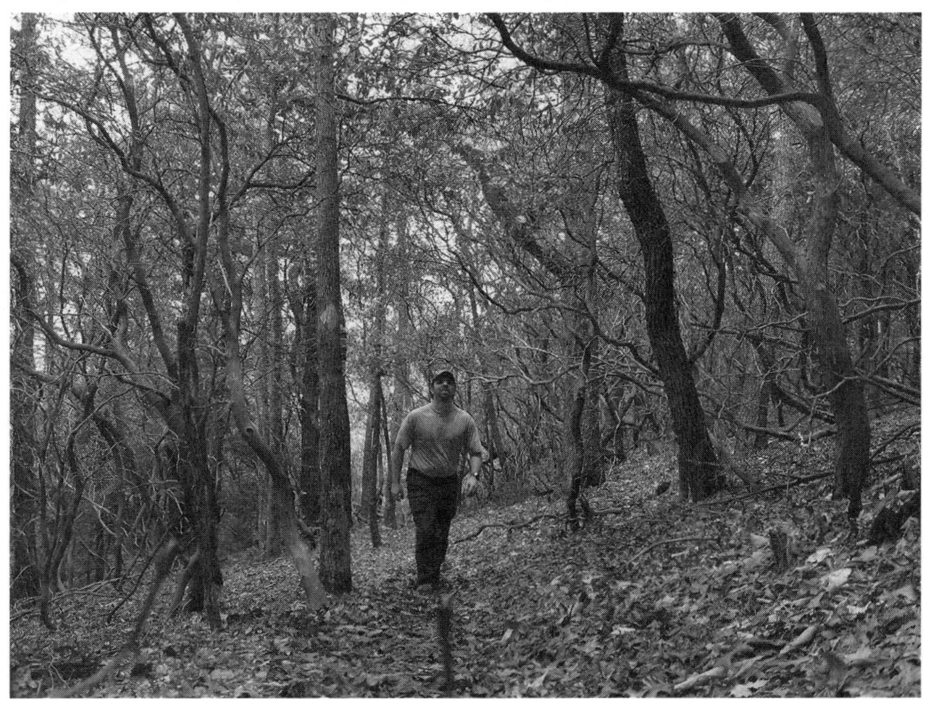

TRIP 1 Cohutta Wilderness: East Cowpen, Hickory Ridge, & Rough Ridge Loop

Distance	15.6 miles, loop
Hiking Time	16 hours
Difficulty	Strenuous
Elevation Gain/Loss	+3480 feet/-3475 feet
Trail Uses	Backpacking and horseback riding
Best Times	Year-round
Agency	Chattahoochee National Forest, Cohutta Ranger District
Recommended Map	U.S. Forest Service *Cohutta and Big Frog Wilderness Georgia-Tennessee*

HIGHLIGHTS The East Cowpen, Hickory Ridge, and Rough Ridge trails form a loop that passes through the heart of the Cohutta Wilderness. Because this is a long trek with some steep climbs, it works best as an overnight trip for experienced backpackers. The best part is that it travels through two distinct types of terrain found in the Cohutta. The trip begins in hardwoods on high ridges that form the western wall of a deep gorge that drops 1500 feet to Rough Creek. If you're backpacking, your first day will likely end with a descent to the banks of Jacks River, which rushes through heath forest of hemlock and rhododendron. There is room on the riverbank for camping, and on clear nights you can gaze at a starry sky undisturbed by city lights. On the second day you climb high again to Rough Ridge where you can look across the gorge and get a real sense of its depth and breadth.

DIRECTIONS From Atlanta, travel north on Interstate 75 to Interstate 575. Take I-575 north to GA Highway 5/515 and take GA 5/515 to East Ellijay. Turn left onto U.S. Highway 76/GA Highway 2 and continue on GA 2 to Ellijay. From the Ellijay town square, go west on GA Highway 52 for 9.5 miles to Forest Service Road 18 and a sign for LAKE CONASAUGA RECREATION AREA. Turn right and go 1.3 miles to where the pavement ends and there is a fork. Bear left at the fork and cross the bridge. Go 2.2 miles and take a sharp right onto Forest Service Road 68. Go 2.5 miles to the three-way junction with Forest Service Road 64. Turn right onto FSR 64 and go 4.4 miles to the Three Forks parking area.

FACILITIES/TRAILHEAD There are no facilities at trailheads within the Cohutta Wilderness. Camping is allowed anywhere in the wilderness, and primitives campsites (usually with nothing more than a fire ring) are right along the trail. Be sure to carry plenty of water as the hiking can be strenuous, and treat all water that you get from streams. Bears and other critters roam the wilderness, so plan to hang your food at night. As an added precaution, give your itinerary to a friend or ranger, especially if you hike solo.

The hike begins at the northwest end of the Three Forks parking lot **(Waypoint 1)**. From here take the East Cowpen Trail, and ascend gradually through mature hardwoods. At 0.4 mile you'll reach the intersection with the Rough Ridge Trail **(Waypoint 2)**. Continue straight (northwest) to cross over Cohutta Mountain. The trail climbs higher than 4000 feet of elevation before descending gradually with hemlocks to your right and seasonal views of distant mountain folds to the left.

At 2.2 miles, on a ridgetop, the Panther Creek Trail intersects on the left, and to the right a large campsite sits among large oaks and hemlocks. Continue straight to

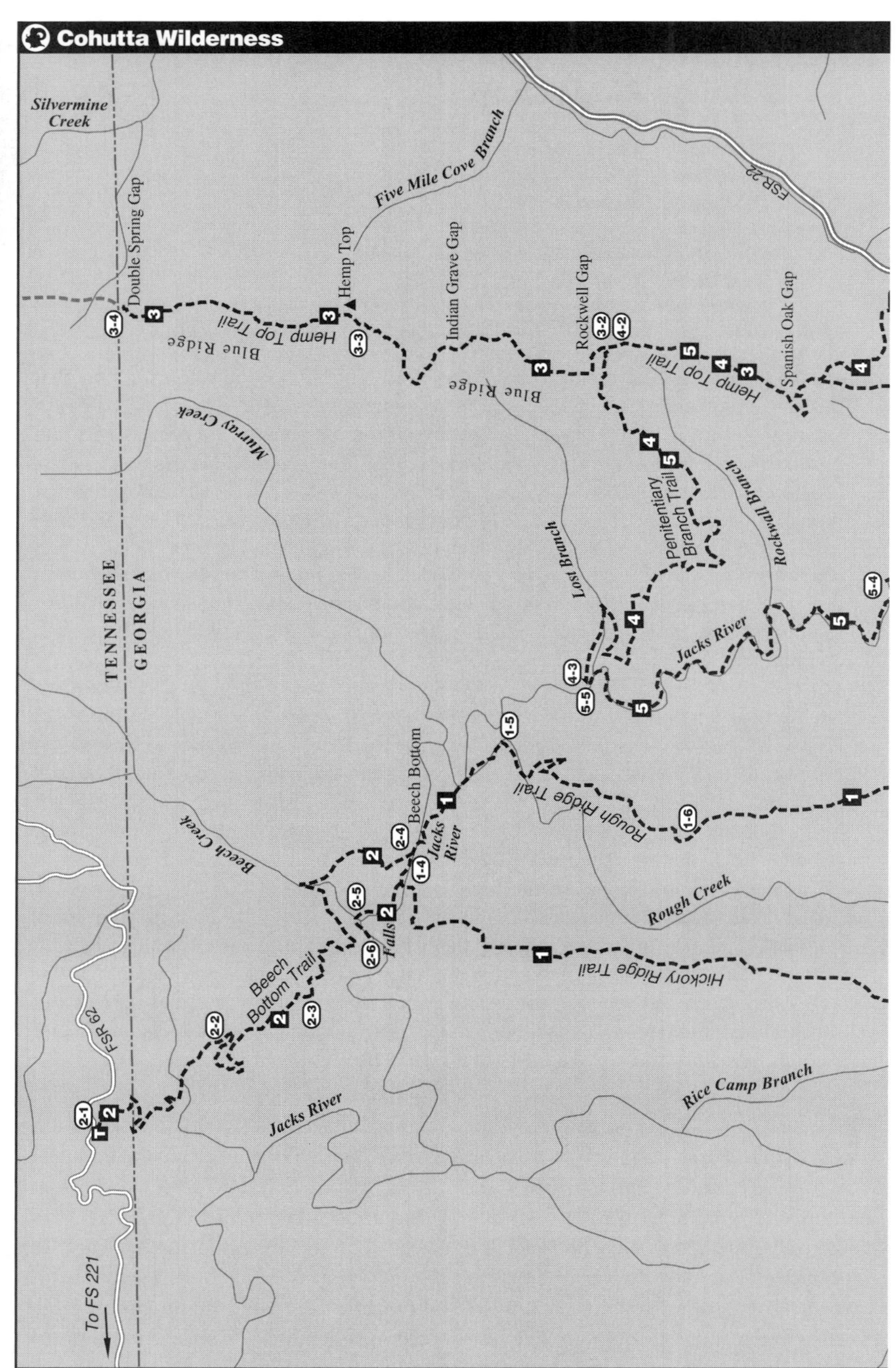
Cohutta Wilderness
Silvermine Creek
Five Mile Cove Branch
FSR 22
Double Spring Gap
Hemp Top
Indian Grave Gap
Rockwell Gap
Spanish Oak Gap
Hemp Top Trail
Blue Ridge
Murray Creek
Penitentiary Branch Trail
Rockwell Branch
Lost Branch
TENNESSEE
GEORGIA
Jacks River
Beech Bottom
Rough Ridge Trail
Beech Creek
Rough Creek
Falls
Beech Bottom Trail
Hickory Ridge Trail
FSR 62
Rice Camp Branch
To FS 221

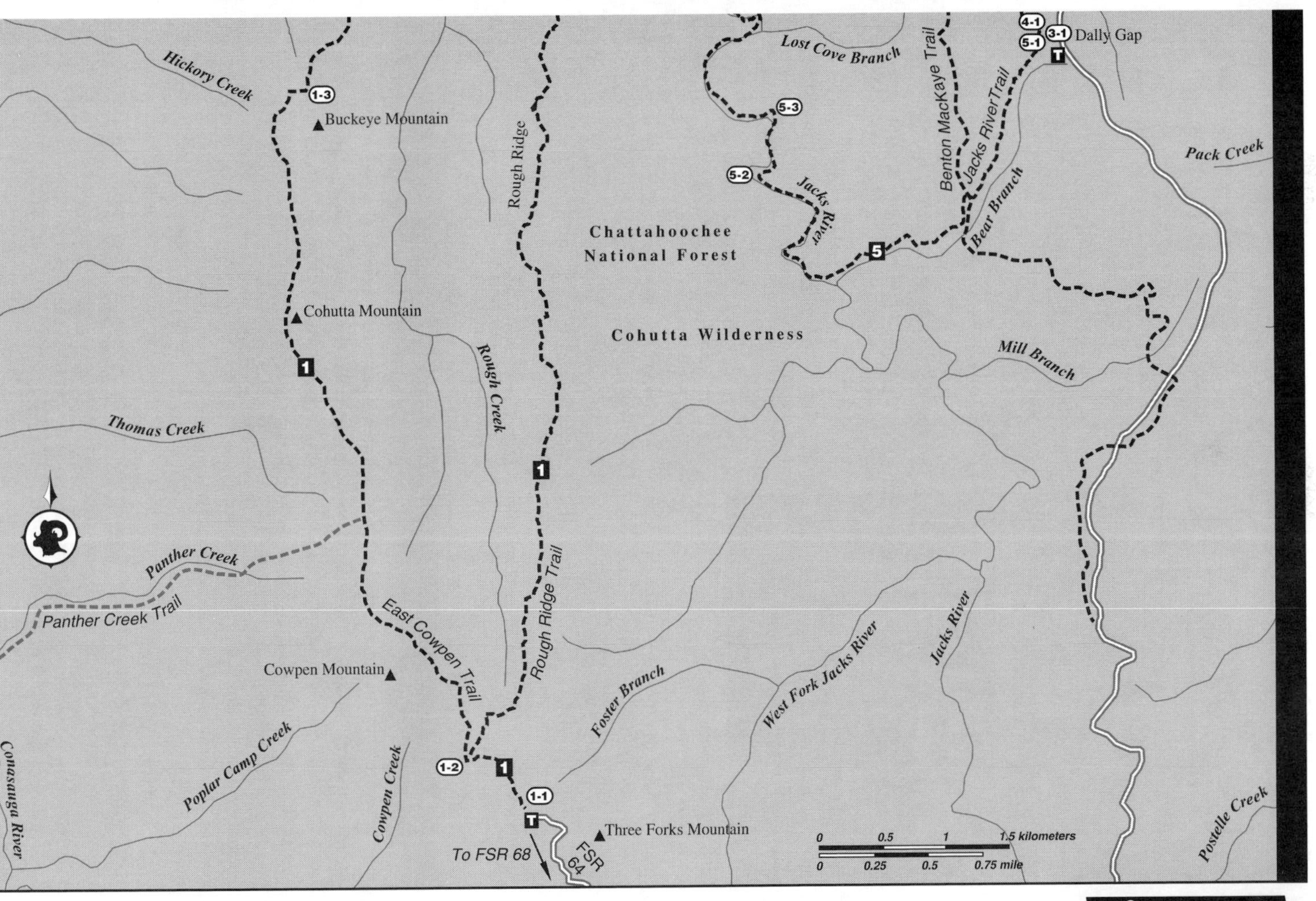

Hickory Creek
1-3
Buckeye Mountain
Rough Ridge
Lost Cove Branch
5-3
5-2
Jacks River
Benton MacKaye Trail
Jacks River Trail
4-1
3-1
5-1
Dally Gap
T
Pack Creek
Bear Branch
Chattahoochee
National Forest
5
Cohutta Mountain
Cohutta Wilderness
Mill Branch
1
Rough Creek
Thomas Creek
1
Panther Creek
Panther Creek Trail
East Cowpen Trail
Rough Ridge Trail
Cowpen Mountain
Foster Branch
West Fork Jacks River
Jacks River
Poplar Camp Creek
Conasauga River
Cowpen Creek
1-2
1
1-1
T
To FSR 68
FSR 64
Three Forks Mountain
0 0.5 1 1.5 kilometers
0 0.25 0.5 0.75 mile
Postelle Creek

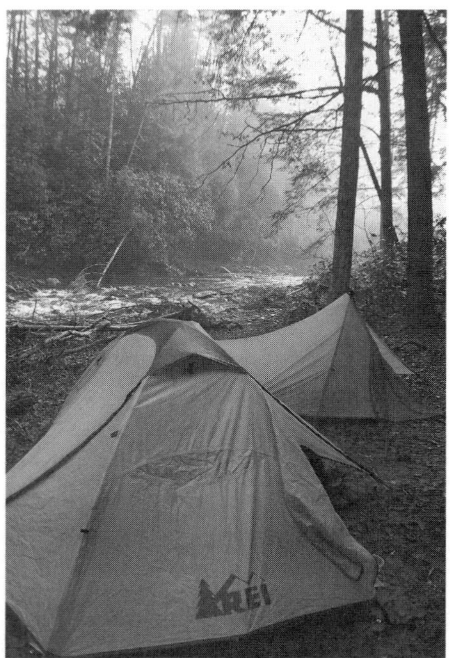

Camping along Jacks River

the northwest to continue on the flat path as it crosses the spine of the ridge. Now, to your left and right, hazy blue bands of faraway mountains stretch across the horizon.

Circle around Buckeye Mountain, and at 3.2 miles the East Cowpen and Hickory Ridge trails intersect at a lofty open space **(Waypoint 3)**. Continue northeast to join the Hickory Ridge Trail (the East Cowpen turns sharply to the southwest) and ascend to a campsite at 3.4 miles. If you're looking for good ridgetop camping in winter, this spot has nice views to each side of this high ground. Just a bit farther, a lone American holly tree (one of the few you'll see on this trail) stands nearly 15 feet high.

At 4 miles the forest puts on a dramatic show as the leafy path drops, while a high forested peak fills the sky to the northeast. The trail rolls along, generally descending as the forest grows thick with mountain laurel, and finally dropping to a stream. Continue to the river **(Waypoint 4)**, and cross to find clearings wide enough to accommodate tents. For those who fish, the Jacks River—often waist-deep in normal flows—holds brown, rainbow, and brook trout.

To complete the loop, travel east on the southwest bank of the river, and at 7.6 miles cross the river. (A trekking pole allows for better balance while crossing.) Turn right and go east for a mile, and then cross the river again, continuing to the east. The forest here is humbling, with massive hemlocks rising 100 feet and measuring 10 to 12 feet around. At 8.3 miles, cross Rough Creek and go straight (east) at the next trail junction to take the Rough Ridge Trail **(Waypoint 5)**. Cross the creek yet again, and at 8.7 miles look carefully for a sharp turn to the east where you ascend through rhododendron.

As you climb, a peak looms large to the north. The path levels momentarily, and you may want to catch your breath before making a hard push up the ridge. Near the 10-mile point, Hickory Ridge comes into view, and suddenly you glimpse the impressive depth of the gorge, though its bottom remains hidden from view **(Waypoint 6)**. The next 3 to 4 miles is a rollercoaster ride on hills and saddles of hardwoods and pines, reaching elevations above 3600 feet, while small campsites dot the area. At 15.2 miles, turn left onto the East Cowpen Trail to return to the trailhead.

UTM WAYPOINTS

1. 16S 722461E 3862612N
2. 16S 722007E 3863015N
3. 16S 720787E 3868275N
4. 16S 721992E 3872409N
5. 16S 723120E 3871653N
6. 16S 722352E 3870251N

TRIP 2 Cohutta Wilderness: Beech Bottom Trail & Jacks River Falls

Distance	9.2 miles, out-and-back
Hiking Time	4–5 hours
Difficulty	Easy
Elevation Gain/Loss	+1635/-1625 feet
Trail Use	Backpacking
Best Times	Year-round (falls run strongest in winter and spring)
Agency	Chattahoochee National Forest, Cohutta Ranger District
Recommended Map	U.S. Forest Service *Cohutta and Big Frog Wilderness Georgia-Tennessee*

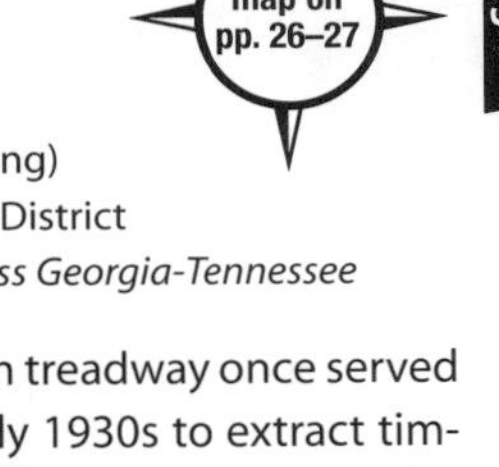

HIGHLIGHTS Conspicuously wide in some stretches, the Beech Bottom treadway once served as a road that logging companies used in the late 1920s and early 1930s to extract timber. Now this gentle descent provides hikers access to Jacks River Falls, the most popular feature in the Cohutta Wilderness. On its way to the river, the trail shifts dramatically as it alternates between dry forests of pine and hardwoods and low, lush ravines with hemlock and mountain laurel. There are some good views during the descent, such as the spot 2.5 miles in where breaks in the trees reveal the soft folds of faraway hills. Even better is the stretch where the path meets Jacks River, and wide spots along the bank can serve as shaded picnic spots or campsites. After walking 4.5 miles, you'll encounter Jacks River Falls where the river surges to whitewater and takes a rough tumble through a rocky corridor and dives into wide pools.

DIRECTIONS From Atlanta take Interstate 75 north to U.S. Highway 411. Go north on U.S. 411 through Chatsworth to the town of Cisco. Just before the Cisco Baptist Church, turn right onto the paved road, Old Highway 2. The pavement gives way to gravel, and Old Highway 2 becomes Forest Service Road 16. Pass the Hopewell Church and then cross a bridge over the Jacks River. Immediately after crossing, turn right and pass the Jacks River Trailhead (on the right). FSR 16 becomes FSR 221. Take FSR 221 for a little more than 1 mile, and turn sharply to the right onto FSR 62. (The road sign is slightly uphill and may be hard to see.) Travel 4.5 miles to the parking area, which is uphill on the left.

FACILITIES/TRAILHEAD There are no facilities at the trailhead. Though camping is generally allowed anywhere in the wilderness, note that the Beech Bottom Trail and Jacks River Falls areas are open for day use only from November 1 to March 31. If you hike from April to November, you will find several clearings suitable for camping along the riverbank. Streams appear frequently along the trail—be sure to treat all water. Also, hang your food to keep it out of reach of bears and other critters.

From the parking area walk downhill to the trailhead at the two kiosks **(Waypoint 1)**. Follow the wide, level path on an easy grade, winding around ravines. Young white pines often line the path, and hardwoods fill the steep slopes. At 0.8 mile, mountain laurel and rhododendron appear, and the shift in foliage is more dramatic as you pass a drainage shadowed by hemlocks. At 1.2 miles look right for a massive hemlock just off the trail **(Waypoint 2)**.

At 1.3 miles, cross a stream and climb to the west. The path rises back to the high, dry ridges with abundant Virginia pines, white pines, and oaks. Look right at 2.3 miles where a stand of dead trees create a window with views of western hills

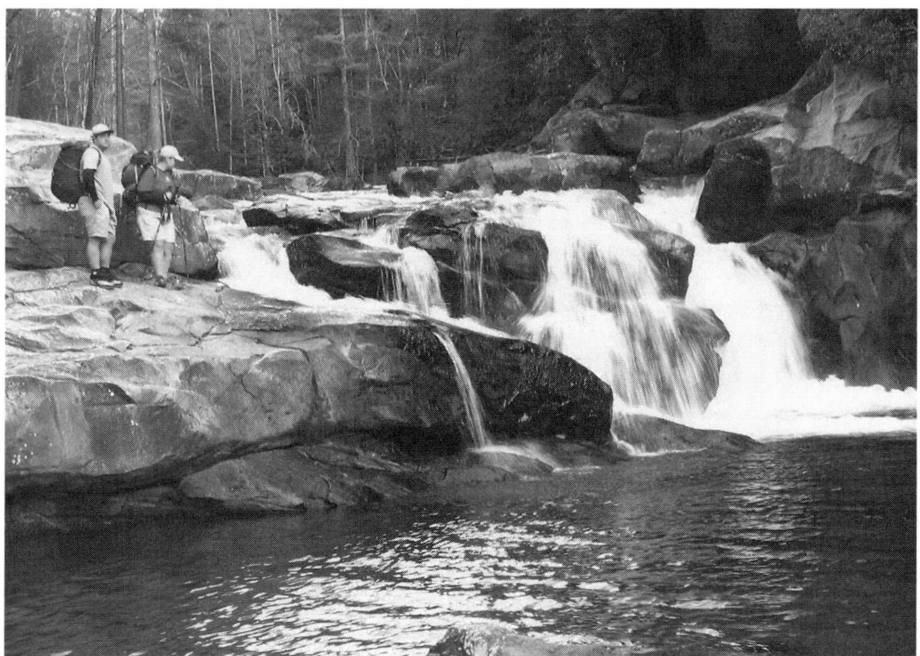

Jacks River Falls

opposite the river basin **(Waypoint 3)**. You can look down a valley to see the folded flanks of a ridge, and you'll get an even better view of this scene as you walk the next 0.2 mile. At 3.3 miles a small, cleared space lies to the right with room for a couple of small tents. The path immediately crosses Beech Creek and becomes a bed of scree in the shade of beech trees, oaks, and pines.

At 3.9 miles, turn right at the trail intersection to go northwest on the Jacks River Trail **(Waypoint 4)**. In a dark hallway of hemlock and pine, the trail runs wide and flat, while Jacks River is visible below on the left. If you're scouting spots to relax or camp, look left for flat clearings along the bank. At 4.4 miles there is an immense clearing to the right where the river bends and Beech Creek feeds into Jacks River **(Waypoint 5)**.

To continue to the falls, go northwest, crossing Beech Creek to walk the rocky path along Jacks River. The path briefly takes a steep climb along the bluff and drops down to a set of falls that feed a large pool. Less than 100 feet farther, at 4.5 miles, are the major falls where whitewater spills over vertical rock until its final leap into a wide pool **(Waypoint 6)**. To return to the trailhead, retrace your steps upstream to cross Beech Creek and take the Beech Bottom Trail back to the trailhead.

UTM WAYPOINTS

1. 16S 720158E 3874648N
2. 16S 720787E 3873773N
3. 16S 721153E 3873061N
4. 16S 722251E 3872326N
5. 16S 721742E 3872764N
6. 16S 721588E 3872610N

TRIP 3 Cohutta Wilderness: Hemp Top Trail

Distance	10.8 miles, out-and-back
Hiking Time	3–4 hours
Difficulty	Easy to moderate
Elevation Gain/Loss	+1855/-2395 feet
Trail Uses	Backpacking and horseback riding
Best Times	Year-round (good views in winter)
Agency	Chattahoochee National Forest, Cohutta Ranger District
Recommended Map	U.S. Forest Service *Cohutta and Big Frog Wilderness Georgia-Tennessee*

see map on pp. 26–27

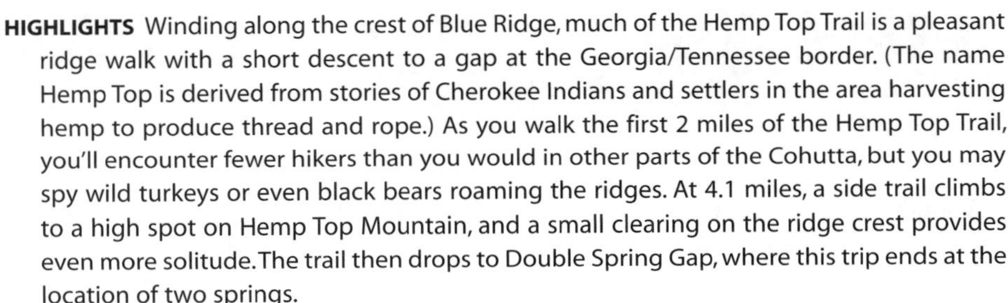

HIGHLIGHTS Winding along the crest of Blue Ridge, much of the Hemp Top Trail is a pleasant ridge walk with a short descent to a gap at the Georgia/Tennessee border. (The name Hemp Top is derived from stories of Cherokee Indians and settlers in the area harvesting hemp to produce thread and rope.) As you walk the first 2 miles of the Hemp Top Trail, you'll encounter fewer hikers than you would in other parts of the Cohutta, but you may spy wild turkeys or even black bears roaming the ridges. At 4.1 miles, a side trail climbs to a high spot on Hemp Top Mountain, and a small clearing on the ridge crest provides even more solitude. The trail then drops to Double Spring Gap, where this trip ends at the location of two springs.

DIRECTIONS From Atlanta, take Interstate 75 north to Interstate 575. Travel north on I-575 to where it becomes U.S. Highway 76. Take U.S. 76 east to the intersection with GA Highway 5 north of Blue Ridge. Take GA 5 north for 3.7 miles to signs for Old State Route 2 and Watson Gap and turn left. Go 10.5 miles to Watson Gap and turn right onto Forest Service Road 22. Continue 3.6 miles to the parking area for the Dally Gap and Jacks River Trailhead.

FACILITIES/TRAILHEAD There are no facilities at the trailhead for Hemp Top. Double Spring Gap is the only location with water, so bring enough for a day's trek. Camping is allowed anywhere in this wilderness area, though this stretch of the Hemp Top Trail has few wide spots for camping. Double Spring Gap is the best bet due to the water source. Black bears frequent the ridges of the Cohutta, so hang your food at night. As an added precaution, give your itinerary to a friend or ranger, especially if you hike solo.

The hike begins on the eastern side of the wilderness at the Dally Gap parking area where you'll find trailheads for the Hemp Top and Jacks River trails. From the parking area, the Hemp Top Trailhead is to the right **(Waypoint 1)**. Pass the metal gate and ascend gradually, traveling north through second-growth forest of hemlocks, pines, and hardwoods. To the right, ferns and oaks fill ravines that run deep, and at 0.6 mile an open spot in the foliage frames a distant ridge—your first clear view to this point.

At 0.9 mile the Benton MacKaye Trail enters on the left and shares the Hemp Top treadway to the border with Tennessee. Continue straight, and take the bend to the north, passing beds of creeping cedar. Steady and easy, the trail rises to the spine of Blue Ridge at 1.4 miles, and you can gaze down slopes to the left and right. Keep alert, as you might encounter a bear along this stretch. I scouted this section following a summer drought that depleted food resources for local animals, and bears were roaming the ridges

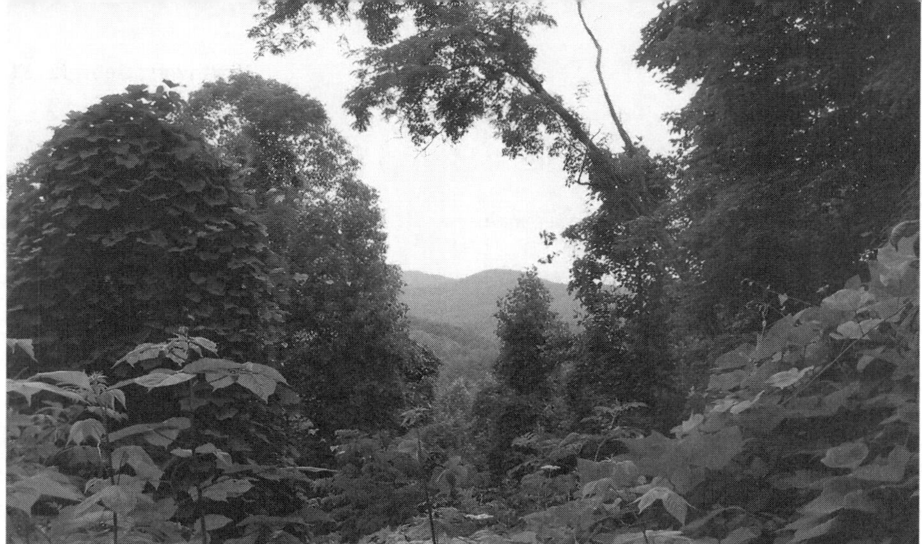

A window to distant mountains on the Hemp Top Trail

scrounging for food. The first evidence of this was the frequent swarms of yellow jackets; spots along the trail were scarred from where bears had dug up their burrows in search of yellow jacket larvae. The surefire evidence was the bear that came cruising around my tent at 2 AM—a heart-pounding moment to say the least.

At 2.3 miles you reach the junction with the Penitentiary Branch Trail **(Waypoint 2)**. Bear right to stay on the Hemp Top Trail, which is flat and bordered by pines and oaks. Traveling this section on a summer morning, I saw sunlight breaching the ridge on my right and setting the woods to the west aglow. From here the path is covered in grass and alternates between flat sections and slight upward grades, and along the trail you can see the tattered, gray trunks of shagbark hickory.

Continuing your ascent, you climb above 3400 feet of elevation at 3.7 miles. At 3.9 miles, a side trail to the right extends 400 feet to the summit of Hemp Top at about 3540 feet **(Waypoint 3)**. On top you'll find a patch of bare ground in the shade of a tree. I paused here and found it to be a peaceful spot with high grasses all around bending in calm wind. As you look down the ridge to the northeast, there is no longer any sign of a fire tower that once stood on this perch.

When you're ready to continue, walk back down to the Hemp Top Trail and turn right to take a moderate descent. The trail crosses a series of hills and saddles, dropping to Double Spring Gap at 5.4 miles **(Waypoint 4)**. The gap lies on the state line and also the Tennessee Valley Divide. The spring to the west eventually joins the river system that drains into the Gulf of Mexico, while waters from the eastern spring eventually flow to the Tennessee River. From the state border, the Hemp Top Trail continues north, up Big Frog Mountain, but for this trip, Double Spring Gap is the turnaround point.

UTM WAYPOINTS

1. 16S 726604E 3868485N
2. 16S 725972E 3869228N
3. 16S 726359E 3872667N
4. 16S 726510E 3874538N

TRIP 4 Cohutta Wilderness: Penitentiary Branch Trail

Distance	11.8 miles, out-and-back
Hiking Time	5 hours
Difficulty	Easy to moderate
Elevation Gain/Loss	+2270/-2280 feet
Trail Uses	Backpacking and horseback riding
Best Times	Year-round (good views in winter)
Agency	Chattahoochee National Forest, Cohutta Ranger District
Recommended Map	U.S. Forest Service *Cohutta and Big Frog Wilderness Georgia-Tennessee*

see map on pp. 26–27

HIGHLIGHTS Isolated in the wilderness for days on end, the men who logged the Cohutta in the 1900s felt as if they were stuck doing time. And this is how the trail known as Penitentiary Branch received its name. But for modern-day travelers, this trail on the east side of the Cohutta Wilderness can be liberating as it provides fairly easy access to the banks of the beautiful Jacks River. Though the trail drops about 1400 feet to the bank of the river, the descent stretches over 5.9 miles, so the going isn't too tough. When the days stretch long in the warmer months, you could soak in the rushing waters or try to reel in a trout, and still have time for the walk back the car. And if you're seeking a night out in the forest, a wide campsite with room for several people lies beneath hemlocks along the riverbank.

DIRECTIONS From Atlanta, take Interstate 75 north to Interstate 575. Travel north on I-575 to where it becomes U.S. Highway 76. Take U.S. 76 east to the intersection with GA Highway 5 north of Blue Ridge. Take GA 5 north for 3.7 miles to signs for Old State Route 2 and Watson Gap and turn left. Go 10.5 miles to Watson Gap and turn right onto Forest Service Road 22. Go 3.6 miles to the parking area for the Dally Gap and Jacks River Trailhead.

FACILITIES/TRAILHEAD There are no facilities at the Dally Gap Trailhead for Hemp Top. On the Penitentiary Trail, water is available at the Penitentiary Branch stream and of course at Jacks River. Be sure to treat water from all streams and the river. Camping is allowed anywhere in the wilderness area; during your trek down Penitentiary Branch you will see a couple of small clearings, though the flat area along Jacks River provides enough room for several people. This is bear territory, so hang your food at night, and before you hike, give your itinerary to a friend or ranger, especially if you hike solo.

Penitentiary Branch is an interior trail in the wilderness that you can reach via the Hemp Top Trail, as detailed below, or the Jacks River Trail. To reach the Penitentiary Trail from the Hemp Top Trail, begin at the Dally Gap parking area on the eastern side of the Cohutta Wilderness. This is the location of trailheads for the Hemp Top and Jacks River trails. Hemp Top is the trail to the right **(Waypoint 1)**. Pass the metal gate and ascend gradually, traveling north through hemlocks, pines, and hardwoods.

Travel on the Hemp Top Trail for 2.2 miles to a Y intersection **(Waypoint 2)**. Bear left to descend on the Penitentiary Branch Trail. At first, you may feel hemmed in as Virginia pines and hemlock trees form green walls on each side of the path. But the 3-mile mark brings slight views of Hickory Ridge to the west. You may detect the pungent odor of galax, a heart-shaped evergreen plant that thrives in shaded forest.

At 3.6 miles, a small opening used as a campsite lies to the right, just before the trail drops briefly and crosses a drainage. The views to the west come and go as you move deeper into the ravine, and at 5 miles you'll hear the first whispers of Jacks River. After another three-tenths of a mile, the forest opens as high-rise hemlocks dominate the land to your right.

Cross the shallow Penitentiary Branch stream at 5.5 miles, and turn to the northwest to parallel with the water. Less than a half mile farther, the trail ends beside Jacks River on a shaded plot of flat ground with wide-open spaces **(Waypoint 3)**. To return to Dally Gap, retrace your steps to the Hemp Top Trail, or you can cross the river to return on the Jacks River Trail (Trip 5).

UTM WAYPOINTS

1. 16S 726604E 3868485N
2. 16S 726197E 3870777N
3. 16S 723587E 3871008N

TRIP 5 Cohutta Wilderness: Jacks River Trail

Distance	14.2 miles, out-and-back (or 12.7-mile loop if returning via Penitentiary Branch Trail)
Hiking Time	4–5 hours
Difficulty	Easy to moderate
Elevation Gain/Loss	+/-1140 feet (+2690/-1850 feet if returning via Penitentiary Branch)
Trail Use	Backpacking
Best Times	Spring, summer, and fall
Agency	Chattahoochee National Forest, Cohutta Ranger District
Recommended Map	U.S. Forest Service *Cohutta and Big Frog Wilderness Georgia-Tennessee*

see map on pp. 26–27

HIGHLIGHTS A massive amount of timber was pulled from the Cohutta Wilderness in the 1900s, with four logging camp employing 300 to 400 men. The effort grew so intense that when logging began along Jacks River in 1929, a railway was built to carry out the lumber. By the late 1930s, the tracks were removed, and now all that remains are a few stone supports and scattered scraps of wood and metal. What thrives now is the popular Jacks River Trail, which follows the old rail bed through magnificent forest of hemlock, oak, hickory, and ferns. The trip outlined below includes 7.1 miles of the Jacks River Trail, though the path totals 16.7 miles on its journey across the wilderness. This can certainly be done as a long dayhike, but ample areas for camping lie along the way.

DIRECTIONS From Atlanta, take Interstate 75 north to Interstate 575. Travel north on I-575 to where it becomes U.S. Highway 76. Take U.S. 76 east to the intersection with GA Highway 5 north of Blue Ridge. Take GA 5 north for 3.7 miles to signs for Old State Route 2 and Watson Gap and turn left. Go 10.5 miles to Watson Gap and turn right onto Forest Service Road 22. Go 3.6 miles to the parking area for the Dally Gap and Jacks River Trailhead.

FACILITIES/TRAILHEAD There are no facilities at the Dally Gap Trailhead for the Jacks River Trail. Water is plentiful, but be sure to treat water from all streams and the river. Camping is allowed anywhere in the wilderness area, and along the way you'll find attractive spots for camping beside the river and in stands of hemlock. This is bear territory, so hang your food at night, and give your itinerary to a friend or ranger, especially if you hike solo.

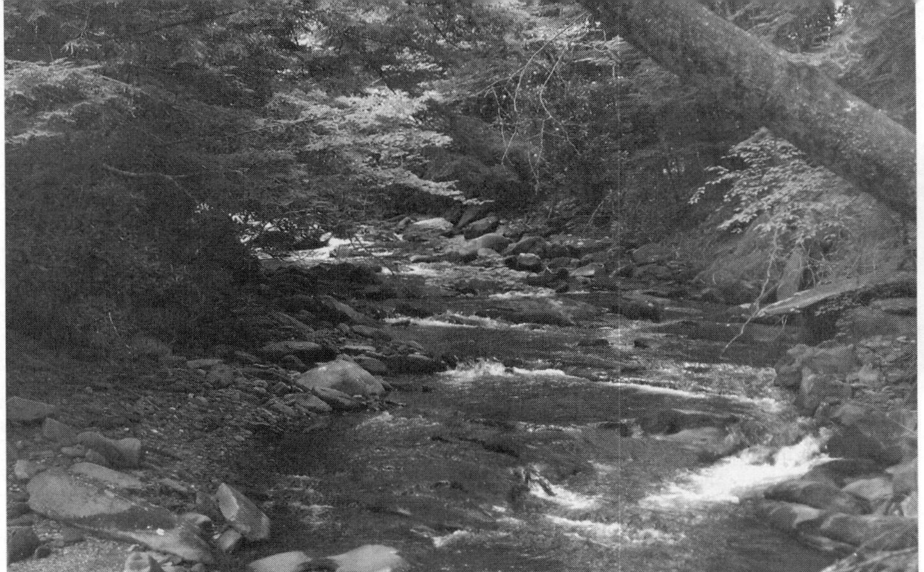

Jacks River

Dally Gap is the trailhead for the Jacks River Trail and Hemp Top Trail. The Jacks River Trail is to the left **(Waypoint 1)**. Follow the wide, shaded path that drops easily through hemlocks, hardwoods, and mountain laurel, which bloom white in spring. The path, with green blazes, runs parallel to the Bear Branch stream, out of view but still a thrumming, distant white noise. At 1.8 miles, Bear Branch flows into Jacks River, which you'll skirt, moving northwest, rolling through low-hanging rhododendron.

When I scouted this section, it seemed quite peaceful until I reached a sandy bluff beside the river. A swarm of fat bees shot in and out of small holes in the sandy earth, and I dashed through the humming cloud like Indiana Jones ducking poison darts. Once you've done the bee dance, the trail drops and crosses Jacks River where it rumbles and crashes through boulders **(Waypoint 2)**.

After topping a hill, the Jacks River Trail takes a long, moderate descent through dense forest with the river roaring at its side. At 3.0 miles **(Waypoint 3)** a spectacular view of the ravine appears and steep green hills overlap in the foreground, while a far ridge stands like a tall gate to this rugged valley.

The trail joins the edge of the river, which keeps a quick pace and grows louder. At 4.0 miles, look right for what may be the best possible spot where you could camp on the trail **(Waypoint 4)**. In the shade of hemlocks, a wide clear section of the bank lies above a large pool, and yards downstream a cascade is just the right size for a water back massage. When you continue down the trail, you'll see a lengthy grove of widely spaced hemlock trees that could also house you for the night. From here, you begin to cross the river umpteen times (you'll probably lose count), until you reach the Penitentiary Branch Trail intersection. At each crossing look sharp to see the green blazes on the opposite bank. The water can be waist deep—trekking poles will help you keep your balance. Also, you might want to pack water shoes for the many crossings to help keep your hiking shoes dry. Because your feet will be dunked frequently, think about traveling in warm weather.

The trail stays mostly flat as it follows the winding path of the river, and at mile 7.1 the trail intersects the river

(Waypoint 5). Across the water, the Jacks River Trail intersects the Penitentiary Branch Trail. Cross here to take the Penitentiary Branch and Hemp Top trails back to the trailhead (see Trip 4), or just retrace your steps on the Jacks River Trail to return.

UTM WAYPOINTS

1. 16S 726604E 3868485N
2. 16S 724384E 3867519N
3. 16S 724508E 3867988N
4. 16S 724373E 3868758N
5. 16S 723583E 3870974N

TRIP 6 Benton MacKaye Trail: Dyer Gap to Watson Gap

Distance	9.0 miles, out-and-back
Hiking Time	4–5 hours
Difficulty	Easy to moderate
Elevation Gain/Loss	+1580/-1585 feet
Trail Uses	Backpacking and horseback riding
Best Times	Winter, spring, and fall
Agency	Benton MacKaye Trail Association and U.S. Forest Service, Cohutta Ranger District
Recommended Maps	USGS 7.5-min. *Dyer Gap* and *Hemp Top GA-TN* and U.S. Forest Service *Cohutta and Big Frog Wilderness Georgia-Tennessee*

HIGHLIGHTS If you're looking for an easy introduction to the Benton MacKaye Trail, Section 9 (running from Dyer Gap to Watson Gap) is a good starting point. The highest elevation for this section is at 2960 feet, while the lowest elevation is about 2500 feet, so there are no extended, difficult climbs. Plus, this is one of the shortest sections of the Benton MacKaye Trail, and with an early start you can do an out-and-back trip in a day without a struggle.

From the western side of the Blue Ridge the trail quickly drops to the South Fork of Jacks River and runs parallel to the stream. At 2.2 miles in Rich Cove the Benton MacKaye Trail splits from the South Fork Trail and turns east, leaving the river to ascend an old logging road. At 3.8 miles you'll leave the old logging road and climb to the crest of Blue Ridge. From the top of a knob, you'll make a gradual descent through large oaks to end at Watson Gap.

DIRECTIONS Parking is available at Dyer Gap as well as Watson Gap. To reach these areas from Atlanta, take Interstate 75 north to Interstate 575. Travel north on I-575 to where it becomes U.S. Highway 76. Take U.S. 76 east to the intersection with GA Highway 5 north of Blue Ridge. Take GA 5 north for 3.7 miles to signs for Old State Route 2 and Watson Gap and turn left. Go 10.5 miles to Watson Gap. To continue to Dyer Gap, turn left onto Forest Service Road 64 and go 3.3 miles to the intersection of FSR 64 and FSR 64A. There is space to park on the right near the road junction.

If you wish to use a shuttle for your hike, you can make arrangements with commercial shuttle operators or members of the Benton MacKaye Trail Association. For a list of commercial vendors or to get contact information for individual volunteers, check out "Hiker Resources" at www.bmta.org.

FACILITIES/TRAILHEAD There are no facilities at the trailhead. There are also no shelters along the trail, but you can camp at any of the several clearings along the way. Water is available at the many stream crossings, but be sure to treat it before using it. If you camp overnight, be sure to hang your food out of reach of bears and other animals.

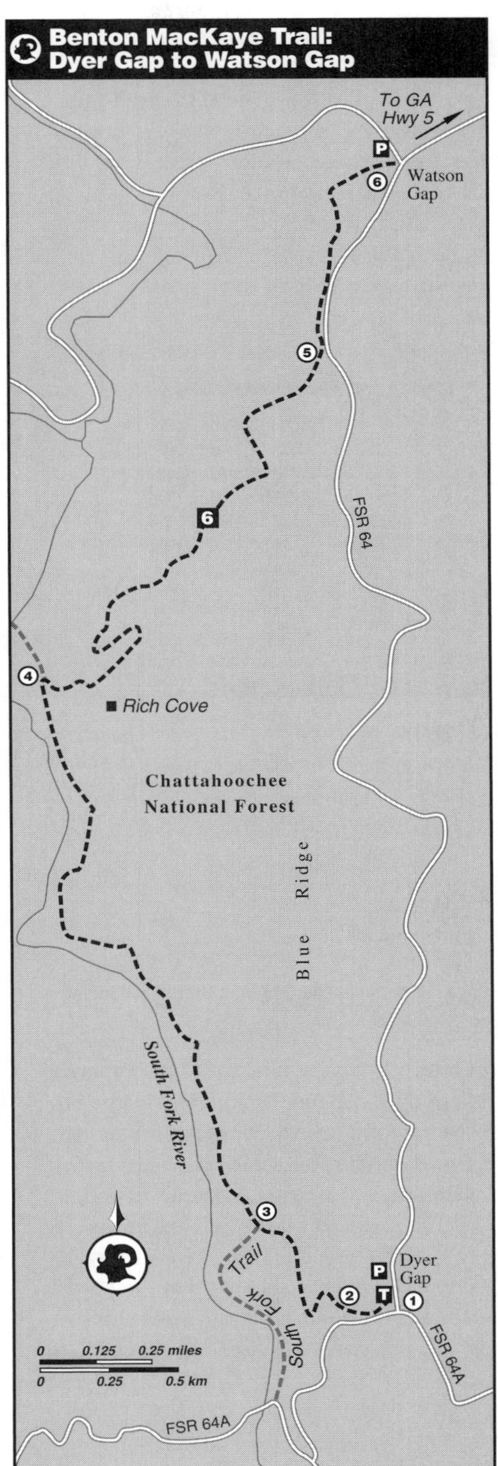

From the parking near the junction of FSR 64 and FSR 64A **(Waypoint 1)**, turn right onto FSR 64 and walk north. At 0.1 mile **(Waypoint 2)**, turn right at a post with double white diamond blazes and enter a narrow path. The path descends gradually through hardwoods and hemlocks and enters shaded forest with mountain laurel and rhododendron.

At the half-mile mark, the trail follows a stream, winds among moss-covered logs, and passes through a striking grove of rhododendron with thick, twisted trunks. At 0.6 mile **(Waypoint 3)** the Benton MacKaye Trail joins the South Fork Trail. (If you turn left onto the South Fork Trail, it proceeds 0.2 mile to Shadow Falls.) To continue the hike from **Waypoint 3**, turn right to travel north and immediately cross a narrow stream. The path visits a scraggly forest that has been heavily logged and then ventures into a mature forest of towering hemlocks and thickets of rhododendron. The South Fork River occasionally comes into view, and you can peer through the heavy foliage to see the wide water sliding through the forest.

The stream crossings continue and spots along the trail can be pretty muddy, so consider wearing waterproof footwear and maybe gaiters. The path is also used by horseback riders, but the trail is not as chewed up as you might expect.

The trail enters Rich Cove, and at 2.2 miles the Benton MacKaye Trail and South Fork Trail split at a marked junction **(Waypoint 4)**. Bear right and ascend to the northeast, following white diamond blazes on an old logging road. The trip continues with an easy walk through hardwoods and hemlocks and then a wide path out of the creek basin. The trail becomes steep as you move through another area that has been logged, and you can see Cohutta Mountain to the west. Though you'll encounter areas of clear-cut forest that are none too attractive, at 3.3 miles the path turns to the northeast and things shift dramatically as you enter a stand of majestic poplars.

At 3.6 miles the trail crosses a ridge, and at 3.8 miles **(Waypoint 5)** bear left to leave the wide treadway and descend a narrow path, walking beneath the low boughs of hemlocks. (The path to the right at **Waypoint 5** continues 300 feet to FSR 64.) The trail drops through a pleasant forest of hardwoods and then climbs to the crest of Blue Ridge. A gradual climb carries you to an elevation of 2960 feet where you'll stand atop an unnamed knob at 4.2 miles with slight views to the east. From this high point the trail takes a hard left turn and moves downward quickly through fern beds shaded beneath oaks and hemlocks.

At 4.5 miles **(Waypoint 6)** the trail intersects with FSR 64. Turn left and walk 100 feet to reach the junction of FSR 64, FSR 22, and Foster Branch Road at Watson Gap. From **Waypoint 6**, retrace your steps to return to Dyer Gap. (You can also walk southwest on FSR 64 to return.)

UTM WAYPOINTS

1. 16S 727186E 3861252N
2. 16S 727051E 3861208N
3. 16S 726727E 3861535N
4. 16S 725973E 3863517N
5. 16S 726973E 3864718N
6. 16S 727260E 3865433N

TRIP 7 Cloudland Canyon State Park: Overlook, West Rim, & Waterfalls Trails

Distance	5.4 miles, semiloop
Hiking Time	3 hours
Difficulty	Moderate to strenuous
Elevation Gain/Loss	+1545/-1550
Trail Use	Leashed dogs and good for kids (Waterfalls Trail)
Best Times	Winter (for canyon views), spring, and fall
Agency	Cloudland Canyon State Park
Recommended Map	*Cloudland Canyon State Park* is available at the ranger station or online at www.gastateparks.org/info/cloudland.

HIGHLIGHTS A thousand feet deep, Cloudland Canyon is truly impressive—an immense gorge with great walls of vertical rock and a floor of lively streams and high waterfalls. Established in 1938, Cloudland Canyon State Park has long been a favorite destination in Georgia, and some trails are quite developed. The Waterfalls Trail, which descends to the floor of the canyon, is comprised of stairs and platforms that allow a wide range of people to safely access the falls, one of which plunges 100 feet into a great pool of turquoise water. (Take note that the hike back up from Falls #2 is strenuous.) Equally inspiring are the views of the canyon from the West Rim Loop Trail, which hugs the lip of the gorge. The hike described below combines the Waterfall and West Rim trails into one extensive dayhike that is mostly moderate but does contain one strenuous ascent on the return trip from Falls #2.

DIRECTIONS From Atlanta take Interstate 75 north to Tennessee and merge onto Interstate 24 west at Exit 2, going toward Chattanooga/Nashville. Travel 17.1 miles and take Interstate 59 south at Exit 167. Travel south on I-59 8.3 miles and take Exit 11 for GA Highway 136, toward Trenton. Turn right onto GA 136 and travel east. Go 4.3 miles and turn into the Cloudland Canyon State Park entrance on the left. Travel 0.1 mile and bear right after the guard shack to go to the ranger station. Or, proceed past the guard shack and go 1.3 miles to the day-use parking lot on the right. From the parking lot, facing the canyon, the trailhead is to the left of the canyon overlook.

FACILITIES/TRAILHEAD There are restrooms and soda vending machines at the day-use area parking lot. Water is not easily accessible along the trail, so carry what you need. The day-use fee is $5. To purchase an annual Georgia State ParksPass for $30, call (770) 389-7401. The park has 73 campsites for tents, trailers, and RVs ($25); 30 walk-in campsites ($12); 11 backcountry campsites ($5 per person); and 16 cottages ($65–$130).

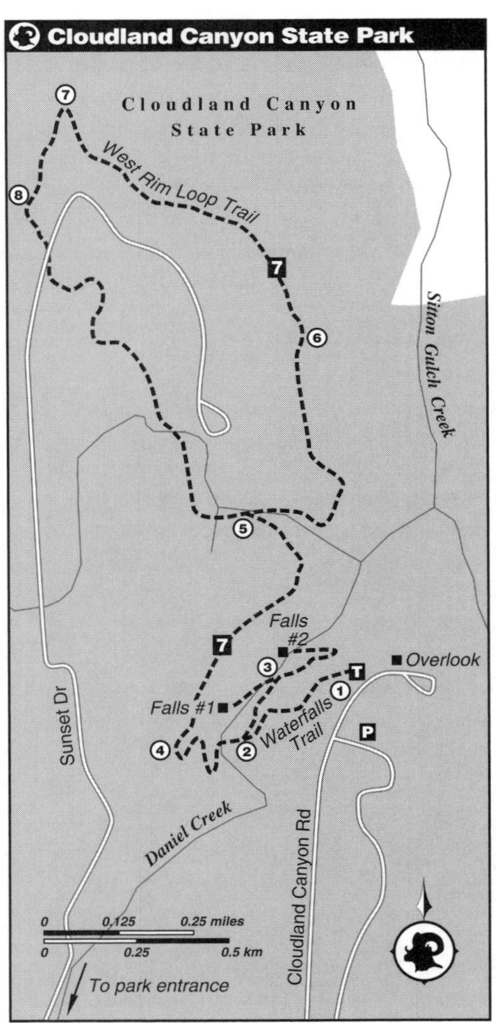

From the day-use parking lot, walk to the canyon overlook for an excellent view to the north, down a long stretch of the gorge. Distinct bands of rock in the limestone and shale walls denote various periods of sedimentation, and the soils here were deposited at the bottom of a sea more than 250 million years ago. After the sea subsided, two streams—Bear Creek and Daniel Creek—cut into the soil, forming two great canyons. Facing the overlook, go to the left (southwest) end of the overlook and enter the Upper Waterfall Trail (**Waypoint 1**). Follow yellow blazes along a wood and stone railing, with the canyon formed by Daniel Creek close on the right. After a tenth of a mile, the trail turns sharply to the right; take the next left down the stairs.

At the bottom of the stairs (**Waypoint 2**), turn right to go to the waterfalls in the bottom of the canyon or turn left to continue to the West Rim Loop Trail. If you turn right for the waterfalls, you'll descend another set of stairs and, at the bottom, turn right to go northeast. The trail runs beneath a massive, undercut rock that has a bench beneath it, and then turns left and descends more stairs. At **Waypoint 3** you can turn left to go to Falls #1 or turn right to go to Falls #2. Falls #2 is the more difficult hike, so you may want to tackle it while you're fresh. After turning right, the path becomes a long boardwalk within reach of a dripping wall of stone. Then, several flights of metal and wood stairs wind down, with landings along the way allowing views of the canyon.

You'll eventually leave the stairs for an earth trail that traverses the moist creek bottom. In a forest of hemlocks, rhododendrons, and mountain laurels, the rushing waters of Daniel Creek grow louder and louder. The path ends at a raised wood platform that stands before the 60-foot falls draped over a wall of rough, grey stone.

Return to **Waypoint 3**, go straight a few feet and turn right to descend the steps toward Falls #1. The payoff at the end of this path is even greater than that of the previous waterfall. Rather than ending at a wood platform that confines you, the trail ends practically at the edge of a large pool that catches water falling 100 feet. From here, retrace your steps to **Waypoint 2**.

At **Waypoint 2**, if you've followed the trip as described so far, you will have hiked a little less than a mile. To continue on the West Rim Loop Trail, turn right, traveling southeast. Walk about 20 feet, and then turn right to descend the steps.

Mountain laurels and oaks border the rocky path, which has a view of the creek below as it bends wide to crash and slide over a floor of rock the color of chocolate. At 1.1 miles, turn right and cross the creek via a wood footbridge. After a hairpin curve to the right, the trail climbs northwest. Then, at 1.2 miles turn sharply left and climb to an obvious, small cave. Continue to the top of the bluff where you will have winter views of the far side of the canyon.

At 1.3 miles **(Waypoint 4)**, bear right at the Y intersection and descend, following

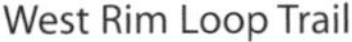
West Rim Loop Trail

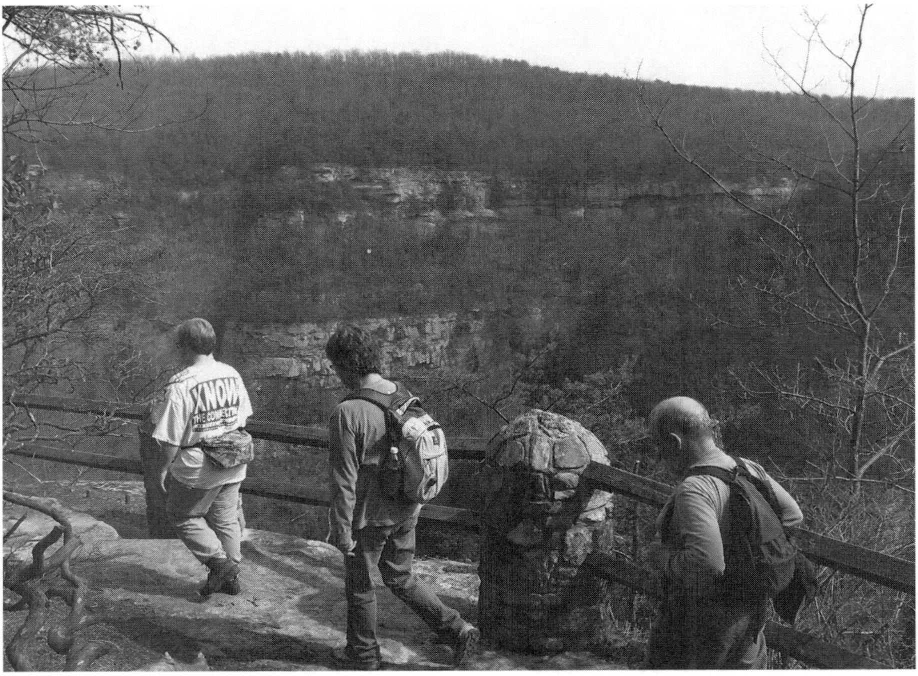

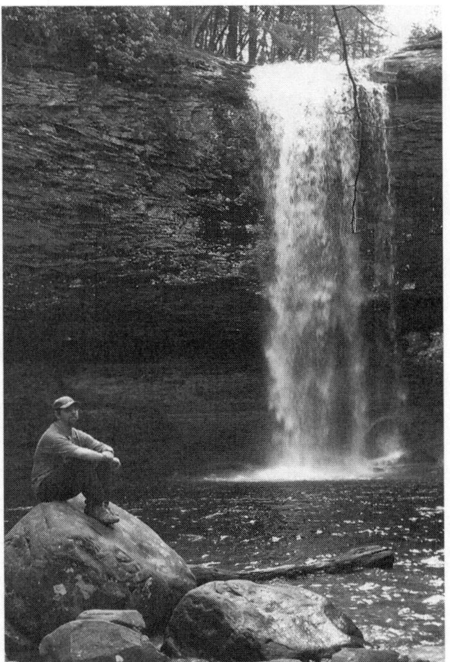

Falls #1 at Cloudland Canyon State Park

yellow blazes. At 1.6 miles, the path crosses wide rock outcrops free of any railings, and you can enjoy stunning views of cliffs opposite the gaping canyon. Here, its enormity is on full display.

The path then drops to a stream. At 1.8 miles **(Waypoint 5)** turn right, cross the wood footbridge and then proceed east back toward the canyon. The path crosses a series of bluff outcrops that are more developed, with railings of stone and wood. But these high stations are still inspiring, offering long views down the great gorge.

At 2.0 miles bear right at the intersection to walk to an overlook. From this perch you can look north down the length of the canyon to where it spills into Lookout Valley. From the overlook, continue northwest on what becomes an easy walk through typical pine and hardwood forest. One of my favorite rest spots lies at 2.4 miles **(Waypoint 6)**. To the right, several yards away from trail there is a rock outcrop surrounded by scrub pine. This spot is less obvious than other overlooks and is free of human-made structures. You can sit on the white stone and have a completely unobstructed view looking north down the canyon.

Farther down the trail at 3.0 miles **(Waypoint 7)**, another overlook lies to the right, down a steep, rooted slope. Here you are closer to the northern end of the canyon and Lookout Valley, and the broad sweep and scope of the scene below is reminiscent of a western U.S. landscape.

From the overlook the trail turns to the south, and at 3.2 miles **(Waypoint 8)**, your route turns left and follow yellow blazes. The trail crosses a road then winds through a pine and hardwood forest that is at first unremarkable but soon transitions to more oaks and crosses a modest stream. Thick heaps of leaves cover the forest floor where oaks are joined by holly trees and hemlocks. On a gradual descent you'll follow a stream drainage, turn right at 4.2 miles **(Waypoint 5)**, and travel southeast to take the West Rim Loop Trail back to the day-use parking area.

UTM WAYPOINTS

1. 16S 638887E 3855773N
2. 16S 638674E 3855622N
3. 16S 638750E 3855770N
4. 16S 638450E 3855582N
5. 16S 638624E 3856224N
6. 16S 638782E 3856765N
7. 16S 638147E 3857363N
8. 16S 638047E 3857083N

TRIP 8 Chickamauga Battlefield Memorial Trail

Distance	8.5 miles, loop
Hiking Time	4 hours
Difficulty	Easy
Elevation Gain/Loss	+/- 70 feet
Trail Use	Horseback riding and good for kids
Best Times	Spring, fall, and winter
Agency	National Park Service, Chickamauga Battlefield
Recommended Maps	*Chickamauga Battlefield Trail Guide* and *Chickamauga and Chattanooga National Military Park* (both available in the visitors center)

HIGHLIGHTS In the 5200-acre Chickamauga Battlefield, trails pass though forests and fields that resemble their condition during the 1863 Civil War battle, allowing you to imagine the challenge of fighting in this formidable terrain. The paths are mostly flat, making it easy to comfortably explore the park with children, and the woods are packed with many memorials and interpretive signs that offer incredible detail—even the specific hours that certain troops occupied spots of land. A unique aspect of the battle is that it claimed the lives of an unusual number of high-ranking officers. The hike detailed below is the Memorial Trail, designed for Boy Scouts, which visits the places where eight brigade commanders fell during battle. Though this hike is 8.5 miles, you can cut it short at several points and walk on roads back to the visitors center.

DIRECTIONS From Atlanta, take Interstate 75 north to Exit 350. Travel west on Battlefield Parkway/GA Highway 2 to Fort Oglethorpe. Turn left at the intersection of Battlefield Pkwy. and Lafayette Rd. Travel 1 mile on Lafayette Rd. to the park entrance and visitors center, which is on the right. The memorial trail begins at the edge of the lower parking area.

FACILITIES/TRAILHEAD Restrooms and a gift shop are available at the Chickamauga Battlefield Visitors Center, which is open daily (except Christmas Day) from 8:30 AM to 6 PM.

At the east side of the visitors center lower parking area, take the path that runs between two trees **(Waypoint 1)**. Just before the wood footbridge, turn left onto the Red Trail and walk beneath the Lafayette Road overpass. Skirt the left side of the field, and look to your left. This dense forest choked with trees and underbrush resembles what the soldiers had to wade through during the battle. At 0.2 mile, the trail leaves the field and enters the forest.

Walk past a line of stone Georgia Regiment markers and turn left on the Red Trail. As you turn, ahead on the left is a monument that looks like a stack of cannonballs; it marks the place where Col. Peyton Colquitt was mortally wounded while commanding the 46th Georgia Infantry Regiment. He was the brother of Alfred Holt Colquitt, who was governor of Georgia from 1876 to 1882.

Continue on the Red Trail east and look left for the cannonball monument for Brig. Gen. Benjamin Helm, Abraham Lincoln's brother-in-law. Helm was a native of Kentucky, which was neutral in the war, and Lincoln offered Helm a position in the Union Army. However, Helm turned it down and chose instead to create the 1st Kentucky Cavalry for the Confederates.

At 1.5 miles, turn right onto the Green Trail and follow the grassy path until it

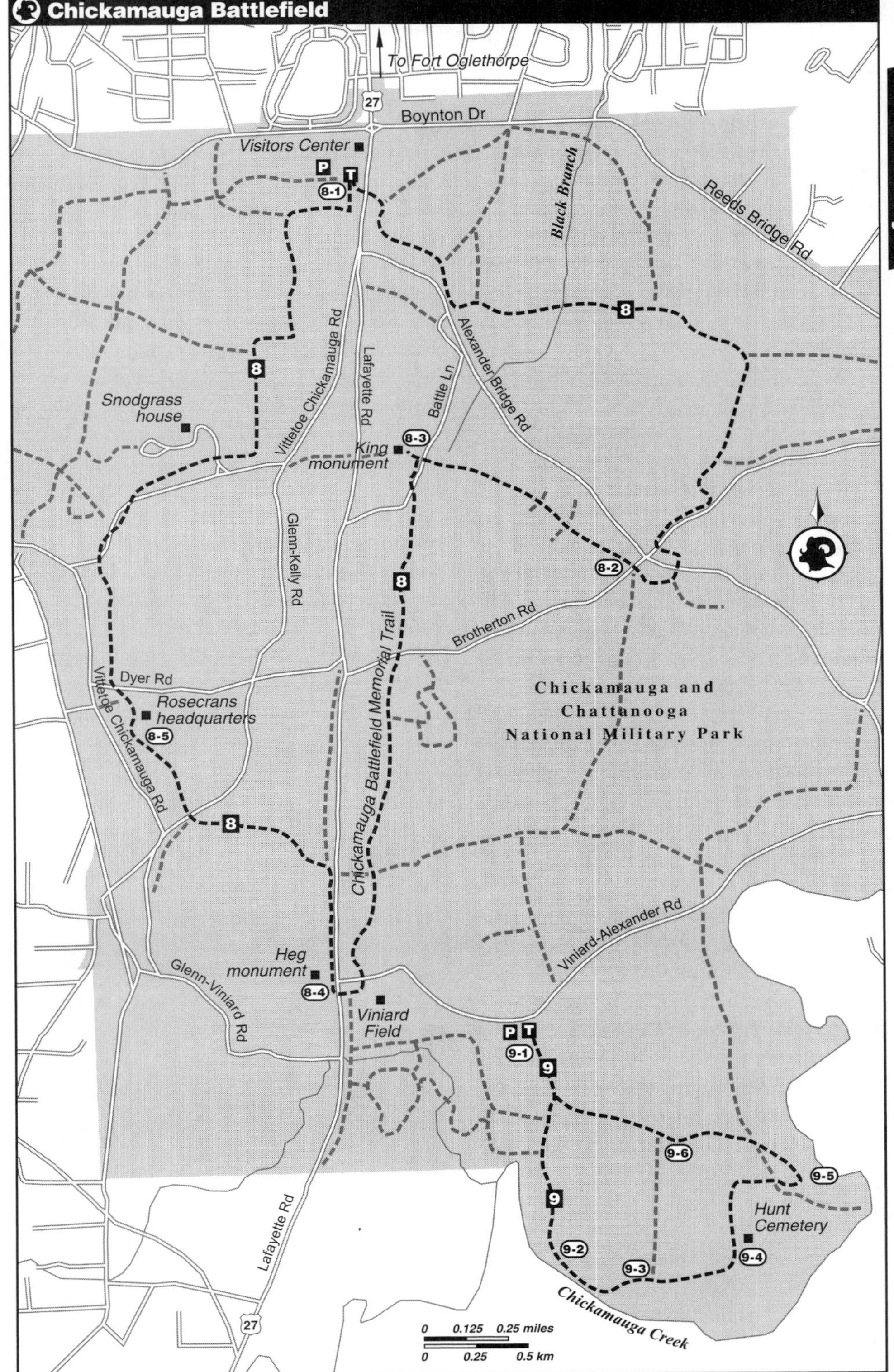
Chickamauga Battlefield
To Fort Oglethorpe
27
Boynton Dr
Visitors Center
P
T
8-1
Black Branch
Reeds Bridge Rd
8
Vittetoe Chickamauga Rd
Lafayette Rd
Battle Ln
Alexander Bridge Rd
Snodgrass house
King monument
8-3
8-2
Glenn-Kelly Rd
Brotherton Rd
Dyer Rd
Rosecrans headquarters
8-5
Vittetoe Chickamauga Rd
Chickamauga Battlefield Memorial Trail
Chickamauga and Chattanooga National Military Park
Viniard-Alexander Rd
Heg monument
8-4
Glenn-Viniard Rd
Viniard Field
9-1
9
9-6
9-5
Hunt Cemetery
9-2
9-3
9-4
Lafayette Rd
Chickamauga Creek
0 0.125 0.25 miles
0 0.25 0.5 km

exits the forest at Winfrey Field. Cannons and hay bales sit in this vast, green opening, which reflects what many have in mind when they imagine a battlefield. Turn right (southwest) and walk along the edge of the field to the monument for Union Col. Philemon Baldwin, a brigade commander for the 6th Indiana. He died on this spot at 7 PM on September 19, 1863. From here, walk south to Brotherton Rd.

At 2.0 miles turn right onto Brotherton Rd. and walk down this tranquil lane to Alexander Rd. Turn left (southeast) onto Alexander Rd. and continue to a spot where cannons sit on each side of the road **(Waypoint 2)**. Turn right and go into the forest to take the Green Trail. At a clearing in tall pines sits the monument for Confederate Brig. Gen. Preston Smith, who died the same hour as Col. Philemon Baldwin. Also, note the striking metal mural on the side of the monument for the Pennsylvania 77th Regiment. One of the more interesting aspects of the battlefield is the great number of elaborate and detailed memorials. Facing Preston's monument, turn right (west) and take the Green Trail and at 2.5 miles cross Brotherton Rd.

Enter the Yellow Trail and go north on a wide, grassy path for a good stretch, passing the monument for Brig. Gen. James Deshler who fell at noon on September 20. In 1861, Deshler had been shot in both thighs during the battle of Allegheny Mountain in West Virginia but recovered. It took an artillery shell to kill him at Chickamauga, and he was hit while inspecting his brigade before an attack.

From Deshler's monument, continue north, cross Battle Line Rd. and look northwest for the cannonball monument resting at the near edge of Kelly Field **(Waypoint 3)**. Here, Union Col. Edward A. King, commander of the 2nd Brigade of the Union's 4th Division, was wounded, and he died two days later. From King's monument, go back to Battle Line Rd., turn right (south) and enter the White Trail. You will reach a four-way trail junction, and go straight to take the Blue Trail.

At 5.0 miles, turn right onto Viniard Rd., traveling northwest, and cross LaFayette Rd. Some of the fiercest fighting took place in this area on September 19—Union Col. John T. Wilder said that men "fell in heaps." From here, turn right and walk north on Lafayette Rd. Immediately to the left downhill is the monument for Union Col. Hans C. Heg, who was born in Norway and immigrated to America with his family in 1840. He died here after he was shot in the abdomen **(Waypoint 4)**. From Heg's monument, walk back toward the road and turn left onto the Yellow Trail.

At 5.5 miles turn left at a T intersection onto the Red Trail and take this across

Helm monument

BENJAMIN H. HELM
BRIG. GEN. C.S.A.
COMMANDING BRIGADE
BRECKINRIDGE'S DIVISION
MORTALLY WOUNDED HERE
ABOUT 10A.M.SEPT.20TH, 1863

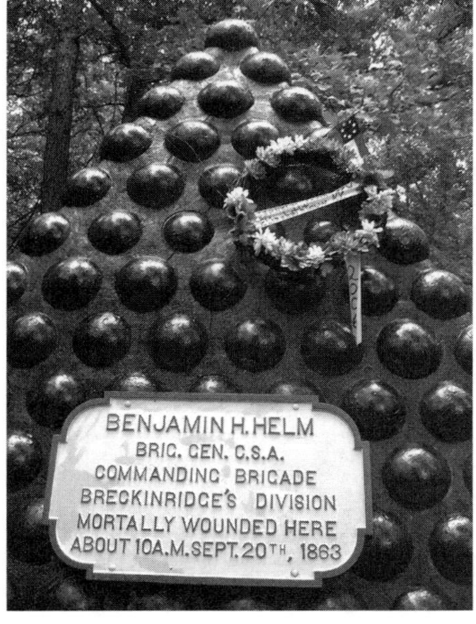

Glenn-Kelly Rd. You will pass the monument for Union Brig. Gen. William H. Lytle, a lawyer and poet who died while leading an attack on horseback. Ahead you'll walk between two large fields and pass the monument marking the headquarters for Maj. Gen. William Rosecrans, leader of the Union Army of the Cumberland **(Waypoint 5)**. Cross Dyer Rd., ascend the low hill, and at 6.9 miles you'll reach a four-way intersection. Turn right onto a dirt road and go northeast.

At 7.5 miles, turn left onto a gravel road and go northwest. Look left for an open field and cabin, which housed the Snodgrass family who lived on this land during the war. From here you'll take an easy walk along small roads heading back to the visitors center.

At 7.9 miles turn left onto an old paved road and go north. At 8.3 miles, turn right and go northeast. Cross the field to the cannons marking Slocum's Louisiana Battery. From the cannons, turn left and return to the visitors center.

UTM WAYPOINTS

1. 16S 658905E 3867699N
2. 16S 660211E 3865794N
3. 16S 659162E 3866397N
4. 16S 658772E 3863759N
5. 16S 657863E 3865075N

TRIP 9 Chickamauga Battlefield Hunt Cemetery Loop

Distance	2.7 miles, loop
Hiking Time	1 hour
Difficulty	Easy
Elevation Gain/Loss	+/-260 feet
Trail Use	Leashed dogs and good for kids
Best Times	Spring, fall, and winter
Agency	National Park Service, Chickamauga Battlefield
Recommended Maps	*Chickamauga Battlefield Trail Guide* and *Chickamauga and Chattanooga National Military Park* (both available in the visitors center)

HIGHLIGHTS During the War of 1812, Helm Hunt served in the South Carolina Militia and fought against the Creek Indians in what is now Alabama. For his service he received 280 acres of land on what is now part of the Chickamauga Battlefield. Hunt and several of his family members are buried in a small cemetery in the southernmost part of the battlefield; their graves date back to the late 1800s. During the battle of Chickamauga, Helm Hunt's home was used as a hospital. Nurse Kate Cumming wrote in her journal "[t]hat there had been fighting in Mr. Hunt's yard, and many killed there." Helm, who was born in 1789—the same year the U.S. Constitution was adopted—was buried in the cemetery in 1870.

DIRECTIONS From Atlanta, take Interstate 75 north to Exit 350. Travel west on Battlefield Parkway/GA Highway 2 to Fort Oglethorpe. Turn left at the intersection of Battlefield Parkway and Lafayette Rd. Travel 1 mile Lafayette Rd. to the park entrance and visitors center on the left. From the Chickamauga Battlefield Visitors Center, travel south on Lafayette Rd. to the intersection with Viniard-Alexander Rd. Turn left onto Viniard-Alexander Rd. and travel east 0.6 mile to the parking area on the right.

FACILITIES/TRAILHEAD There are no facilities at the trailhead. Restrooms and a gift shop are available at the Chickamauga Battlefield Visitors Center, which is open daily (except Christmas Day) from 8:30 AM to 6 PM.

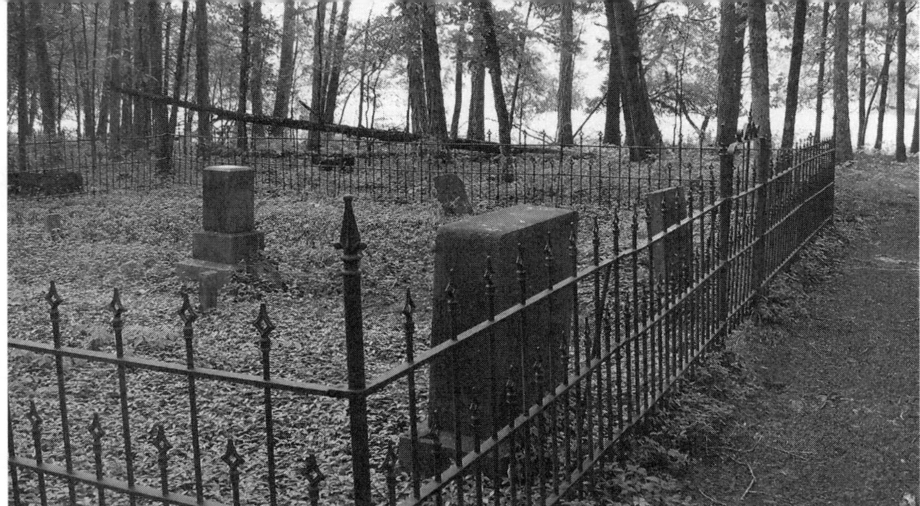

Hunt Cemetery

From the parking area enter the wide gravel path and travel southeast **(Waypoint 1)**. After traveling a little more than 1000 feet, turn right onto the Yellow Trail, a dirt and gravel path that goes south. As you approach Chickamauga Creek, the forest transitions from pines to hardwoods. This part of the park sees relatively few visitors; a group of six deer scampered away as I hiked here in summer.

At 0.7 mile, the trail bends left near the bank of Chickamauga Creek and runs east **(Waypoint 2)**. Along the next section I had an unexpected encounter with a small group of cattle on the trail, no doubt escapees from a nearby farm. The leader sported horns, though I suspect it was a female rather than a male. Still, horns are horns, so I gave them a wide berth as they passed.

The trail crosses a massive field, bearing slightly to the right (east) and continues in the trees at the opposite side of the opening **(Waypoint 3)**. At 1.2 miles, the path leaves the forest and turns sharply left, running north along the edge of a field.

At 1.3 miles, Hunt Cemetery lies a few yards inside the forest **(Waypoint 4)**. The small, square plot is surrounded by an iron fence; you can enter through a gate, but tread lightly and do not disturb the tombstones. Some of the stone markers are quite weathered and difficult to read, but some clearly date back to the 1800s. One family member buried in the cemetery, Jeptha Hunt, served in the 12th Georgia Cavalry from 1863 to 1865, survived the war, and lived until 1895.

From the cemetery, continue into the forest, traveling north through a corridor of brambles and thickets. At 1.7 miles **(Waypoint 5)**, turn left onto a gravel road and continue north in a quiet and much more attractive forest of pines and hardwoods.

You'll reach a road intersection at 2.1 miles **(Waypoint 6)**. Turn right on the gravel road to go north briefly before bending to the west. Along this road, Maj. Gen. Benjamin Cheatham assembled his troops; they served as reserve forces for General Braxton Bragg's front line. Continue on this road to return to the parking area.

UTM WAYPOINTS

1. 16S 659743E 3863515N
2. 16S 659868E 3862415N
3. 16S 660213E 3862377N
4. 16S 660680E 3862545N
5. 16S 660970E 3862882N
6. 16S 660435E 3863010N

TRIP 10 Chickamauga Creek Trail

Distance	6.2 miles, loop
Hiking Time	3 hours
Difficulty	Moderate
Elevation Gain/Loss	+800/-820 feet
Trail Use	Leashed dogs
Best Times	Spring, fall, and winter
Agency	U.S. Forest Service, Armuchee Ranger District
Recommended Maps	USGS 7.5-min. *Catlett* and *Trails of the Chattahoochee-Oconee National Forests*

HIGHLIGHTS The Chickamauga Creek Trail is easy to access, but traffic tends to be light, and the trail is set deep enough in national forest that you'll feel as if you've found a hidden corner of the world. The trail explores terrain that is a bit unusual because it crosses two ridges that are closer together than most in northwest Georgia, making the valley separating the ridges seem deeper and more secluded than it is. In the valley, clear streams wind among American beech trees, and in spring, trilliums, dwarf irises, and other wildflowers lie near the trail. On the ridges, the forest is much different, with open hardwood forests of hickory and oak. You may encounter deer and wild turkeys.

DIRECTIONS From Atlanta take Interstate 75 north to Exit 320. Turn left onto GA Highway 136 and go to Villanow. From Villanow, continue west on GA 136 for 3.4 miles and turn right onto Ponder Creek Road. Go 0.6 mile and bear right onto Forest Service Road 219. Go 1.8 miles to where FSR 219 ends at the parking area.

You can also access the Chickamauga Creek Trail by driving to the parking area at Waypoint 4, where Forest Service Road 250 crosses the Tennessee Valley Divide. To get to there from Atlanta, take I-75 north to Exit 320. Turn left onto GA 136 and go to Villanow. From Villanow continue west on GA 136 for 5 miles to the top of Taylor Ridge at Mattox Gap. Here, turn north onto FSR 250 (not paved) and take it 2.6 miles to the junction with FSR 250A. Park in the small clearing on the side of the road. The trail is at the northeast end of the parking area marked with a FOOT TRAVEL WELCOME sign.

FACILITIES/TRAILHEAD There are no facilities at the trailhead, and there is no fee to use the area. Stream levels are unpredictable, so carry enough water for the day. Be aware that hunting takes place in this area from October through December (deer season) and March through May (turkey season), so during these times stay on the path, wear orange clothing, and avoid hiking in early morning or late in the day. For hunting season dates, visit the Georgia Department of Natural Resources website at www.gadnr.org.

At the east side of the parking area there is a road with a gate (**Waypoint 1**). Take the trail that begins on the right side of the gate, and follow white blazes. After a short distance, take a wood footbridge over Ponder Branch.

At the power line break, the loop begins. The hike can be done in either direction, and this description goes counterclockwise. Turn right (south) and take the gentle ascent through the hardwoods and pines. After cutting across the slope of a hill, the trail drops into a ravine and then climbs Rocky Ridge, which boasts nice stands of oak.

At 1.5 miles, travel northeast across a power-line clearing and enter the forest on the opposite side of the clearing. The trail levels and turns left onto an old, grass-covered roadbed that leads to the top of Dick Ridge. At 2 miles you begin an appealing trek across the east face of a slope where grasses, mountain laurel, and oak trees thrive.

The land to each side of the trail falls away dramatically as you ascend to an elevation of about 1630 feet on Dick Ridge to cross the Tennessee Valley Divide (**Waypoint 2**), which separates the watershed for the Tennessee and Mississippi rivers from the Alabama River watershed. East Chickamauga Creek, north of the divide, eventually flows to the Tennessee and Mississippi rivers, while Ponder Creek, south of the divide, eventually joins river systems that flow to the Gulf of Mexico. From the ridge summit, the path goes left, and a series of switchbacks wind down the western slope of the ridge. As you drop, the forest becomes a tangle of vines and underbrush.

The trail again follows an old road at 3.5 miles and you'll reach a Y intersection (**Waypoint 3**). Bear right to descend more switchbacks through an area with heaps of blown-down trees. A little farther on, look west in winter to see Taylor Ridge.

At 5.3 miles, the trail crosses FSR 250, and this marks your second passage over the Tennessee Valley Divide line (**Waypoint 4**). This is also the alternate parking area. Take the narrow dirt path down to the East Chickamauga Creek drainage and prepare to hop the narrow stream a handful of times. The last mile of the hike is a rolling tour of hills and ravines lavished with hickory, white oak, and tulip trees.

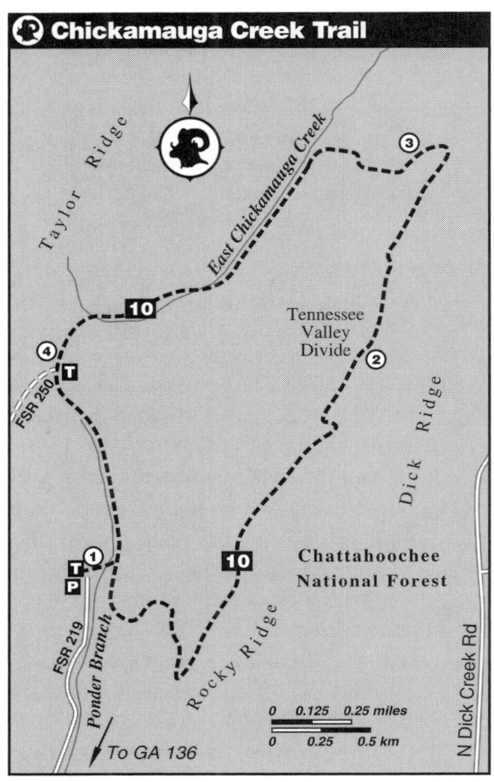

At 5.5 miles you'll cross Ponder Branch, which may just be a trickle here, and continue across the power line break to complete a loop. Turn right to go west to the parking area.

UTM WAYPOINTS

1. 16S 668275E 3842694N
2. 16S 669719E 3843927N
3. 16S 669900E 3844888N
4. 16S 668105E 3843872N

TRIP 11 Rocktown Trail

Distance	2.0 miles, out-and-back
Hiking Time	1 hour
Difficulty	Easy
Elevation Gain/Loss	+/-15 feet
Trail Use	Climbing and good for kids
Best Times	Year-round (winter is best for climbing)
Agency	Georgia Department of Natural Resources, Wildlife Resources Division
Recommended Maps	USGS 7.5-min. *Cedar Grove* and *Lafayette* or visit www.drtopo.com for a downloadable PDF of the bouldering problems.

HIGHLIGHTS The Rocktown Trail leads to a sprawling jumble of rock formations that offer some of the finest bouldering in the Southeast, with problems that range in difficulty from V0 to V8. Even those who don't climb will find Rocktown fascinating, because it seems as if you're walking through a village ruin where ancients lived among houses of sandstone. Heightening the effect are narrow alleys with steep walls that snake between boulders some 30 feet high. The hike to the Rocktown boulder field is brief, but pleasant, as ferns and hardwoods surround the path. Once you reach the boulders you'll find that the rocks have eroded in curious ways—some with scooped out, round pockets, others with vertical furrows that make the rock face appear like rows of bones. The lower portions of some boulders have eroded more quickly than their tops, so some appear to be balanced precariously, defying gravity by not toppling. In the Rocktown labyrinth, you will also find arêtes and an overhanging roof.

DIRECTIONS From Atlanta take Interstate 75 north to the exit for GA Highway 136 (Exit 320) toward Resaca/Lafayette. Take GA 136 west for 26.8 miles to E. Villanow St./GA Highway 193. Take GA 193 west, and in Lafayette take GA 193 north for 2.8 miles. Turn left onto Chamberlain Road at the CROCKFORD-PIGEON MOUNTAIN WILDLIFE MANAGEMENT AREA sign. Travel 3.4 miles on Chamberlain Road and turn right onto Rocky Lane at a WMA sign. Go 3.5 miles, passing a DNR check-in station, and at the next road intersection, turn right. Travel another 1.3 miles and turn left onto Rocktown Road. Take this 0.6 mile until it ends at the parking area.

FACILITIES/TRAILHEAD There are no facilities at the parking area for Rocktown. The nearest camping area is Sawmill Lake. To get there, go to the junction of Rocky Lane and Rocktown Road, continue on Rocky Lane (about a quarter mile), and turn onto the first road on the right. There are no facilities at Sawmill Lake and no water source other than the lake itself. Groups of 10 people or more should seek permission to visit Rocktown by calling the office of the Georgia Department on Natural Resources at (706) 695-6041. Rocktown is closed to nonhunters for 10 days each year during a limited firearm deer-hunting season. For exact dates, visit www.gohuntgeorgia.com.

At the north end of the gravel parking area, enter the trail **(Waypoint 1)**. Soon you will cross a branch of Allen Creek and take an easy, pleasant walk over fairly flat ground populated with Virginia pines, oaks, and hickory trees. The forest is fairly open with ferns, as well as stands of mountain laurel, lining the path. At 0.5 mile **(Waypoint 2)** you'll soon pass between two rock formations. Keep going because the main area known as Rocktown is a half mile ahead.

At 1 mile you'll reach the first stone formations in the main Rocktown collection **(Waypoint 3)**. The sandstone and conglomerate stones display a variety of colors, from dull grays to shades of red and brown. The rust color in some of the stones hints at the fact that iron ore was once mined in the surrounding area.

Continue ahead to further explore the many "streets," or trails, that wind among the stones. Those interested in climbing should download the Rocktown map at www.drtopo.com, which includes sketches of the various rock formations and identifies the locations of many bouldering problems, such as the Scoop (V3), Croc Block (V5), Bermuda Triangle (V7), and the Orb (V8). The topo provides unofficial names for many problems as well as difficulty ratings.

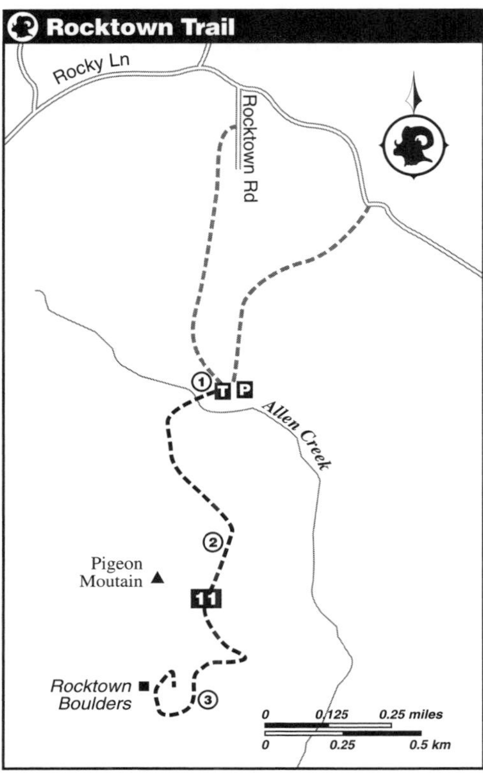

UTM WAYPOINTS

1. 16S 647557E 3836402N
2. 16S 647600E 3835859N
3. 16S 647483E 3835330N

The strange stone "buildings" of Rocktown

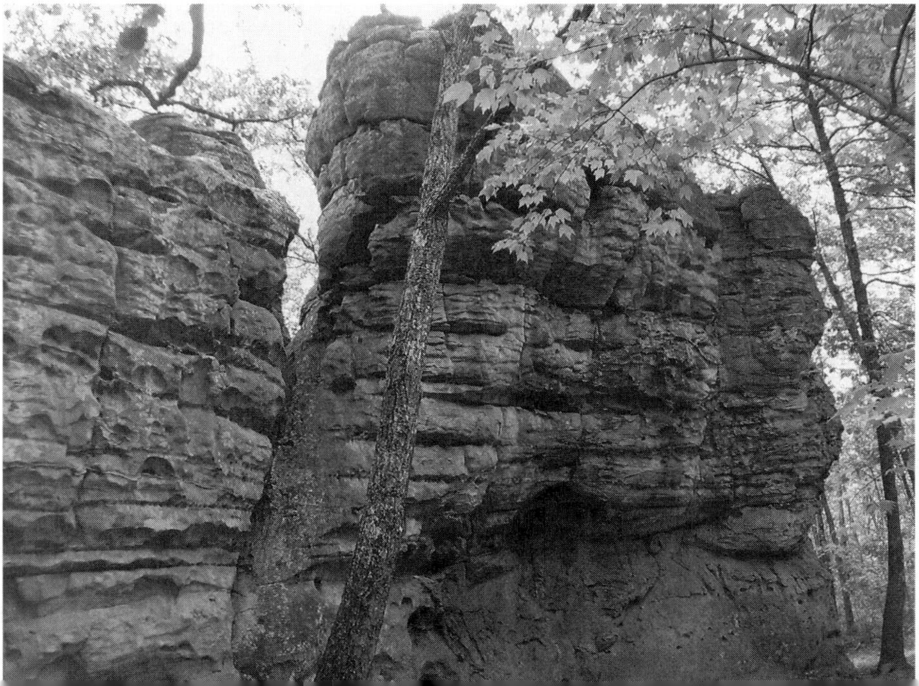

TRIP 12 Pocket Recreation Area

Distance	2.6 miles, main loop
Hiking Time	1 hour
Difficulty	Easy
Elevation Gain/Loss	+150/-120 feet
Trail Use	Leashed dogs
Best Times	Spring and fall
Agency	U.S. Forest Service, Armuchee Ranger District
Recommended Map	USGS 7.5-min. *Sugar Valley*

HIGHLIGHTS On a topographic map, Mill Mountain and Horn Mountain appear as two long spines that connect to form a U. Their steep slopes wrap around an area of low land, known as the Pocket. The Pocket Loop Trail heads through forest where spring-fed streams and other rivulets support a rich variety of trees and wildflowers. In the lower forest, American beech and sycamore trees thrive in the moist soil, while surrounding hills are thick with white oaks, hickory trees, and shortleaf and loblolly pines. In spring you'll also see dogwoods in bloom. The paths here are easy, and the campground is pleasant, making it a good place to combine overnight camping with a relaxing walk. A real gem here is the Aquatic Viewing Area, a wetland about a half mile into the hike. Set in a broad clearing, it allows excellent views for birding.

DIRECTIONS Take Interstate 75 north to Resaca. Take GA Highway 136 west for 15 miles. East of Villanow, turn south onto Pocket Road and travel 7 miles to the entrance of the Pocket Recreation Area. Go 0.3 mile on the one-way loop road to a parking area on the right.

FACILITIES/TRAILHEAD Restrooms (with handicapped facilities), water sources, and picnic tables are available in the camping area. You can hike year-round, though the campground, with 27 sites, is closed from November 1 through April 1.

Begin at the southeast end of the paved parking area and enter the path marked with green blazes **(Waypoint 1)**. Walk south to take a footbridge across a creek and pass the sign for the Pocket Loop Trail.

Walk a little more than 500 feet to reach the beginning of the loop **(Waypoint 2)**. Turn left to follow the trail marked with green blazes. This dirt path crawling with roots and moss takes you through oak and beech trees, which are called out on an interpretive sign near the beginning of the loop. The downed trees in the dense forest ahead lay as reminders that drought and southern pine beetles have put this forest under stress.

Some of the interesting points along this path are subtle, such as a sinkhole at about 0.3 mile. This slight depression was dry as I passed by in summer, but it actually fills with water in wet times of the year.

Just ahead is the Pocket's more obvious attraction. At the half-mile mark, bear right at the Y intersection and go east about 400 feet to the Aquatic Viewing Area **(Waypoint 3)**. On a bright summer day, this wetland is striking, as tall trunks of dead trees cast long reflections across the still pond. Georgia birding expert Giff Beaton recommends that you visit this spot in spring to hear migrant songbirds, while the summer months draw breeding waterbirds. "Red-winged blackbirds

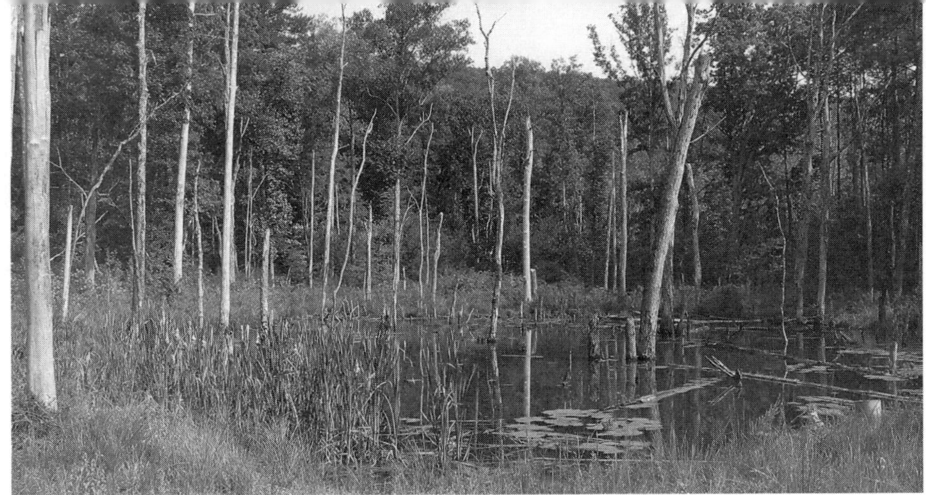

Aquatic Viewing Area

breed here," Beaton says. "And keep your eyes open for green or great blue herons in summer."

When you're set to depart, retrace your steps to the intersection and turn right to continue on the main loop. Just beyond 0.8 mile is a trail intersection **(Waypoint 4)**. The Interpretive Trail goes to the left (southwest) for 0.4 mile and allows you to complete a short loop back to the beginning of the Pocket Loop Trail. (The mileage listed in the summary information doesn't include this connector trail.) To continue on the Pocket Loop Trail, go straight at **Waypoint 4** and travel north, ascending a hill. (Be careful not to trample the bulbous mushrooms in the path.) After a gentle descent, you'll skirt another small hill and pass over a long wood walkway, which takes you across a bog **(Waypoint 5)**. More beech trees, pines, and oaks dominate the forest ahead, and your stroll ends at a paved campsite road. Turn left on the road to return to the parking lot.

UTM WAYPOINTS

1. 16S 675909E 3828729N
2. 16S 676025E 3828654N
3. 16S 676707E 3828694N
4. 16S 676499E 3828897N
5. 16S 676137E 3829620N

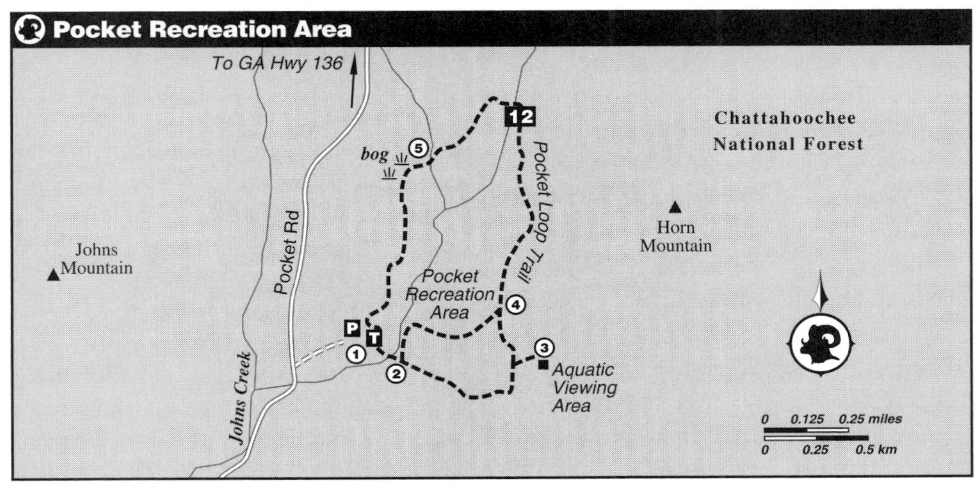

TRIP 13 New Echota Cherokee Capital

Distance	1.5 miles, loop
Hiking Time	1–1½ hours
Difficulty	Easy
Elevation Gain/Loss	+/- 65 feet
Trail Use	Good for kids
Best Times	Year-round
Agency	New Echota Cherokee Capital State Historic Site
Recommended Map	A trail map with interpretive information is available at the museum and visitors center.

HIGHLIGHTS When most people imagine a Native American village, they don't picture Colonial-style buildings or a courthouse, but the New Echota Cherokee Capital, established in 1825, looked much like a European farm settlement. This walk through the reconstructed village includes stops at farmstead houses, a town square, a tavern, and even a print shop. According to an interpretive pamphlet for the site, in 1835 more than 90 percent of the Cherokees in the area "lived in small cabins on farms and tilled an average of eleven acres of land" per household. There were about 50 residents in the settlement, though the capital drew many visitors during annual tribal council meetings. In the early 1800s, the demand for land in Georgia increased greatly, and the U.S. government forced the Cherokee to leave the land in the 1830s.

DIRECTIONS From Atlanta, travel north on Interstate 75 and take Exit 317. Go east on GA Highway 225 1 mile. The entrance to the New Echota site is on the right.

FACILITIES/TRAILHEAD There are restrooms in the visitors center. The park is open Tuesday–Saturday 9 AM–5 PM and Sunday 2–5:30 PM. Admission costs between $2.50 and $4.

Before taking this easy walk through the New Echota village, pick up a trail map brochure at the visitors center and museum. It has detailed interpretive information about each building on the site. On-site there is also a nature trail that passes through bottomland forest and one of the lowest areas of elevation in north Georgia.

At the south side of the museum and visitors center, begin at the Cherokee Farmstead **(Waypoint 1)**. The cabin, corn crib smoke house, and barn represent the typical farmstead of an upper-middle-class Cherokee family in the 1800s. Though these actual structures were built in the 1800s, they were relocated from other sites in Georgia and Tennessee. Be sure to check out the interpretive signs in the building, including one that provides good details about the Cherokees' use of corn cribs.

Beyond the farmstead, turn left to go to the Town Center and the Council House **(Waypoint 2)**. In 1819, the seat of the Cherokee Nation moved to New Town (renamed New Echota in 1825), and the reconstructed building here was the Cherokee Nation's headquarters. Rather than having a traditional, single chief, the Cherokees had a legislature with two houses, elected council members, and an executive branch that included a principal chief and vice-principal chief.

From the Council House, continue southeast to the nearby Supreme Courthouse (another reconstructed building), which has an impressive, raised bench where the three judges on the Cherokee Supreme Court would sit. Following the removal of the Cherokees, the original buildings on this land were destroyed and the fields were used for farming.

Walk east to the Common Cherokee Farmstead, turn right and walk south to the wide dirt path. Turn left onto the path and walk southeast toward the Worcester House.

At 0.3 mile on your walk, the entrance to the New Town Creek Nature Trail lies on the left **(Waypoint 3)**. Soon after entering the trail, turn left at a T intersection and travel northeast. This 1-mile path passes through lowland forest of sweetgums, shagbark hickory trees, and river cane near the bank of New Town Creek. The path runs along at an elevation of 630 feet, making this one of the lowest areas of land in north Georgia. Local park employees can tell you some pretty entertaining stories about how this land gets so flooded that it's possible to traverse much of the site via canoe.

The path rises slightly, and at 0.7 mile New Town Creek comes into view on the left. Not far ahead, a wood platform **(Waypoint 4)** looks over the modest creek as it bends through heavy bottomland woods. Look for the interpretive sign that explains how this was likely a recreation spot for the Cherokee.

The trail then climbs between pine forest and mixed hardwoods, and at 0.8 mile the woods are so overgrown you would never know that a farm once sat in this very spot. Now covered in pines and thickets, this land supported crops until the 1940s. As you continue, look for interpretive signs for a variety of trees, including red maple, sugar maple, and black cherry.

Just beyond the 1-mile mark, the path runs alongside the wood rail fence of the Worcester House, the only building on the New Echota site that is an original structure. Walk around to an opening in the fence at the front of the house **(Waypoint 5)** to more closely inspect this home built in 1828 by the Rev. Samuel A. Worcester. He not only set up a New Echota church but a school as well. When Worcester lost his house and property in an 1832 land lottery, he moved West to further serve the Cherokees.

To continue, go to the dirt path that leads up to the house and walk west to the Vann Tavern. Rustic, with a tight interior, this was an actual Cherokee tavern constructed around 1805. Notice the slate

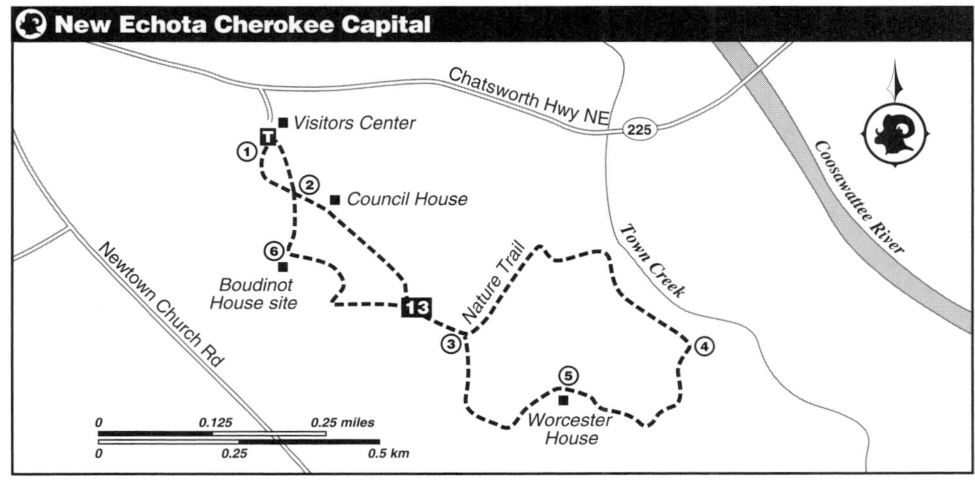

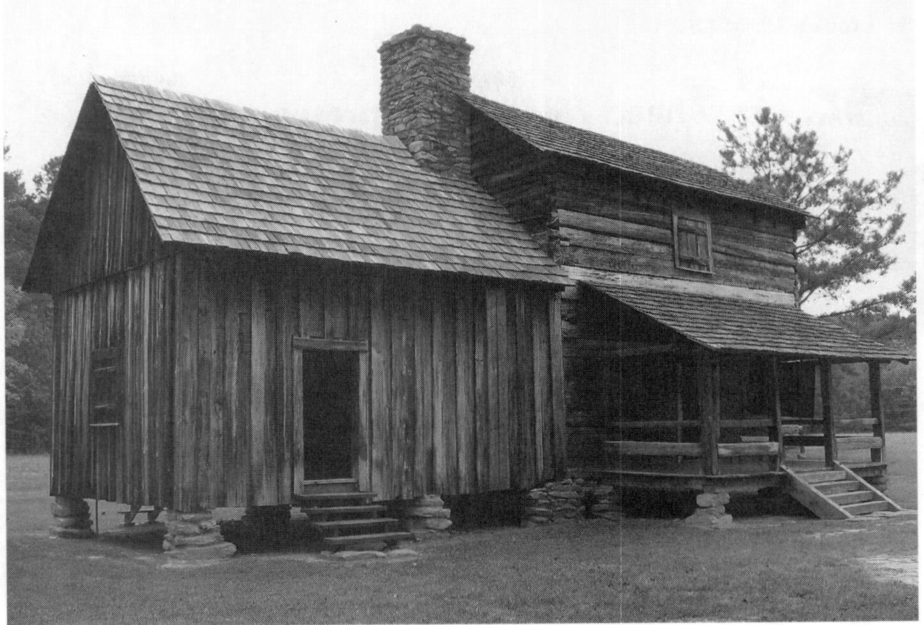

The rustic Vann Tavern at New Echota

menu on the wall advertising whiskey for $1.60 a gallon.

Walk north to see the one-room print shop, which began publishing the *Cherokee Phoenix* newspaper in 1828. From the left side of the print shop turn left to walk west to the Boudinot House site **(Waypoint 6)**. The first editor of the *Cherokee Phoenix*, Elias Boudinot, built a two-story house here in 1827. In 1830, the U.S. Congress passed the Indian Removal Act, and two years later much of the Cherokee land was given to Georgia citizens in a lottery. At the Boudinot house, a small group of Cherokees signed the controversial Treaty of New Echota in 1835, which gave up all of their lands in exchange for improvements to be made on resettlement lands out West. This treaty effectively killed the town of New Echota, and in 1838 federal and state troops forcibly removed any Cherokees remaining in Georgia.

From the Boudinot House site, walk northwest, passing the old town square to return to the visitors center.

UTM WAYPOINTS

1. 16S 691817E 3824060N
2. 16S 691872E 3823976N
3. 16S 692147E 3823732N
4. 16S 692528E 3823706N
5. 16S 692150E 3823654N
6. 16S 691832E 3823877N

TRIP 14 Arrowhead Wildlife Interpretive Trail

Distance	2–2.9 miles, loop
Hiking Time	1–2 hours
Difficulty	Easy
Elevation Gain/Loss	+/-90 feet
Trail Use	Good for kids
Best Times	Fall and spring
Agency	Georgia Department of Natural Resources, Wildlife Resources Division
Recommended Map	A rough map is available in the Georgia DNR office.

HIGHLIGHTS Drive fast enough and blink twice, and you could easily miss the Arrowhead Wildlife Interpretive Trail. It lies off a country road in a patch of former farmland. But the 377 acres of forest, ponds, and wetlands surrounding the trail are absolutely hopping with wildlife. Since 1980, the Department of Natural Resources has used this area to demonstrate methods of managing animals and their habitats, and an environmental education center on-site serves local schools. The flat and easy trails make this natural lab accessible to young and old hikers, and you can turn to interpretive signs to identify and better understand the surprisingly vast and diverse plant and animal species. The area was once a fish hatchery, and the old water collection areas, or impoundments, are flooded during seasonal migrations of herons, egrets, and other waterfowl.

DIRECTIONS From Atlanta, take Interstate 75 north to Exit 306 for GA Highway 140, Adairsville. Turn left onto GA 140 and travel west for 15.2 miles. Turn right onto Floyd Springs Rd., go 4 miles, and turn right into the gravel parking area before reaching the sign for NORTHWEST REGION HEADQUARTERS GEORGIA DEPARTMENT OF NATURAL RESOURCES, WILDLIFE RESOURCES GAME MANAGEMENT.

FACILITIES/TRAILHEAD The Northwest Region Headquarters for the Georgia Department of Natural Resources is located on Floyd Springs Rd. just north of the trailhead parking area. Here you can obtain a map of the area and get information about local wildlife. There are no public restrooms at the headquarters or trailhead. The Arrowhead Wildlife Trail is open year-round.

The Arrowhead Interpretive Trail begins at a kiosk on the east side of the parking area **(Waypoint 1)**. As you walk east on the flat, grassy path, the depression areas on the left are impoundments, which are left dry to allow certain grasses to grow, and then flooded for waterfowl to use. After walking a little more than 480 feet, turn right at the trail junction to go south toward the edge of the forest, and immediately look to the left. The hollow gourds suspended from the pole are houses for purple martins. Native Americans were actually the first to create such houses when they recognized that martins would nest in gourds that were hung up when not in use. The Native Americans may have welcomed the martins and used them like scarecrows or to reduce the insect population.

From the gourds, continue south, following blue blazes into a forest where some trees have small tags that identify their type, including southern red oaks, mockernut hickorys, and shagbark hickorys. When I scouted this area in summer, the air was still and quiet save for the hollow thunk of a woodpecker. The

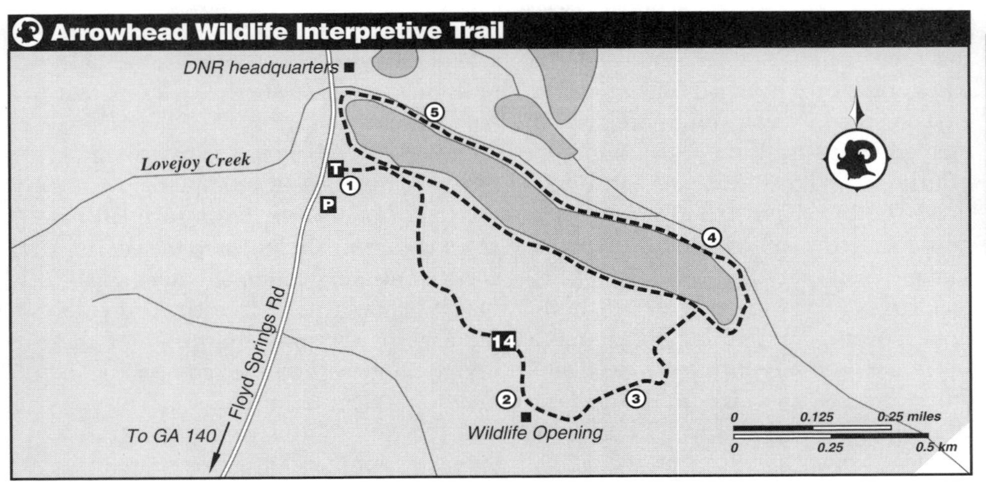

wildlife opening at 0.5 mile **(Waypoint 2)** had been plowed over, and land managers were preparing to put down a mix of clover and grass so animals could forage on some cool-weather greens. As you approach the opening, an interpretive sign to the right explains how the "soft-mast" plants, such as beech and hickory, also provide animals with food that's rich in fat and protein.

Turn left at the opening (southeast) and skirt the left side of the field. At 0.6 mile turn left to leave the field and enter the trees. Walk a tenth of a mile, and

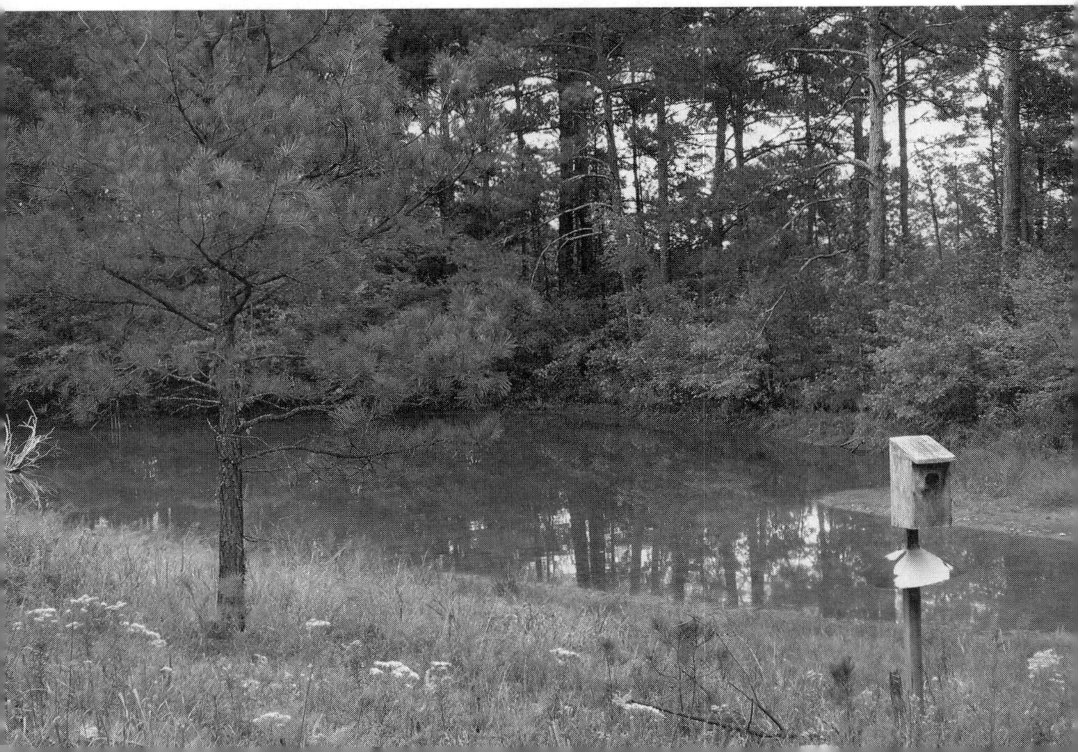

Wood duck box along the Arrowhead Wildlife Interpretive Trail

you'll notice that there is much more space between the pines here, and the bases of the trees are charred **(Waypoint 3)**. Certain sections of the forest are burned every three years to prevent a build-up of fuel, which could lead to catastrophic fires. The prescribed burns also deliver nutrients to the soil and thin the trees so sunlight can spur the growth of plants that serve as food for animals. In addition, burning creates "edge habitats," which are necessary for turkey, deer, and other animals to thrive. At 0.8 mile a clearing appears, and a wood duck box sits near a small pond to the right. The metal cone beneath the wood box is actually a predator guard to keep out snakes and other possible invaders.

At 0.9 mile you can bear left or right to walk along the impoundments. Bearing right, you go northeast and the trail soon bends to the left. As you walk between hedges, you may see birds darting back and forth across the trail, and Johns Mountain stretches across the sky ahead of you **(Waypoint 4)**. If the impoundments to your left are dry, you might catch a glimpse of wild turkeys strutting through high brush. If you wish to cut to the other side of the depressions, there are passable trails on some of the berms that separate the impoundments.

At 1.5 miles there is a four-way intersection, and the DNR headquarters is on the right **(Waypoint 5)**. If you turn left or go straight, you can return to the parking area. Continuing straight (northwest), the trail soon bends left to circle around the edge of the impoundments. At the next trail intersection keep going straight. Then, at 1.9 miles, there is a four-way trail junction. If you go straight (east), the path continues for a little more than a half mile along the impoundments; along the way there is a wood box made for bats. Or you can turn right at the four-way intersection, walk another 45 feet, and take a right to travel west back to the trailhead.

UTM WAYPOINTS

1. 16S 669882E 3812469N
2. 16S 670270E 3811869N
3. 16S 670541E 3811912N
4. 16S 670712E 3812253N
5. 16S 670010E 3812578N

Chapter 2
North Central Georgia

Atlanta residents are fortunate to live in a state with an abundance of well-maintained state parks, and north central Georgia holds some of the most popular destinations. The many lakes in the region, such as Carters Lake and Allatoona Lake, draw large crowds during peak travel times. However, if you visit a place such as Red Top Mountain State Park midweek or during less popular weekends, you can hike lakeside trails in peace and picnic on a quiet spot by the water. Farther north is Lake Conasauga. Nestled in the high mountains, this is the state's highest lake, and the still body of water lies near trails that wander rich bird habitat and climb to inspiring views. Georgia also offers several state parks with easy access to backcountry trails. Fort Mountain State Park and Vogel State Park are good options for beginner backpackers looking for a place to hike and camp overnight.

Fort Mountain State Park

It's quite the mystery. Archaeologists and historians aren't really sure who built the curious stone wall that sits atop Fort Mountain, a towering peak in the southern Appalachians. The mountain is named for the spine of rock that stretches 855 feet, and some believe that Native Americans constructed the wall around 500 AD as a defensive structure. However, the stonework may have served some ceremonial purpose, and no artifacts have been found to support a solid conclusion one way or the other. As with any mystery, people have offered a host of alternate theories about the wall's origin. Perhaps Welsh explorers constructed the wall while exploring this area in the 14th century, or maybe Hernando de Soto and his conquistadores built it as a fortification to repel Native Americans. A series of short trails in the northwest corner of Fort Mountain State Park allow people to see the wall themselves and contemplate its history. The park's other major draw is the lengthy Gahuti Trail, which loops around the crown of the mountain. As a dayhike, the trail is a rewarding challenge as it tops ridges with inspiring views and dives into creek ravines. But the Gahuti Trail also has four backcountry campsites, making this a good option for an overnight backpacking trip.

Carters Lake

"You don't beat it. You don't beat this river," wrote James Dickey, describing the mythical and powerful Cahulawassee in *Deliverance.* The actual river that the book is based on is the Coosawattee, which flows into Carters Lake. Paddlers say that the Coosawattee once held one of the greatest whitewater runs east of the Mississippi River, and Dickey's book was

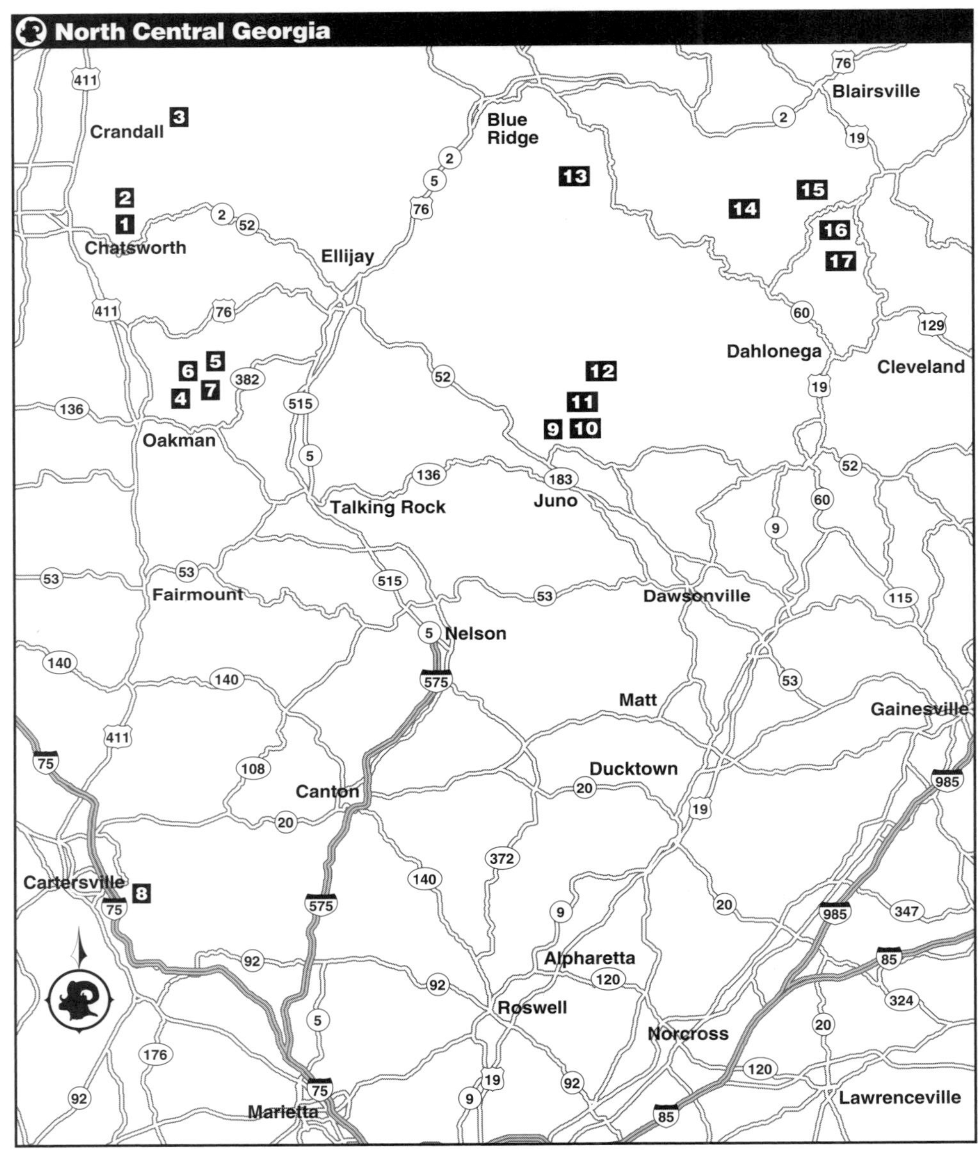

based on his own attempt to canoe these rapids right before the river was to be dammed. The experience led him to fashion his tale about man's futile attempt to tame nature, but the Coosawattee was indeed put under man's yoke.

In 1962, the U.S. Army Corps of Engineers began constructing a dam to control the river's flooding, harness its energy for hydroelectric power, and create a recreation area. Carters Lake was also formed to serve as a watershed for the river. Covering more than 3000 acres, the lake and the surrounding forest now draw hikers, bikers, campers, boaters, and hunters. Several hiking trails here allow relatively easy access to ridges, lakeshore, and creeks.

While this is now a popular destination for modern outdoor lovers, from Prohibition into the 1970s this was a secluded place that drew a different kind of folk—moonshiners. In fact, Dickey's run-in with whiskey makers inspired portions of *Deliverance*. But, once the dam was built, the moonshiners abandoned their stills, and you can now wander this place without fear of running into the Griner Brothers. If you hear the distant twang of a banjo, don't fret, it's probably just your imagination running wild.

Amicalola Falls State Park

The tallest cascading waterfall east of the Mississippi River, Amicalola Falls drops 729 feet. This spectacle makes Amicalola (Cherokee for "tumbling waters") one of the most-visited state parks in Georgia. On a sunny spring day, the parking lots here are jam-packed, but the falls and other trails in the park are well worth a visit. At the visitors center in early spring you'll likely see backpackers hanging their packs on a scale to weigh them, as this is a jumping-off point for Appalachian Trail hikers. The 8.3-mile Appalachian Approach Trail begins behind the visitors center and runs to Springer Mountain, which marks the southern terminus of the Appalachian Trail. Also, the 5-mile trail to the rustic Len Foote Hike Inn begins in the state park. But for day visitors, the most popular path is the Base of Falls Trail, which climbs to a narrow bridge that stands before the massive cascade. A little less crowded are several short trails in the western side of the park. These pass through the Amicalola Falls watershed below the falls and also explore the dry western slopes of the ravine.

Amicalola Falls, Base of Falls Trail (Trip 9)

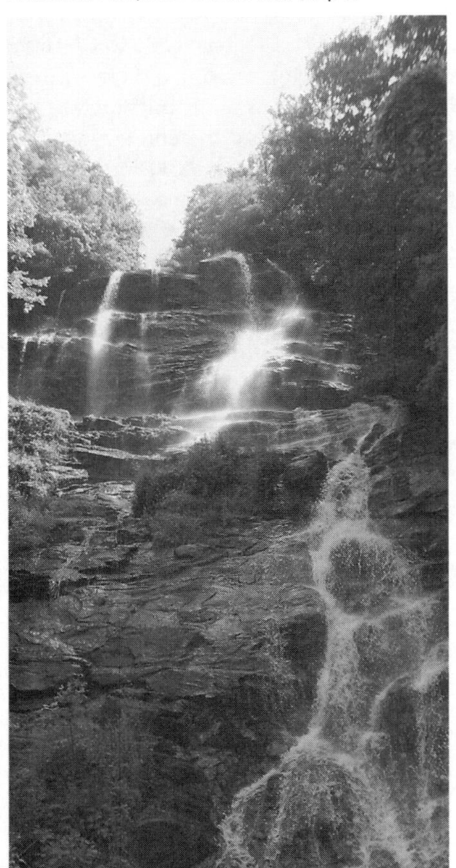

Vogel State Park

In the fall, when scarlet oaks and hickory turn north Georgia red and gold, people flock to Vogel State Park. Sitting at about 2300 feet of elevation near the base of Blood Mountain, the popular park is a prime destination for fall leaf watchers, but it also remains relatively cool in spring and summer, offering a respite from the heat. Established in the 1930s, Vogel is Georgia's second-oldest state park. One of its central attractions is the 20-acre Trahlyta Lake, which is popular for fishing. However, the park also provides easy access to excellent trails that reach beyond the state park boundaries to explore surrounding wilderness areas. The 3.6-mile Bear Hair Gap Trail serves dayhikers, while the 12.9-mile Coosa Backcountry Trail delves deep into wilderness for those seeking a night out under the stars.

TRIP 1 Fort Mountain State Park: Gahuti Trail

Distance	8.2 miles, loop
Hiking Time	5 hours
Difficulty	Moderate to strenuous
Elevation Gain/Loss	+/-1495 feet
Trail Uses	Leashed dogs and backpacking
Best Times	Year-round
Agency	Fort Mountain State Park
Recommended Map	A *Fort Mountain State Park Trail Map* is available in the park office and online at www.gastateparks.org.

HIGHLIGHTS The elevation profile of the Gahuti Trail looks like a healthy cardiogram, with frequent and regular peaks and valleys that will definitely get your heart pumping. The upshot is that it covers diverse terrain, from ridges with awesome views to jungle creek bottoms and windy hilltops. It's possible to complete the trail in a single day, but you should be in very good condition to try it. If you choose to make this a two-day backpacking trek, there are four backcountry campsites, two of which lie near water sources. You can hike the loop in either direction; it's described clockwise. A little less than halfway in, there is a good resting spot where you can sit in the sun on a bench that overlooks mountains to the south. And the trek ends at the Cool Springs Overlook, which provides a grand view of the Cohutta Mountains.

DIRECTIONS From Atlanta take Interstate 75 north to Interstate 575. Take I-575 to GA Highway 5 north and continue to East Ellijay. Turn left on U.S. Highway 76/GA Highway 2, go 0.1 mile and turn left onto GA Highway 2/52. Go 0.9 mile to a roundabout and take the second exit onto GA 2/52. Travel west on GA 2/52 17.3 miles to the entrance for Fort Mountain State Park on the right. Take the park road north toward the "Old Fort" area; the parking area for the Cool Springs Overlook and Gahuti Trailhead is on the right.

FACILITIES/TRAILHEAD There are no facilities at the trailhead. Pack plenty of water for a full day of vigorous hiking. There is a $3 parking fee for the park, and you can purchase an Annual ParkPass for $30 by calling (770) 389-7401. Backcountry campsites on the Gahuti Trail are available by permit ($5 per person).

At the southeast side of the Gahuti Trail parking area, enter the trail marked by the large GAHUTI MOUNTAIN TRAIL sign and walk southeast following orange blazes **(Waypoint 1)**. The rocky path lined with moss is surrounded mostly by oaks, and then the trail drops into a stretch dominated by pines. Though the path initially parallels a park road, in less than a mile it moves away to seem very remote. You'll descend steeply and then rollercoaster between drainages filled with ferns and slopes of poplars, oaks, and pines.

At 1.5 miles **(Waypoint 2)** you reach the site of the first backcountry campsite. Turn left at the tree with double orange blazes to descend east along Mill Creek in a tunnel of rhododendron. Cross a wood footbridge and turn right (to the left the path ends at a stop sign). Ascend along the creek where very little light hits the tea-colored water that flows beneath dense foliage.

At 1.8 miles, a trail and a wood footbridge lie to the right. Continue straight, following orange blazes on the Gahuti Trail and climb to a higher, dry forest of

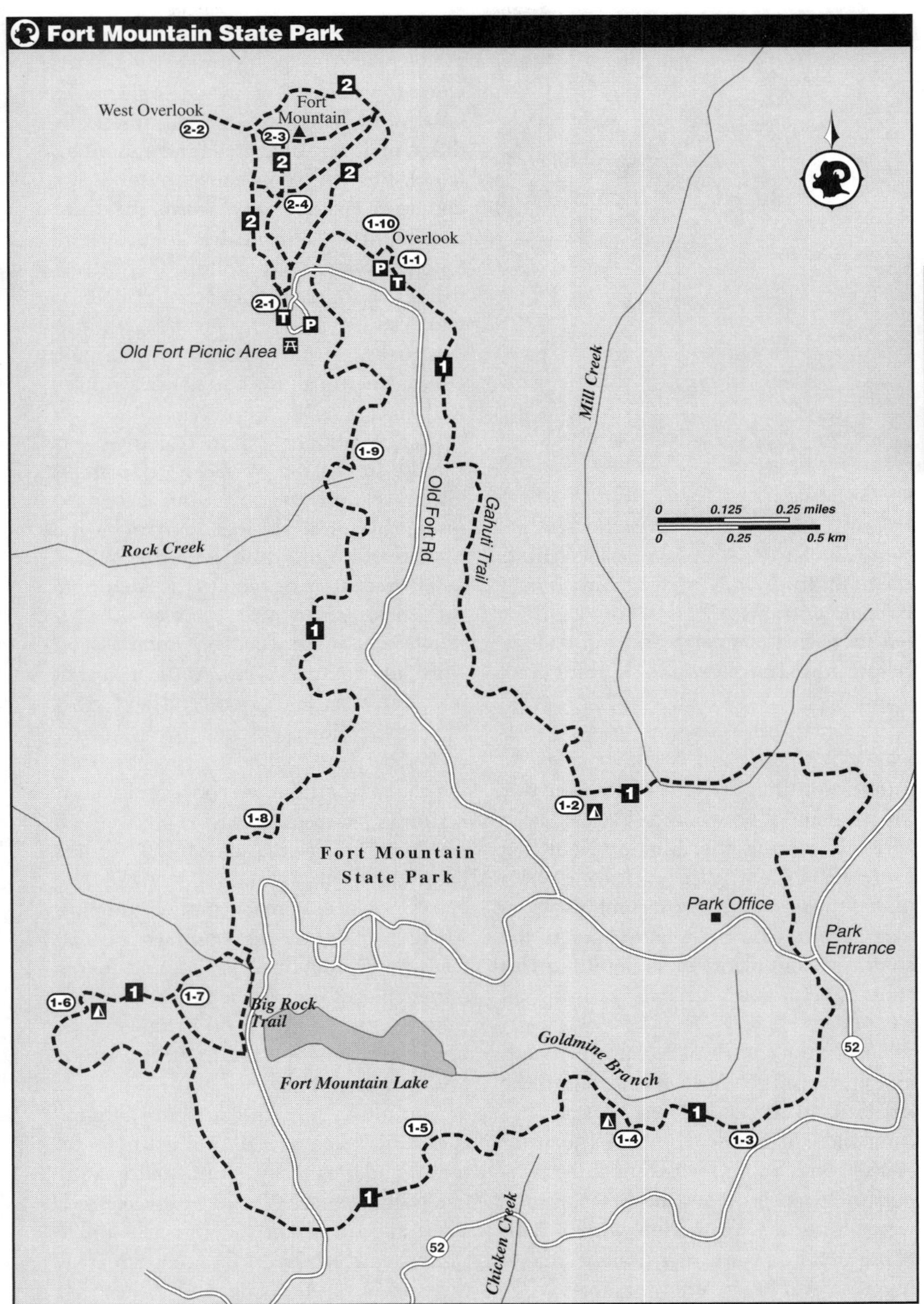
Fort Mountain State Park
West Overlook
Fort Mountain
2-2
2-3
2-4
2-1
1-10
Overlook
1-1
Old Fort Picnic Area
1-9
Rock Creek
Old Fort Rd
Gahuti Trail
Mill Creek
0 0.125 0.25 miles
0 0.25 0.5 km
1-2
1-8
Fort Mountain State Park
Park Office
Park Entrance
1-6
1-7
Big Rock Trail
Goldmine Branch
52
Fort Mountain Lake
1-5
1-4
1-3
Chicken Creek
52

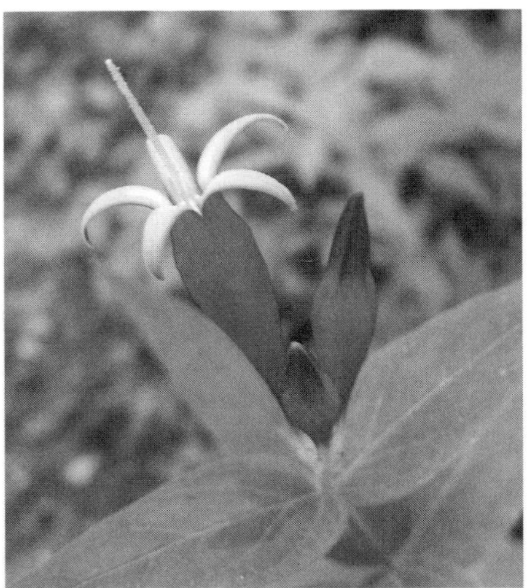

Indian pink

pines and hardwoods. After a steep climb, the path drops and crosses the road near the park entrance. Cross the road and jog left to walk down earth and wood steps. Before you know it, you're climbing once again.

The path joins a wider, grassy treadway at 2.7 miles and crosses a ridge. At 3 miles continue straight at the four-way junction and follow orange blazes. About 250 feet beyond the junction, look left for a bench sitting in a clearing on a bluff **(Waypoint 3)**. This overlook provides a great view of a ridge and valley to the southeast, and plenty of sunlight hits this spot, so it's a good place to warm up on a cool day.

From the overlook, continue west, and at 3.4 miles **(Waypoint 4)** a trail to the left leads to the Gold Mine backcountry campsite. This is a dry campsite (no water source) with room for two or three two-person tents. From **Waypoint 4** continue west and reach a junction with a path blazed red and white. Go straight, traveling west, and follow orange blazes.

At 3.9 miles **(Waypoint 5)** turn left, leaving the wide path to take the orange-blazed trail southwest. Cross a ridge and then roller coaster through pine-hardwood forest. Laughter from people on the lake rises as you drop into a dramatically different forest of poplar and mountain laurel. But you soon gain ground again, and at 5.3 miles **(Waypoint 6)** the third backcountry campsite lies to the right. Situated on an airy hilltop, this attractive site can accommodate a couple of tents, and a fire ring sits beneath two large oaks. A little farther down the trail, a rock outcrop allows you to see for miles to the west.

At 5.5 miles the Gahuti Trail intersects the Big Rock Trail **(Waypoint 7)**. Turn left and travel northeast following yellow and orange blazes. To the west you can see the Chatsworth Valley and miles beyond. A quick descent brings you to the Goldmine Branch stream, which tumbles down a staircase of stone. Turn right and ascend alongside the steep creek. At the next trail junction, turn left to descend and cross the creek, following orange blazes.

Watch your footing as you climb on the rocky trail up a west-facing slope. At 6.1 miles **(Waypoint 8)** turn right, walk 50 feet to a Y junction and bear left ascending to the southeast and following orange blazes. You'll soon reach another junction where you'll turn right and go east 30 feet to a Y junction. Bear left and follow orange blazes into dense forest. The trail traverses the headwall of a draw, passes between large boulders, and then winds down through pines.

You move through consecutive drainages where ferns and mountain laurel thrive, and the musky odor of galax plants hangs in the air. At 7.3 miles **(Waypoint 9)**, a side trail leads to the fourth backcountry campsite, which has two decent flat areas for tents, a big fire ring, and stones that form chairs with backs. These features, plus the fact that a stream runs nearby, make this one of the best campsites along the trail.

The trail climbs through oak, sourwood, and laurel, crosses the road, and meets the Tower Trail at a T intersection, Turn right and follow orange blazes to the Cool Springs Overlook **(Waypoint 10)**. From this wood platform you have an amazing view of a massive, forested tract of the Cohutta Mountains. From the overlook take the paved pathway back to the parking area.

UTM WAYPOINTS

1. 16S 709967E 3850909N
2. 16S 710544E 3849263N
3. 16S 711060E 3848235N
4. 16S 710683E 3848251N
5. 16S 710087E 3848201N
6. 16S 708994E 3848618N
7. 16S 709295E 3848651N
8. 16S 709555E 3849163N
9. 16S 709826E 3850333N
10. 16S 709973E 3851010N

TRIP 2 Fort Mountain State Park: Stone Wall, Tower, & West Overlook Trails

see map on p. 63

Distance	1.6 miles, loop
Hiking Time	1 hour
Difficulty	Easy
Elevation Gain/Loss	+/-405 feet
Trail Use	Leashed dogs and good for kids
Best Times	Year-round
Agency	Fort Mountain State Park
Recommended Map	A *Fort Mountain State Park Trail Map* is available in the park office and online at www.gastateparks.org.

HIGHLIGHTS This series of short paths on the crest of Stone Mountain takes you to the ancient stone wall, the impressive West Overlook, and a stone observation tower built by the Civilian Conservation Corps in the 1930s. You can hike these trails in a number of ways, and the sequence you choose depends on which features you'd like to visit first. As described here, the hike forms a loop that tours each major feature.

DIRECTIONS From Atlanta take Interstate 75 north to Interstate 575. Take I-575 to GA Highway 5 north and continue to East Ellijay. Turn left on U.S. Highway 76/GA Highway 2, go 0.1 mile and turn left onto GA 2/52. Go 0.9 mile to a roundabout, and take the second exit onto GA 2/52. Travel west on GA 2/52 17.3 miles to the entrance for Fort Mountain State Park on the right. Take the park road north toward the "Old Fort" area, and continue to the loop road at the Old Fort Picnic Area.

FACILITIES/TRAILHEAD There is a restroom at Old Fort Picnic Area. There is a $3 parking fee for the park, or you can purchase an Annual ParkPass for $30 by calling (770) 389-7401. The park has 70 tent, trailer, and RV campsites ($25), 4 backcountry campsites on the Gahuti Trail ($5 per person), 6 platform campsites ($10), and 15 cottages ($110–$130).

Near the entrance to the parking area, on the west side, enter the yellow-blazed Stone Wall Trail **(Waypoint 1)**. At the next Y junction, bear right to follow the Stone Wall Trail and continue past an intersection with the Gahuti Trail. The

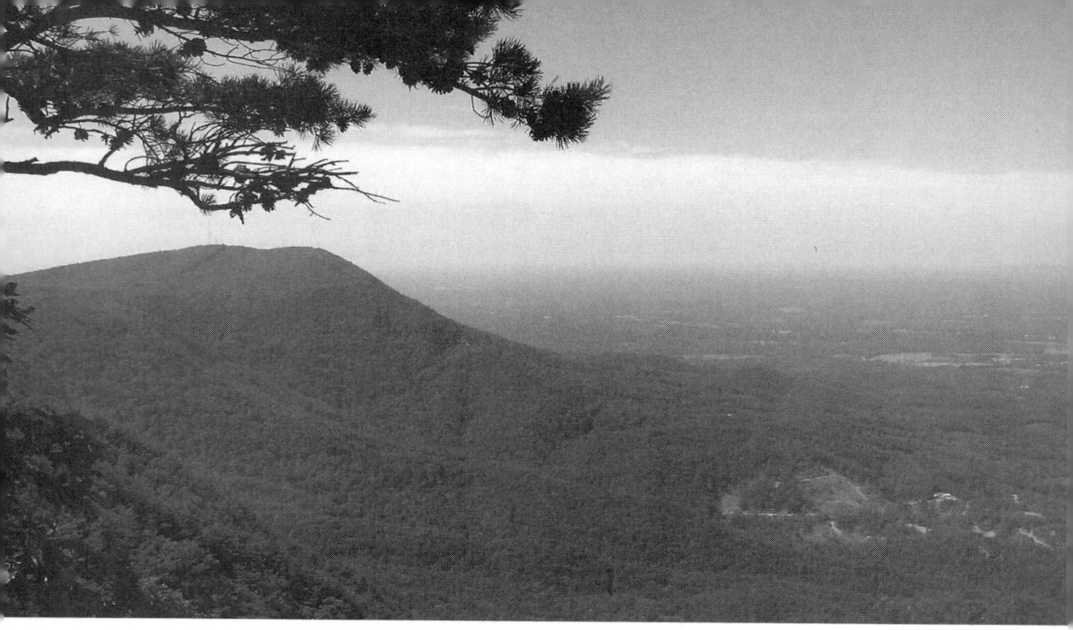

West Overlook

path circles the mountaintop where views of high ridges to the east provide a good sense of your high elevation. Proceeding past stacks of boulders, you circle to the south and reach a junction with the red-blazed Tower Trail. Turn right to descend to the West Overlook (**Waypoint 2**). This platform boasts a remarkable, sweeping view of the north Georgia mountains where a succession of ridges and valleys extend to the horizon.

Walk back up to **Waypoint 2** and continue straight to reach the stone tower (**Waypoint 3**), which sits atop the mountain at 2832 feet of elevation. From the tower you can take the red-blazed trail to the stone wall, or backtrack to the West Overlook Trail. From the West Overlook Trail, turn left and travel south to the junction with the blue-blazed Rock Wall Trail on the left.

Turn left onto the Rock Wall Trail and ascend to the southeast to reach the wall (**Waypoint 4**). A plaque on a stone relates some of the legends that surround this prehistoric site. The wall snakes across the mountaintop, intersecting first with the Tower Trail and finally with the Stone Wall Trail. You can turn right onto either of these paths to return to the trailhead.

Civilian Conservation Corps tower atop Fort Mountain

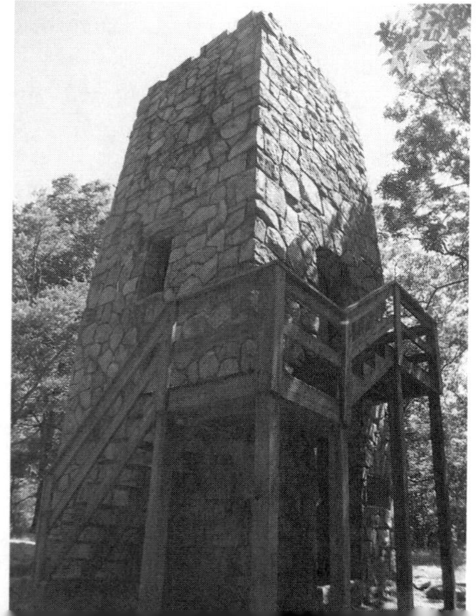

UTM WAYPOINTS

1. 16S 709628E 3850858N
2. 16S 709425E 3851402N
3. 16S 709599E 3851351N
4. 16S 709615E 3851188N

TRIP 3 Lake Conasauga Recreation Area: Lake, Songbird, & Tower Trails

Distance	6.0 miles, semiloop
Hiking Time	3 hours
Difficulty	Easy to moderate
Elevation Gain/Loss	+970/-900 feet
Trail Use	Good for kids
Best Times	Spring is best for birding.
Agency	U.S. Forest Service, Conasauga District
Recommended Map	USGS 7.5-min. *Crandall*

HIGHLIGHTS Sitting at an elevation of 3150 feet, Lake Conasauga is the highest lake in Georgia. Spanning 19 acres, the lake is off-limits to gas-powered motorboats, making this a serene place to hike, paddle, swim, or fish for bass and trout. The lake also lies near extensive wildlands, including portions of the Cohutta Wilderness and large areas of forest managed to provide habitat for a wide array of songbirds. This hike begins on the 1-mile lake loop, and then follows the Tower Trail for 2 miles to the top of Grassy Mountain (3600 feet). There you can ascend a fire tower to get an almost-360-degree view of farmland and surrounding ridges. After walking back down the mountain, you can turn onto the Songbird Trail, which lies within the 120-acre Songbird Management Area. Here, there is a large pond formed by a beaver dam and a wood platform that serves as a prime spot for viewing wildlife.

DIRECTIONS From Atlanta take Interstate 75 north to Dalton. From Dalton, travel east on U.S. Highway 76 to Chatsworth. From Chatsworth travel north on U.S. Highway 411 about 4 miles to Eton. In Eton, turn right at the traffic light onto old CCC Camp Road, which becomes Forest Service Road 18. Travel east on FSR 18 about 10 miles to the intersection with Forest Service Road 68. Turn left onto FSR 68, go 6 miles to an intersection, and turn left at a sign for Lake Conasauga Recreation Area. Travel 5.3 miles, passing the road to Camping Loop A. Just past the sign for the swimming and picnic area, turn right into a paved parking loop.

FACILITIES/TRAILHEAD From the parking area, a restroom lies about 280 feet down the trail. Around the lake are 35 family camping units, and an overflow area has 6 sites for tents. The fee is $8 per night, and it's open from April to October (call for exact dates).

At the north end of the parking lot **(Waypoint 1)**, descend the wide dirt and gravel path to the lake and turn right to travel southeast. You circle the lake on an easy, mostly flat path, passing through corridors of hemlocks and rhododendron and a wide field of ferns. As the trail goes through a portion of the camping area, look left for a sign for the Songbird Trail, and take this path to continue around the lake.

At 0.6 mile, at the northwest end of the lake, turn right onto the trail marked TOWER TRAIL/SONGBIRD TRAIL **(Waypoint 2)**. Poplars surround the rocky path, which takes you through long, dim hallways of heath forest where rhododendron produced great white blooms when I passed through here on a June morning.

At 0.9 mile you reach a WELCOME TO LAKE CONASAUGA sign. Turn right to travel northwest on the Tower Trail. To your left

Lake Conasauga Recreation Area: Lake, Songbird, & Tower Trails

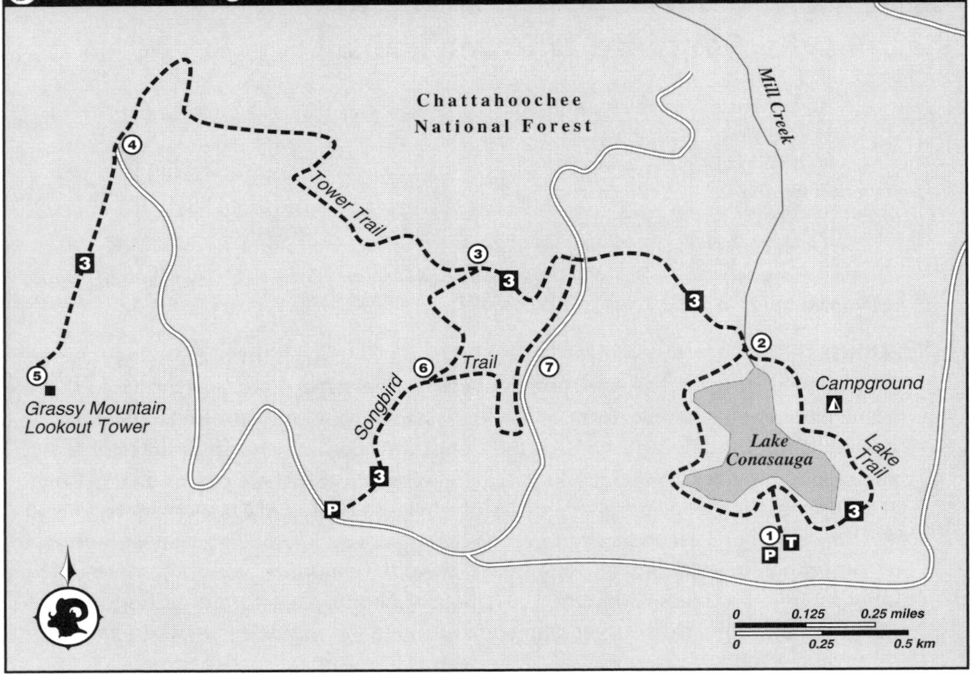

Chattahoochee National Forest
Mill Creek
Tower Trail
Songbird Trail
Grassy Mountain Lookout Tower
Campground
Lake Conasauga
Lake Trail
0 0.125 0.25 miles
0 0.25 0.5 km

is one of the many beaver ponds dotting the area, and the path goes over a wood footbridge and heads into dense forest. At 1.1 miles, the Songbird Trail intersects to the left in a shaded stand of hemlocks **(Waypoint 3)**. Keep right to continue on the Tower Trail, ascending to the northwest. Lining the trail are great beds of galax, and the forest transitions to hardwoods and white pines.

At 1.5 miles the trail turns sharply to the right (east)—don't be fooled by the path that turns to the left (west). As you climb, pines become more abundant, the path is heavily rooted, and the skunky smell of galax permeates the place. As the trail climbs onto a ridgeback, look left for flaming azalea, with orange petals that appear brilliant amid the green brush. Traverse the ridge and at 2 miles **(Waypoint 4)** intersect with a gravel road. A sign directs you toward Grassy Mountain

Grassy Mountain Lookout Tower

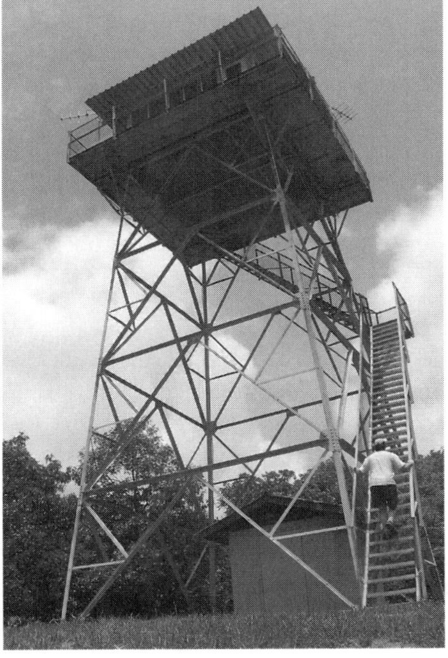

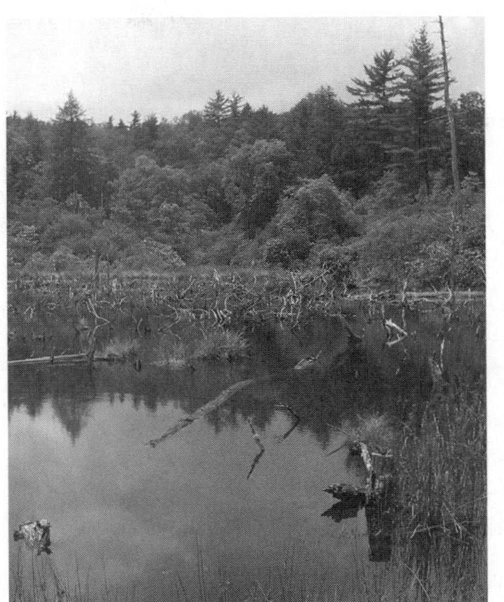

Beaver pond along the Songbird Trail

Lookout Tower; continue straight, traveling southwest on the gravel road.

At 2.5 miles the tall metal lookout tower stands in a wide clearing **(Waypoint 5)**. I climbed to the tower's first platform on a hazy summer day, yet still had good views of impressive features near and far. A hulking ridge to the east appeared much like a camel's back, with hills and saddles forming great humps. The Cohutta Wilderness rolled endlessly to the northeast, and Fort Mountain dominated the sky to the southwest. This is one of the most stunning mountain views in northwest Georgia.

To continue, retrace your steps to **Waypoint 3** (3.8 miles), and turn onto the Songbird Trail, traveling southwest. The single-track path cuts across a moderate slope into rhododendron thickets, and a footbridge passes over a small stream. The dense foliage through here is an ideal environment for birds, offering them protection from weather and animals on the hunt.

At 4 miles, cross a stream with boulders blanketed by moss. On the opposite bank is a trail junction where you can turn either left or right onto the Songbird Trail **(Waypoint 6)**. To the right (west) the trail continues for another 0.2 mile to its terminus at a gravel road. If you turn left onto the Songbird Trail and travel east, open sky greets you as you pass through areas with fewer trees, though thickets crowd the path. At 4.7 miles an interpretive sign explains how controlled burns have created this brushy habitat to provide shelter for birds such as the indigo bunting and rufous-sided towhee. About 300 feet farther, turn left at a T intersection with a gravel path and travel north.

At 4.8 miles the beaver pond lies to the left **(Waypoint 7)**. When I reached this spot at midday, a bright sun stood high and flashed across the still water. As I walked down the wood observation platform, the heat seemed to have lulled everything to sleep, save for the plop, plop of diving frogs and the hollow knock of a woodpecker. Georgia birding guru Giff Beaton says that this spot offers great birding from spring through fall. "Many high-elevation breeders, such as blackburnian and black-throated blue warblers breed here," he says. "And it's a good site for landbird migrants also."

From the pond, return to the trail, and go left to return to the junction with the WELCOME TO LAKE CONASAUGA sign (5 miles). Turn right to return to the lake and **Waypoint 2**. At **Waypoint 2**, turn right to complete your loop of the Lake Trail and return to the parking area.

UTM WAYPOINTS

1. 16S 714757E 3859778N
2. 16S 714695E 3860221N
3. 16S 714056E 3860441N
4. 16S 713210E 3860780N
5. 16S 713006E 3860197N
6. 16S 713936E 3860165N
7. 16S 714175E 3860218N

TRIP 4 Carters Lake: Talking Rock Nature Trail

Distance	2.1 miles, out-and-back
Hiking Time	1 hour
Difficulty	Easy to moderate
Elevation Gain/Loss	+325/-230 feet
Trail Use	Good for kids and leashed dogs
Best Times	Year-round
Agency	U.S. Army Corps of Engineers, Carters Lake
Recommended Maps	USGS 7.5-min. *Oakman*; a very basic map is available at http://carters.sam.usace.army.mil/bike.htm

HIGHLIGHTS Talking Rock is one of the more satisfying hikes in the Carters Lake area for a few reasons. First, it gives you a good opportunity to hear songbirds and observe a wide range of wildlife, from wood ducks to deer. And though it covers a modest distance, the path takes you through a great mix of terrain from wetlands to ridges of pines and hardwoods. This hike is particularly engaging because interpretive signs highlight various habitats and the types of animals that dwell there. For most of the hike you are enveloped by forest, but the trail reaches a high clearing with a good view of a reregulation reservoir, a pool where water is held until it is fed back into the main reservoir for energy production and recreation use, or simply released to flow downstream.

DIRECTIONS From Atlanta, take Interstate 75 north to Exit 293 for Chatsworth/U.S. Highway 411. At end of ramp turn right and take U.S. 411 north 25.5 miles. Turn right onto GA Highway 136, travel east 2.6 miles and turn left onto Carters Dam Road. Go 1.9 miles to a fork. Go right to reach the visitors center, or go left for the hiking pay station ($4). From the pay station continue 0.1 mile to trailhead parking on the left. Look downhill for a prominent TALKING ROCK NATURE TRAIL sign.

FACILITIES/TRAILHEAD There are no facilities at the trailhead. You can obtain a map and trail and campground information at the visitors center. The closest camping is at the Harris Branch Campground, located about 3 miles off GA Highway 382 on the south side of the lake. It has 10 primitive campsites open May–September ($14 per night). There are also hot showers and coin-op laundry facilities.

The hike begins beneath the TALKING ROCK NATURE TRAIL sign where a wide path begins a moderate descent through oaks and pines **(Waypoint 1)**. The grade becomes gentle as you begin to see the first of many bird boxes affixed to trees along the trail. An interpretive signs explains that the eastern bluebird and Carolina chickadee are two of the songbirds living in these woods. Also, look for a small clearing, or food plot, where grasses and grains such as sorghum, wheat, and rye have been planted as a food source for a host of animals,

Virginia pines destroyed by pine beetles

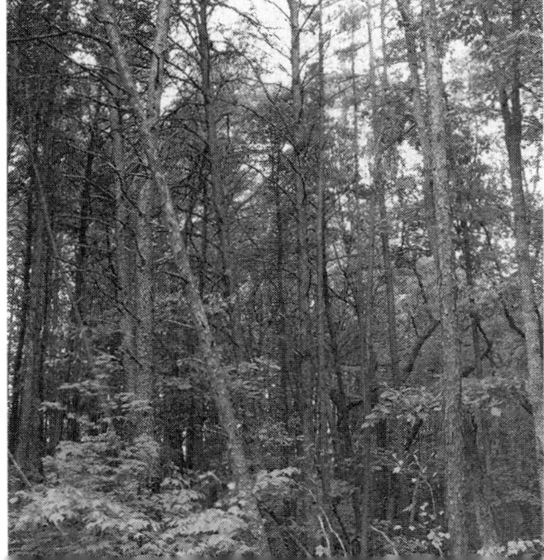

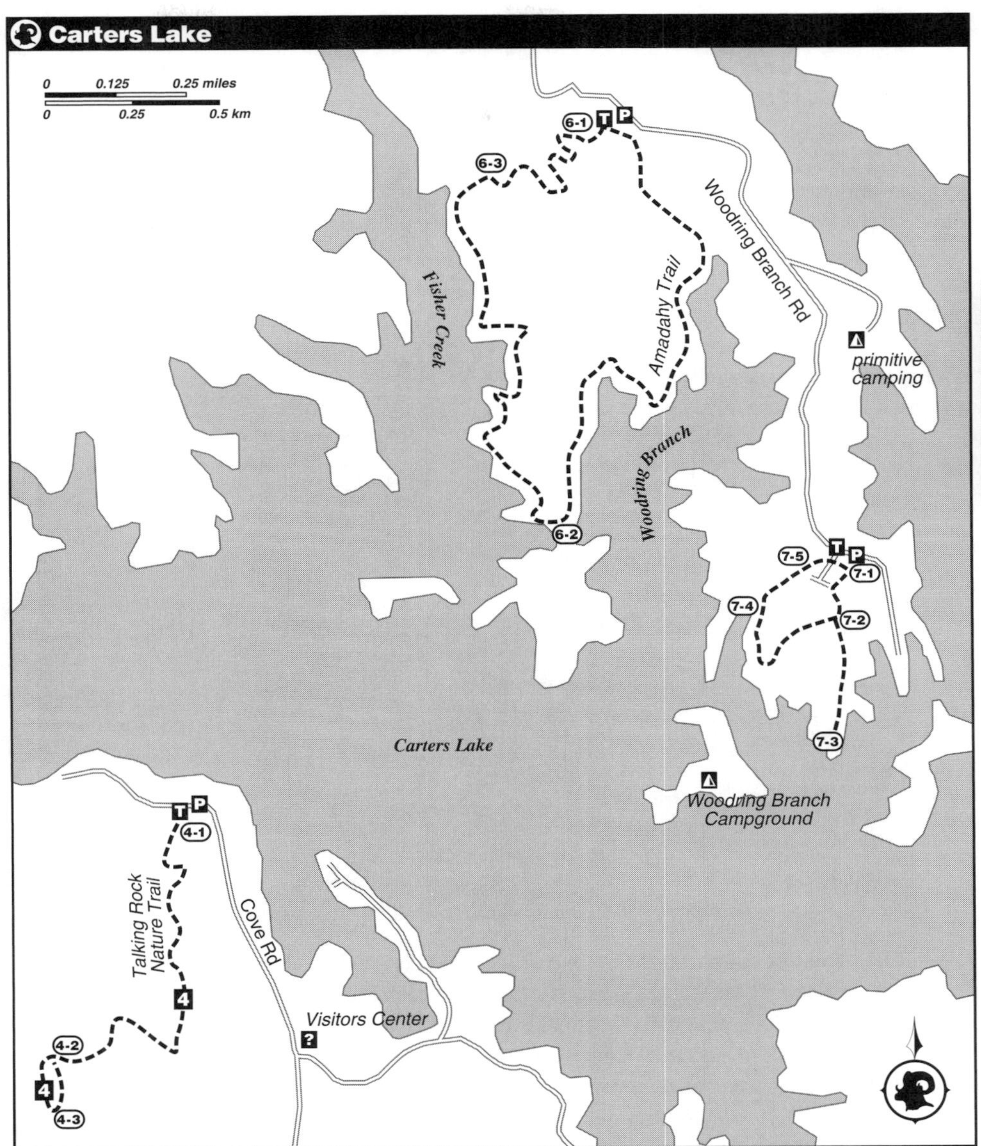

including turkeys, rabbits, and waterfowl. Within a few hundred feet, you reach a wetland created when Carters Lake was formed. To the right is a bench that sits slightly higher than the watery clearing, allowing you to survey the scene. Turn left here to travel south.

Climb gradually, and at 0.2 mile go through a creek drainage where moss and ferns sprout from the forest floor. As you ascend, you'll pass a "site selection" interpretive sign that suggests that you try to identify the difference between the lowland trees and those on the higher ridge. If you're hiking with kids, this could be a good exercise to tune them into their surroundings. You'll keep gaining elevation as the path circles a hill and the path of loose rock turns steep. If you are hiking in winter, to the left (southwest) you will be able to see Carters Lake through the curtain of trees.

At 0.8 mile turn right at the T intersection and go southwest into Virginia pines that have suffered from pine beetle infestations since 1987 **(Waypoint 2)**. An interpretive sign on the left offers details on the beetle and its effect on trees.

At 0.9 mile continue straight at the trail junction and you will soon arrive at a power line clearing **(Waypoint 3)**. To your right (west) is a clear view of the reregulation reservoir, which appears as a small lake encircled by forest.

From here, turn left and go east along the left side of the clearing for 115 feet, and then turn left at the trail marker. As you climb gradually through pines, the land to your right falls away to a draw filled with oaks. At 1.2 miles, turn right at the trail junction to travel east back to the trailhead.

UTM WAYPOINTS

1. 16S 714119E 3832169N
2. 16S 713790E 3831388N
3. 16S 713713E 3831234N

TRIP 5 Carters Lake: Tumbling Waters Nature Trail

Distance	1.4 miles, out-and-back
Hiking Time	1 hour
Difficulty	Easy
Elevation Gain/Loss	+/-270 feet
Trail Use	Leashed dogs
Best Times	Year-round
Agency	U.S. Army Corps of Engineers, Carters Lake
Recommended Maps	A *Carters Lake Hiking Trails* map is available at the Carters Lake Visitors Center; USGS 7.5-min. *Webb*

HIGHLIGHTS The Tumbling Waters Nature Trail leads to Tails Creek, a remote stream that slides through a pocket of hemlock forest that is easily accessible but has the air of a hidden gem. A wood bridge spanning the creek sits high above a long stretch of cascades, and observation platforms on each side of the creek also provide elevated views. If you would like to play in the creek or relax on the bank, the bridge leads to a path that descends to the water's edge, while another path climbs the bluff that overlooks the creek. The trails provide access to a fairly limited portion of Tails Creek, but the stellar forest and rushing water make this a spot worth visiting for a few hours of serenity.

DIRECTIONS From Atlanta, take Interstate 75 north to Exit 293 for Chatsworth/U.S. Highway 411. At the end of the ramp turn right and take U.S. 411 north 25.5 miles. Turn right onto GA Highway 136 and travel east 0.4 mile to Old Highway 411. Turn left and travel north on Old Highway 411 6.2 miles. Turn right onto U.S. Highway 76/GA Highway 282 and travel east 8.5 miles to the RIDGEWAY sign at Dotson Road. Turn right onto Dotson Road, travel 3 miles (following signs to the boat ramp parking area), and turn right onto the road leading to boat ramp parking. The trailhead is on the right.

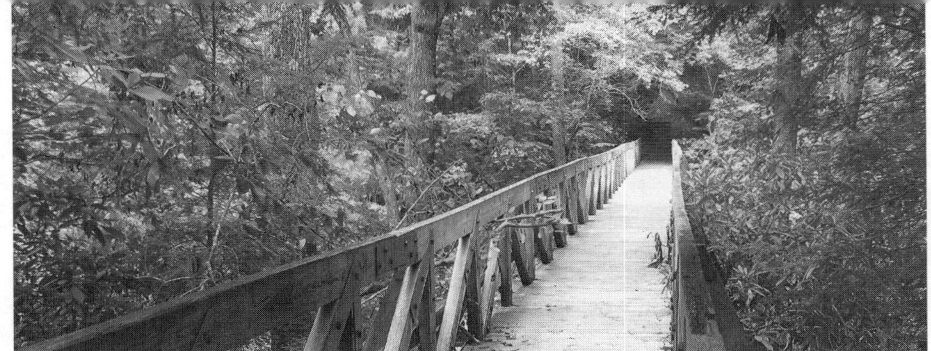

Crossing Tails Creek on the Tumbling Waters Nature Trail

To reach the visitors center, take Interstate 75 north to Exit 293 for Chatsworth/U.S. 411. At the end of the ramp turn right and take U.S. 411 north 25.5 miles. Turn right onto GA 136, travel east 2.6 miles, and turn left onto Carters Dam Road. Go 1.9 miles to a fork, and take the right branch to reach the visitors center.

FACILITIES/TRAILHEAD A restroom is located in the parking area. Also, there is a pay box for day use ($4). The Ridgeway Campground, located less than a half mile from the trailhead, has primitive campsites ($4 per night). Maps and trail information are available at the Carters Lake Visitors Center.

At the north side of the parking area, enter the trail at the TUMBLING WATERS NATURE TRAIL sign and descend the wood steps **(Waypoint 1)**. As you walk beneath the low limbs of hemlocks, you get your first glimpse of water to the left. White pines and ferns also grow along this path, which is surrounded by greenery. The path dips into a low area briefly and climbs to a hillside where the sound of gurgling water rises. As you descend, with the creek growing ever louder, look for mushrooms that have sprouted up in the trail.

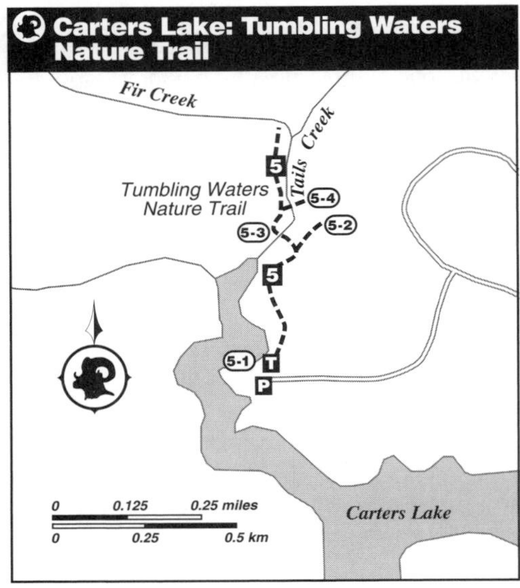

At 0.3 mile go straight at the trail junction, and travel another 360 feet to the wood overlook platform on the left **(Waypoint 2)**. This is a high perch with a good view of the falls upstream. The low boughs of a large hemlock form a shaggy roof over the platform, so you might imagine that you're in a great tree house. From here, retrace your steps, and turn right at the next trail junction to cross the wood bridge. In each direction, the creek bends in the distance and disappears among the trees.

After crossing the bridge, ascend the steep bank and walk to a trail junction **(Waypoint 3)**. To reach the creek from here, turn right and walk northeast on a trail with high sidewalls. This path continues for about 500 feet to a 10-foot-square wood platform that sits above the water and allows a good sight line to the cascades **(Waypoint 4)**. As you walk to the platform, look for side trails that access the water's edge below.

From **Waypoint 2** you can also ascend to the northwest on a steep path through slight pines and substantial hemlocks. Streaks of sunlight filter through layers of feathery canopy, and through the timber, low to the right, you can see flashes of whitewater in the tan creek. Unfortunately, this trail is pretty short and soon ends at an intersection with a dirt road. From the road, retrace your steps back across the bridge to return to the trailhead.

UTM WAYPOINTS

1. 16S 719126E 3836861N
2. 16S 719289E 3837396N
3. 16S 719178E 3837330N
4. 16S 719286E 3837432N

TRIP 6 Carters Lake: Amadahy Trail

Distance	3.4 miles, loop
Hiking Time	1½ hours
Difficulty	Easy
Elevation Gain/Loss	+/-270 feet
Trail Uses	Mountain biking and leashed dogs
Best Times	Year-round
Agency	U.S. Army Corps of Engineers, Carters Lake
Recommended Maps	A *Carters Lake Hiking Trails* map is available at the Carters Lake Visitors Center; a very basic *Amadahy* map is available at http://carters.sam.usace.army.mil/bike.htm.

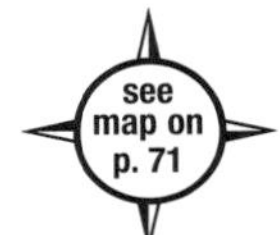

HIGHLIGHTS One of the newest trails near Carters Lake, the Amadahy Trail was constructed in 2006. Volunteers from the Ellijay Mountain Bike Association played a key role in building the trail, and while the path primarily draws bikers, it has become much more popular with hikers. *Amadahy* is a Cherokee word meaning "forest water," and much of the gently rolling path runs within sight of Carters Lake whose shores are free of boathouses and other human-made structures. In some spots, you walk right near the water, and in others the trail runs high through forests of chestnut oak and hickory. The wooded slopes in some areas are free of underbrush, as prescribed burns have reduced the fuel load to prevent extremely hot fires. The burns also supply nutrients to the soil, which will support vegetation that provides habitat for deer, songbirds, and other animals.

DIRECTIONS From Atlanta, take Interstate 75 north to Exit 293 for Chatsworth/U.S. Highway 411. At the end of the ramp turn right and take U.S. Highway 411 north 25.5 miles. Turn right onto GA Highway 136 and travel east 0.4 miles to Old Hwy 411. Turn left and travel north on Old Hwy 411 6.2 miles. Turn right onto U.S. Highway 76/GA Highway 282 and travel east 3.5 miles to Woodring Branch Road. Turn right onto Woodring Branch Road, go 3 miles. A short distance past the campground entrance, turn into the gravel parking lot on the right.

FACILITIES/TRAILHEAD There are no facilities at the trailhead. The most convenient camping is at the Woodring Branch Campground primitive sites, which are open year-round ($8 per night). It has sites for cars near restrooms, showers, water, and other facilities ($14 without hookups). The campground is located about 4 miles off U.S. 76 on the north side of the lake.

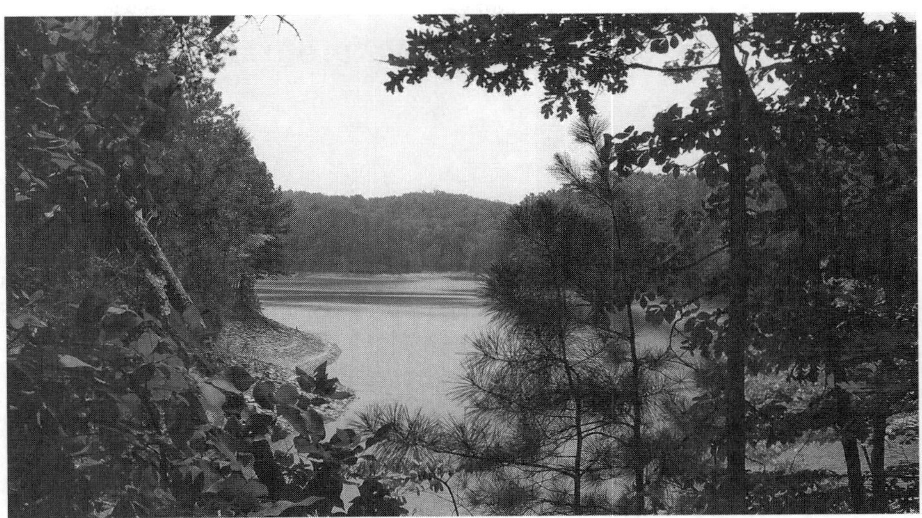
A glimpse of Carters Lake from the Amadahy Trail

At the south end of the gravel parking area, walk past the metal gate and turn left to go north **(Waypoint 1)**. The trail begins in an extremely dense forest that can best be described as scraggly. At 450 feet you skirt the west side of a clearing and then walk beside a heavily silted creek. You finally get your first glimpse of the lake at 0.4 mile. The path then hugs the lake for a long while, and to your right is much more attractive hardwood forest with little to no underbrush.

Other than the sound of the occasional motorboat, the lakeshore is quite peaceful, and the far shores of light brown sand are free of houseboats or other structures you typically see on Georgia lakes. As you're lulled into a quiet state of mind, be aware that you need to remain alert for mountain bikers cruising through here. Step aside to allow them to pass safely.

At 0.8 mile the lake extends far ahead in your field of view, while trees on the slopes to your right have visible signs of charring from prescribed burns. Ample sunlight splays across the leafy ground beneath widely spaced pine, oak, and hickory trees.

At 1.5 miles, go straight at the four-way trail junction **(Waypoint 2)** to travel north toward a lake cove. You'll soon descend to a point near lake level, and there's easy access to the water. Farther ahead, the path again hugs the lake in a series of mellow ups and downs with the lake ever visible beyond thin stands of trees.

There's a notable shift at 2.9 miles **(Waypoint 3)**, where the forest floor is no longer swept clean of brush, and mountain laurel creeps up the slopes. You'll leave the lake behind, as the trail presses inland and passes a series of cuts that are increasingly deep and steep.

At 3.1 miles, take a horseshoe turn to the north, and make your way through the undulating terrain, winding among the cuts, to return to the trailhead.

UTM WAYPOINTS

1. 16S 715595E 3834607N
2. 16S 715504E 3833235N
3. 16S 715191E 3834444N

TRIP 7 Carters Lake: Oak Ridge Nature Trail

Distance	1.2 miles, semiloop
Hiking Time	1 hour or less
Difficulty	Easy to moderate
Elevation Gain/Loss	+355/-325 feet
Trail Uses	Leashed dogs and good for kids
Best Times	Year-round
Agency	U.S. Army Corps of Engineers, Carters Lake
Recommended Maps	A *Carters Lake Hiking Trails* map is available at the Carters Lake Visitors Center; USGS 7.5-min. *Oakman*

HIGHLIGHTS With only short stretches of moderate or steep terrain, the Oak Ridge Trail is one of the easier walks in the Carters Lake area. Beginning on a ridge in shady hardwood forest, the path descends to the bank of Carters Lake where a peninsula provides a broad view of the water and forested shoreline. The trail then climbs back up the ridge and passes an odd natural feature that is the subject of debate. Beside the path is an "Indian trail tree," or a tree whose trunk bends dramatically near the base and runs horizontally before stretching skyward. Some say Native Americans altered trees into such odd shapes to serve as directional signs, but some experts say there's no evidence to support this. Check it out for yourself and join the debate.

DIRECTIONS From Atlanta, take Interstate 75 north to Exit 293 for Chatsworth/U.S. Highway 411. At the end of the ramp turn right and take U.S. Highway 411 north 25.5 miles. Turn right onto GA Highway 136 and travel east 0.4 mile to Old Highway 411. Turn left and travel north on Old Highway 411 6.2 miles. Turn right onto U.S. Highway 76/282, and travel east 3.5 miles to Woodring Branch Road. Turn right onto Woodring Branch Road, continue 4.3 miles, and park on the right shoulder of the road just beyond the DEVELOPED CAMPING area. The trailhead lies 130 feet to the left where an OAK RIDGE NATURE TRAIL sign is suspended.

To reach the Carters Lake Visitors Center from Atlanta, take Interstate 75 north to Exit 293 for Chatsworth/U.S. Highway 411. At the end of the ramp turn right and take U.S. Highway 411 north 25.5 miles. Turn right onto GA Highway 136, travel east 2.6 miles and turn left onto Carters Dam Road. Go 1.9 miles to a fork, and take the right branch to reach the visitors center.

FACILITIES/TRAILHEAD There are no facilities at the trailhead. Nearby Woodring Branch Campground has restrooms, hot showers, 42 campsites ($14, including 11 tent-only sites), and a primitive camping area with 12 tent sites ($8). For more information or reservations, call the campground at (706) 276-6050.

Begin beneath the large, suspended trail sign **(Waypoint 1)** and amble along the wide path through pines and hardwoods that shade leafy ground. Look up and you will see birdfeeders attached to tree trunks, and also scan the ground for bright white and brilliant red mushrooms dotting the trail.

At 700 feet you reach a Y intersection **(Waypoint 2)**. Bear left and travel south to descend from the ridge, with dense stands of young pines on each side of the path. At 0.3 mile, the lake comes into view on the left, and after another tenth of a mile the trail reaches the shore of the lake **(Waypoint 3)**. On this peninsula, the land is clear, with just a few pines keeping you company, so you have an excellent view of the lake to the south.

From the lakeshore, retrace your steps to **Waypoint 2**, turn left and travel west. The wide, grassy path briefly runs through more young pines, but after about 360 feet the trees are more mature and tall oaks appear. In the open forest ahead, you can clearly see the terrain sloping downward, and the lake shimmers in the distance. The path drops moderately, makes a horseshoe bend to the northeast, and continues downward to the bank of a narrow lake inlet (**Waypoint 4**) at 1 mile.

The trail is narrow and rises steeply to the northeast. You cross a creek drainage, and the trail widens and becomes lined with moss. Continue climbing, following the drainage up through an especially inviting stretch of oaks and other hardwoods.

At 1.2 miles, notice the tree with a bent lower trunk that runs horizontally (**Waypoint 5**). This is a supposed "Indian trail tree." It's believed that Native Americans altered the growth patterns of certain trees so that they would serve as markers to point the way for traveling, or to indicate the way to a resource, such as shelter or water.

From the Indian trail tree, continue northeast for about 200 feet to return to the trailhead.

UTM WAYPOINTS

1. 16S 716427E 3833100N
2. 16S 716396E 3832909N
3. 16S 716355E 3832451N
4. 16S 716122E 3832979N
5. 16S 716399E 3833058N

TRIP 8 Red Top Mountain State Park: Homestead Loop, Sweetgum, & White Tail Trails

Distance	5.3–6.1 miles (add another 0.75 mile for Lakeside Trail), loop
Hiking Time	3 hours
Difficulty	Easy to moderate
Elevation Gain/Loss	+585/-290 feet
Trail Use	Wheelchair accessible (The 0.75-mile wheelchair-accessible Lakeside Trail begins in the lodge parking lot.)
Best Times	Year-round
Agency	Red Top Mountain State Park and Lodge
Recommended Map	A *Red Top Mountain State Park* trail map is available at the visitors center.

HIGHLIGHTS Covering 12,000 acres, Allatoona Lake draws crowds of boaters and anglers, but it's also surrounded by a rolling forest of pines and hardwoods with more than 15 miles of trails. The best path in the park is the Homestead Loop Trail, which winds through cool, shaded ravines and skirts the lakeshore where you can swim, fish, and picnic in coves located just off the path. The trail rises high into a diverse forest of loblolly and Virginia pines mixed with hardwoods and the lake below forming a bright, shining backdrop.

Another notable trail is the White Tail Trail, which starts near the park lodge and crosses a peninsula to a secluded point of land where a grove of trees and a large black boulder frame a postcard view of the water. The Lakeside Trail, located behind the park lodge, is a wheelchair-accessible paved loop that follows the lakeshore and is a good route for observing hummingbirds and other wildlife.

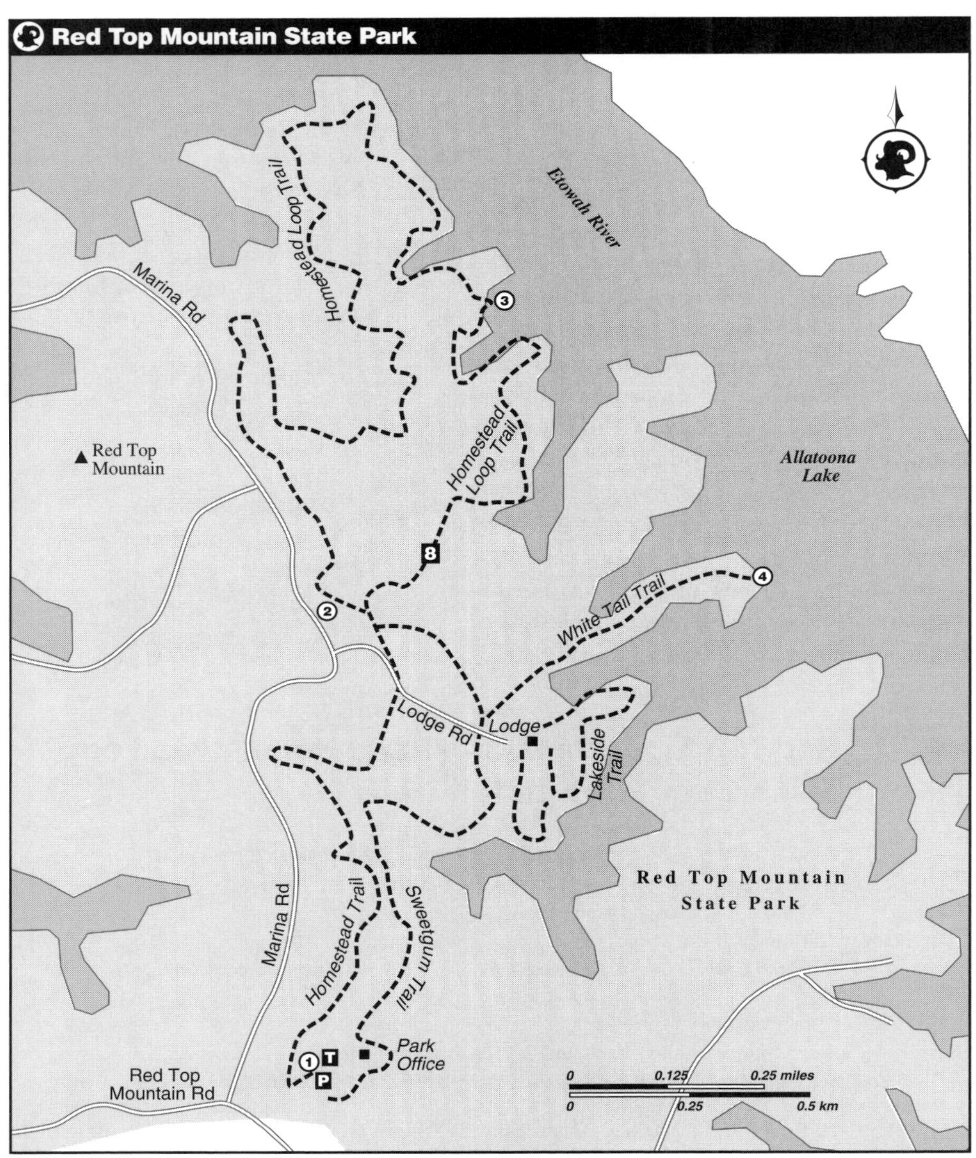

DIRECTIONS From Atlanta, take Interstate 75 north to Exit 285. Go right or east on Red Top Mountain Road and cross Allatoona Lake. Continue on Red Top Mountain Road to the visitors center parking lot on the left. To reach the lodge and the Lakeside Trail, just before reaching the visitors center, turn left onto Marina Road. Take this to Lodge Road and turn right.

FACILITIES/TRAILHEAD There are restrooms at the visitors center next to the trailhead and at the lodge. Camping facilities include tent and RV sites ($20–$24), plus there are cottages and a lodge. There is a $3 daily parking fee, and you can purchase a $30 Annual ParkPass by calling (770) 389-7401.

From the visitors center pass the HOMESTEAD sign **(Waypoint 1)** and follow the trail that descends to the west through tall poplars and sweetgum trees. At 0.3 mile look to the right for a sign explaining that the surrounding trees have been attacked by pine beetles, which bore into the trunks, inhibiting the flow of water through the trees.

At 0.4 mile, turn left at the trail intersection to take the Homestead/Sweetgum Trail. You'll cross low ground and briefly follow a small stream before the trail veers away. At the next intersection, bear left to take the Homestead Trail and follow the yellow blazes. A series of switchbacks takes you up into hardwoods where leaves blanket the open forest floor. As you traverse the slope of a hill, look right and you can peer deeply into the sloping, clear forest.

At 0.9 mile turn left to take the Homestead/Sweetgum Trail across another slope of a hill, and ahead cross a wood footbridge. At 1.1 miles, cross Lodge Road and bear left at the next trail intersection to take the Homestead Trail. When I scouted this route, I interrupted a snake here that was trying to swallow his lunch. Although it wasn't a rattlesnake, it rattled its tail at me and backed away, all while continuing to down his catch—impressive multitasking.

Just ahead is a Y intersection **(Waypoint 2)**. Bear right to begin the Homestead Loop, traveling east. The trail returns to low ground where a lawn of high grass lines a clear stream and poplars stand straight and tall. A bench offers a good opportunity to rest and enjoy the scene, but don't be surprised if a crowd of noisy crows protest your presence. Also, this is one of many places along the hike where you may spot deer. Though deer are common in the park, their steadily growing population has wreaked havoc on many plant species, and due to their grazing, you're much less likely to spy the many wildflower species that were once abundant in this area. Though the park vegetation can support about 50 deer, there were once as many as 400. The park

Quiet beach cove just off the Homestead Loop Trail

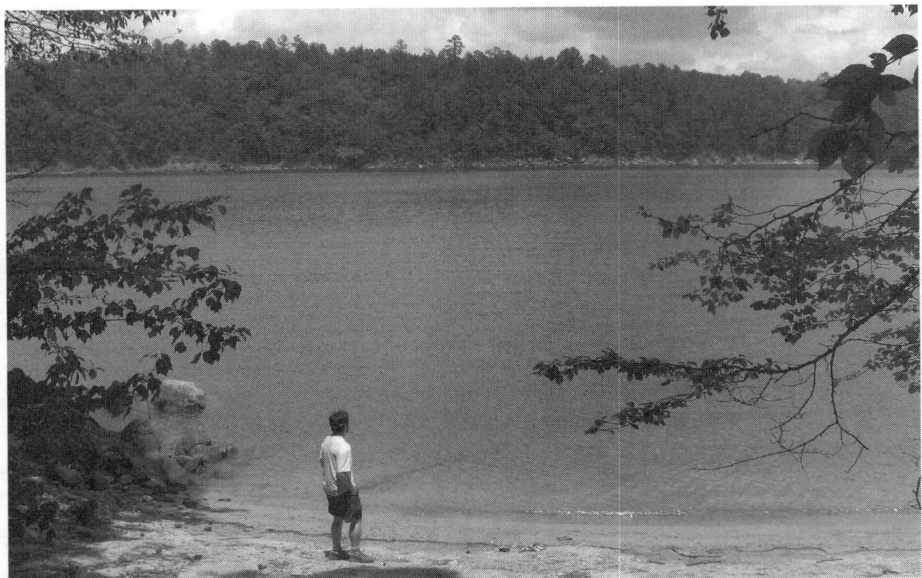

recently held a controlled and limited hunt to cull the population; the deer population is now under control, and many plant species are just now recovering.

Continuing on, the trail climbs to high ground. In winter you will have intermittent views of the lake, which is just a distant gleam in the summer. Farther on, a descent leads to the tip of a finger of land, and a bench rests in a spot with a good view of a lake inlet.

At 2 miles **(Waypoint 3)**, look to the right for a lake cove. There are several little inlets along the trail, but this may be the best spot because of its wide, clear beach and broad view of the lake to the east. This makes a good rest spot before continuing your long trek through the forest.

Traffic can be high in the park, but the next section of the Homestead Loop is relatively secluded as it winds around inlets, tops 900 feet of elevation on quiet hills, and takes frequent twists through stands of deciduous trees and pines. At 3.8 miles, the path is less remote and runs near Marina Road before dropping back down to the beginning of the loop.

From the beginning of the loop, either retrace your steps to the trailhead, or explore a secluded peninsula via the White Tail Trail. To reach the White Tail Trail, walk back to the junction of the Yellow Trail and Red Trail (just before reaching Lodge Road). Turn left and take the red-blazed Sweetgum Trail southeast for 0.2 mile to the junction with the White Tail Trail. Turn left and take the White Tail Trail to the end of the peninsula **(Waypoint 4)**. At the very tip, trees huddle around a large boulder to beautifully frame the wide lake channel. You'll be tempted to hop up on the rock and stay awhile. Shaded and secluded, with a postcard view of the water, this is a prime spot in the park to relax and have a snack.

Walk back to the junction with the red-blazed Sweetgum Trail. Turn left to follow the Red Trail south (crossing the parking lot) for 0.3 mile. At the trail junction, turn left to continue south on the Sweetgum Trail, following red blazes, for 0.5 mile to return to the parking area.

UTM WAYPOINTS

1. 16S 711391E 3780985N
2. 16S 711519E 3781439N
3. 16S 711750E 3782646N
4. 16S 712303E 3782058N

Looking out over Allatoona Lake from the end of the White Tail Trail

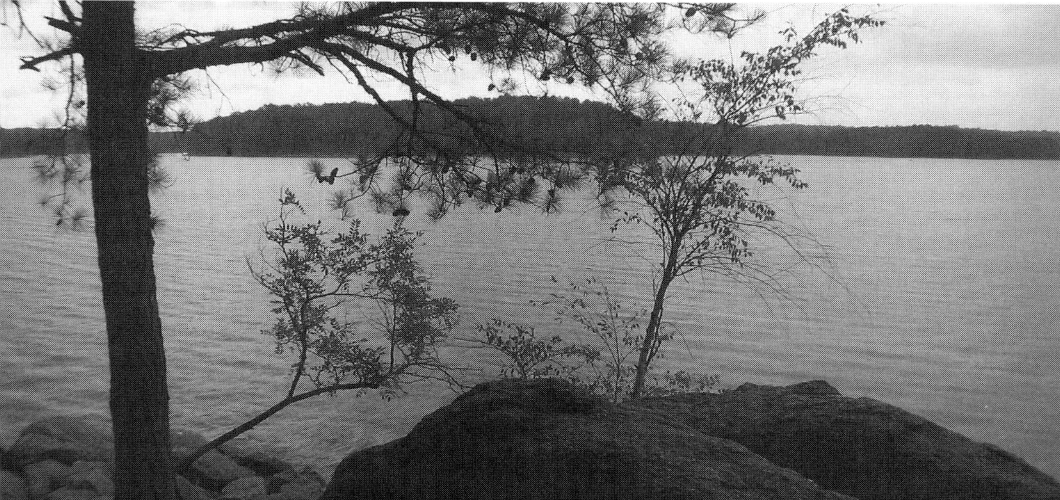

TRIP 9 Amicalola Falls State Park: Base of Falls Trail

Distance	1.5 miles, out-and-back (from visitors center)
Hiking Time	1 hour
Difficulty	Moderate
Elevation Gain/Loss	+/-485 feet
Trail Use	Leashed dogs
Best Times	Year-round
Agency	Amicalola Falls State Park
Recommended Map	A trail map is available at the visitors center and online at www.gastateparks.org.

HIGHLIGHTS Beginning at the visitors center, the Base of Falls Trail runs through a corridor of sweetgum trees, maples, and blueberry bushes, and crosses the entrance road to skirt Little Amicalola Creek. Rainbow trout inhabit this clear, cold stream, and fishing is popular in the park. The trail then continues to a reflecting pool where people often fish, and you get a view of the distant Amicalola Falls. A paved trail then rises steadily to meet wood steps, which carry you to a platform that puts you close to the falls.

DIRECTIONS From Atlanta take Interstate 75 north to Interstate 575. Travel north on I-575 to GA Highway 5/515. Go north on GA 5/515 through East Ellijay, and turn right onto GA Highway 52 to go east. Take GA 52 east 19 miles to the Amicalola Falls State Park entrance on the left. Take the entrance road to the parking area near the visitors center.

FACILITIES/TRAILHEAD There are restrooms at the visitors center. There is a $3 parking fee for the park. You can purchase an Annual ParkPass for $30 by calling (770) 389-7401. Accommodations include 24 tent, trailer, and RV campsites ($25); 14 cottages ($69–$199); and a 56-room lodge ($89–$189).

At the rear (or east side) of the visitors center enter the Appalachian Approach Trail at the stone arch **(Waypoint 1)**. Walk a few yards and turn left off of the Appalachian Approach Trail to take a dirt path that runs beside a series of picnic shelters and the amphitheater. Along the trail are blueberry bushes that serve as a food source for birds, deer, opossum, and squirrels. Scan the ground and you'll see the small, spiked fruit of sweetgum trees, while poplars and maples fill out the forest.

After walking 0.2 mile, passing the amphitheater, the trail jogs left. Cross the road to the trail at the east side of Little Amicalola Creek **(Waypoint 2)**. The clear water of the creek has plenty of oxygen to support breeding trout, whereas muddy water would suffocate their eggs. As you walk northeast along the creek, watch out for poison ivy plants. You can see their vines climbing the trees (and you'll recognize the leaves by the single notch on one

Falls Access for People with Disabilities

The 0.3-mile West Ridge Falls Access Trail runs from an upper parking area in the park to the bridge at the base of the falls. To reach the upper parking area, take the entrance road and turn left at the visitors center, just before the Appalachian Trail parking lot. Go 0.9 mile to the parking lot on the right. The West Ridge Falls Access Trail begins on the east side of the lot.

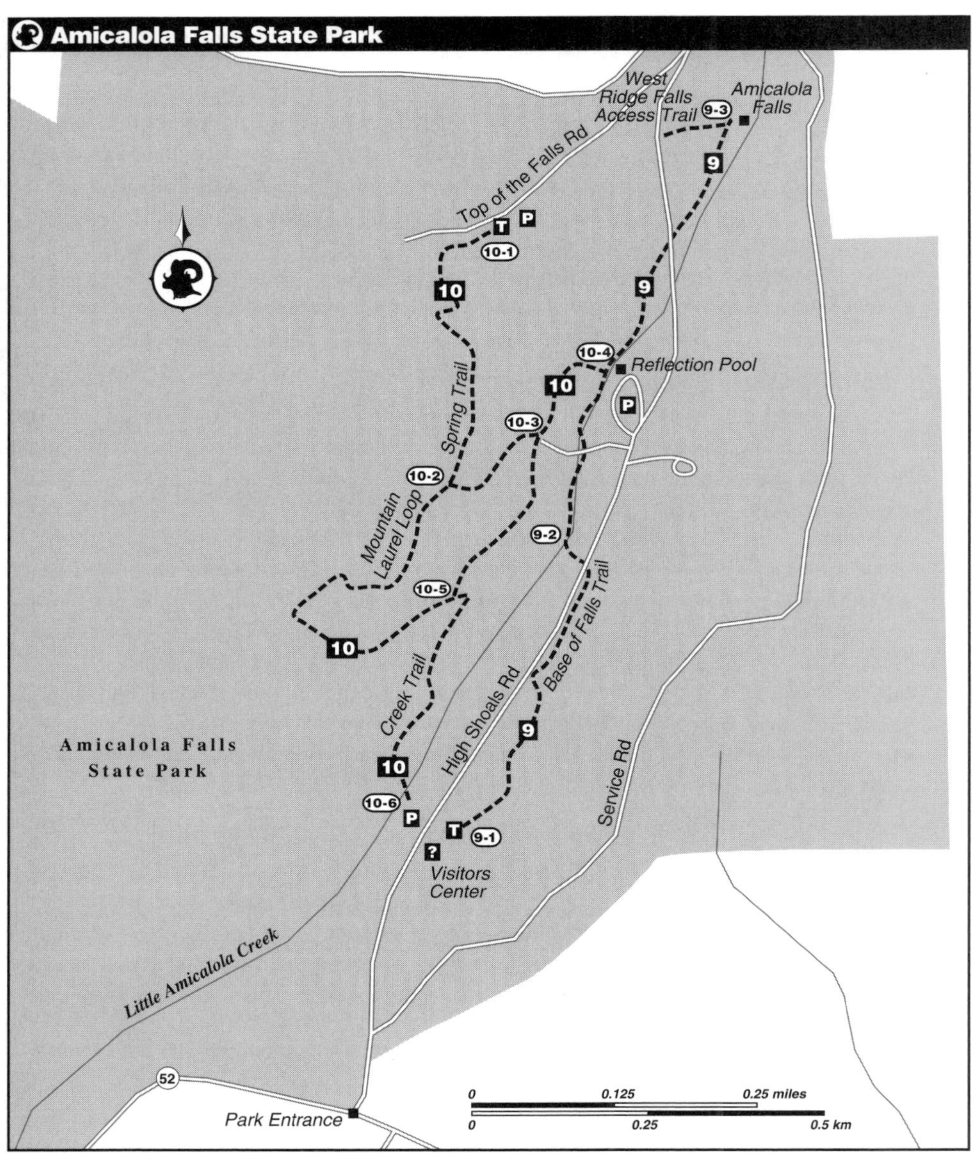

side of each leaf). Also, growing along the trail are May apple plants whose ripe fruit is used to make jam and jelly, though the stem and leaves are highly toxic. There are also muscadine vines in this area.

At 0.4 mile bear left to cross the creek on a wood footbridge, and see if you can spy water snakes that frequent this stretch of the stream. Not far ahead is the reflecting pool where you can look northeast for a view of the distant falls. Circle the left side of the pool and continue northeast on a paved path beside the creek.

At 0.7 mile you reach a set of wood steps that climb to a bridge **(Waypoint 3)**, which stretches across the face of the falls. To return to the Base of Falls trailhead, retrace your steps.

If you were to continue west across the bridge, at the end is a set of 475 steps that climb steeply to the falls overlook. From the base of the steps you can also continue west on the wheelchair-accessible West Ridge Falls Access Trail, which ends at a parking lot.

UTM WAYPOINTS

1. 16S 752377E 3827419N
2. 16S 752529E 3827837N
3. 16S 752762E 3828461N

TRIP 10 Amicalola Falls State Park: Spring Trail, Mountain Laurel Loop, & Creek Trail

see map on p. 82

Distance	2.4 miles, semiloop
Hiking Time	1 hour
Difficulty	Moderate
Elevation Gain/Loss	+515/-480 feet
Trail Use	Leashed dogs
Best Times	Year-round
Agency	Amicalola Falls State Park
Recommended Map	A trail map is available at the visitors center and online at www.gastateparks.org.

HIGHLIGHTS Three relatively short trails, the Spring Trail, Mountain Laurel Loop, and Creek Trail, explore the western slopes of the Amicalola Creek watershed. While these paths are popular, they might not be as crowded as the uber-popular Base of Falls Trail. From the upper parking area, you begin on the Spring Trail, descending moderately to steeply on a ridge covered with hardwoods. This path intersects the Mountain Laurel Loop, which winds through the twisted trunks of high laurel and drops to the reflection pool where Amicalola Falls is visible to the distant northeast. Backtracking along the Mountain Laurel Loop, you reach the short Creek Trail, which rolls through thick foliage just above Amicalola Creek and ends at the Appalachian Trail parking area. From the parking area, walk back up the Creek Trail to turn west and finish the Mountain Laurel Loop, climbing steeply back to the upper parking area.

DIRECTIONS From Atlanta take Interstate 75 north to Interstate 575. Travel north on I-575 to GA Highway 5/515. Go north on GA 5/515 through East Ellijay and turn right onto GA Highway 52 to go east. Take GA 52 east 19 miles to the Amicalola Falls State Park entrance on the left. Take the entrance road and turn left at the visitors center, just before the Appalachian Trail parking lot. Go 0.9 mile to the parking lot on the right.

FACILITIES/TRAILHEAD There are no facilities at the trailhead. There is a $3 parking fee for the park. You can purchase an Annual ParkPass for $30 by calling (770) 389-7401. Accommodations include 24 tent, trailer, and RV campsites ($25); 14 cottages ($69–$199); and a 56-room lodge ($89–$189).

Begin at the west side of the parking area and enter at the sign for the Spring Trail, visitors center, Mountain Laurel Loop, and Creek Trail **(Waypoint 1)**. Follow orange blazes, descending moderately on the rocky, rough path through

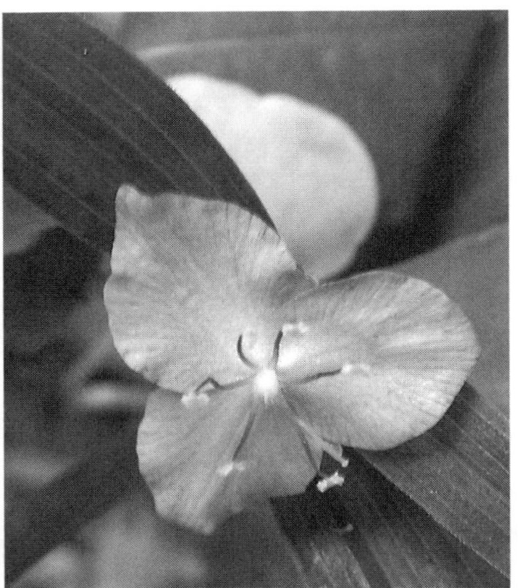

Spiderwort

oak, sourwood, mountain laurel, and pine.

At 0.3 mile **(Waypoint 2)**, bear left onto the Mountain Laurel Loop Trail and travel east following green blazes. As the narrow path winds downward, mountain laurel becomes more prevalent and envelopes the trail.

At 0.5 mile you'll reach a T junction **(Waypoint 3)**. Turn left onto the yellow-blazed trail, which runs level on the flank of a hill before dropping to the reflection pool **(Waypoint 4)**. There tends to be lots of activity at the pool because it's popular for fishing and has an open view of Amicalola Falls. From the pool, retrace your steps to **Waypoint 3**. Continue straight, traveling southwest on the Mountain Laurel Loop Trail.

After walking another tenth of a mile there is a trail junction **(Waypoint 5)**. Turn left to descend the Creek Trail blazed yellow. You might have to duck to walk beneath the dense mountain laurel that lines this narrow, rooted path. You'll drop close to the creek and pass through rhododendrons as campsites are visible just across the stream. The trail ends at a footbridge **(Waypoint 6)**, which you can cross to reach the parking area across from the visitors center.

From **Waypoint 6**, walk back up the Creek Trail to **Waypoint 5**. Turn left onto the Mountain Laurel Loop and walk southwest, climbing gradually on a wide path in pines and hardwoods. You'll notice many damaged and downed trees that have suffered attacks of pine beetles. The trail turns sharply to the northeast and climbs gradually through overhead mountain laurel and high oaks. As the trail steepens a bit, your elbows brush the elbows of crooked laurel trunks.

The path steadily climbs up the spur to the junction with the Spring Trail **(Waypoint 2)**. Bear left onto the orange-blazed Spring Trail to make the steep climb back to the parking lot.

UTM WAYPOINTS

1. 16S 752436E 3828304N
2. 16S 752355E 3827914N
3. 16S 752508E 3828000N
4. 16S 752579E 3828085N
5. 16S 752377E 3827764N
6. 16S 752298E 3827493N

TRIP 11 Len Foote Hike Inn Trail

Distance	9.8 miles, out-and-back
Hiking Time	3–4 hours each way
Difficulty	Moderate
Elevation Gain/Loss	+2070/-2020 feet
Trail Use	Leashed dogs are allowed on the trail but not at the Hike Inn.
Best Times	Spring and fall (winter is least crowded)
Agency	Len Foote Hike Inn and Amicalola Falls State Park
Recommended Map	A *Len Foote Hike Inn* trail map is available at Amicalola Falls State Park Visitors Center.

HIGHLIGHTS A trek to the Len Foote Hike Inn with an overnight stay is a unique experience that I highly recommend. Accessible only by trail (a little less than 5 miles), the inn is comfortable yet rustic with rooms that have no electrical outlets. This is a place where you can escape ringing cell phones and enjoy the company of fellow travelers while feasting on delicious meals in a comfortable dining hall. You can also relax and read while sitting beside the wood-burning stove in the community room. Not only is the inn a tranquil retreat, but it is also a fascinating facility that is LEED certified (meaning it is officially recognized as being extremely energy efficient).

The trail to the inn is only moderately difficult, and in spring many species of wildflowers grow along the path. This trail is also popular with women because it is considered quite safe. There is some built-in security because people staying at the inn check in at the Amicalola Falls State Park Lodge before hiking, and the inn personnel are on the lookout for their guests' arrival.

DIRECTIONS From Atlanta take Interstate 75 north to Interstate 575. Travel north on I-575 to GA Highway 5/515. Go north on GA 5/515 through East Ellijay, and turn right onto GA Highway 52 to go east. Take GA 52 east 19 miles to the Amicalola Falls State Park entrance on the left. Take the entrance road and turn left at the visitors center, just before the Appalachian Trail parking lot. Go about 1.2 miles to the Top of Falls parking lot.

FACILITIES/TRAILHEAD There are no facilities at the trailhead. There is a $3 parking fee for the park. You can purchase an Annual ParkPass for $30 by calling (770) 389-7401. There are 20 rooms at the inn ($70–$97), and each has bunk beds. The inn has a dining facility, hot showers, and eco-friendly (and odor-free) composting toilets. Before hiking, check in at the Amicalola Falls State Park Visitors Center. For more information on rooms, meals, amenities, and such, visit the Len Foote Inn website (http://hike-inn.com) .

At the southeast side of the parking area enter the trail at the sign marked TRAIL TO LODGE **(Waypoint 1)**. Ascend to a junction with a path that leads to the East Ridge Trail and visitors center. Bear left and travel north following blue and yellow blazes.

After about 700 feet cross a road, and at 0.2 mile bear right at the Y junction to take the Hike Inn Trail and ascend slightly. The trail passes through a mix of hardwoods and then crests a ridge where a log bench looks over the forested valley to the southeast. A descent takes you through corridors of mountain laurel, and then a long, steady climb leads to a ridgetop where the path hairpins to the north.

Len Foote Hike Inn Trail

Len Foote Trail
Bee Bar Rd
Nimblewill Creek
Cochrans Creek
Len Foote Hike Inn
Frosty Mountain
Anderson Creek
Appalachian Approach Trail
Amicalola Mountains
High Shoals Rd
Len Foote Hike Inn Trail
Cochrans Falls
Chattahoochee National Forest
Amicalola Lake
Amicalola Falls State Park
Visitors Center
0 0.25 0.5 miles
0 0.5 1.0km

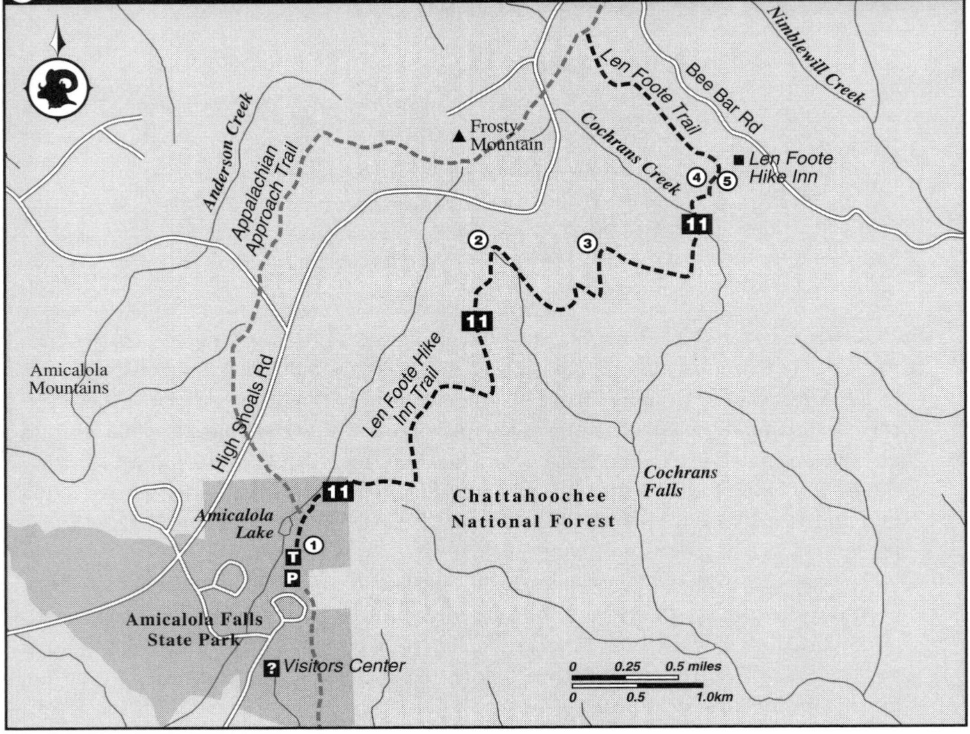

At 2.6 miles **(Waypoint 2)** cross a creek on a wood footbridge and climb through rhododendron and mountain laurel with galax at your feet. You might pick up the sweet fragrance of trailing arbutus through here and see the white blooms of serviceberry. In spring, also look for dwarf irises, flame azaleas, and trillium. The forest is diverse, with dogwoods and sourwood gathering beneath the canopy of oaks, pines, and tulip poplars. This large tract of wild land also provides habitat for bears, turkeys, and deer.

The trail passes through a hemlock heath at 3.6 miles before descending through thick rhododendrons that shroud a stream to transform the woods into something ancient and exotic **(Waypoint 3)**. At 4.3 miles scan the ground for beds of running ground pine, or "running cedar," a plant that has a history dating back to the Paleozoic era.

You'll climb up and over a ridge, dropping to the intersection with the Cove Trail at 4.7 miles **(Waypoint 4)**. Continue straight, traveling northwest, to reach the Len Foote Hike Inn **(Waypoint 5)**. When you check in, ask about joining a tour of the grounds. Inn personnel will point out

Len Foote Hike Inn

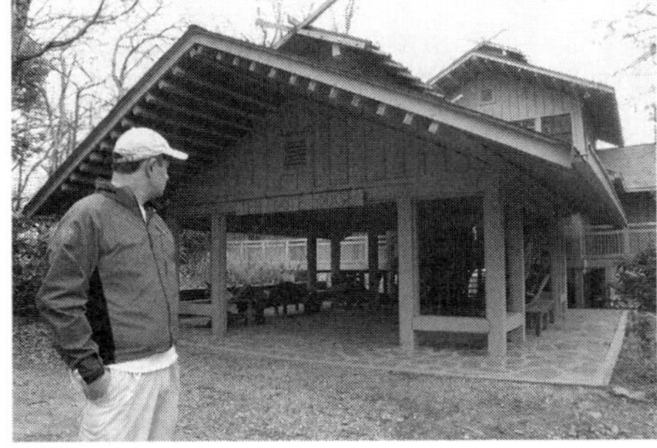

the inn's "green" features and explain how the facility uses solar panels, composting toilets, and a rainwater catch to conserve energy and reduce waste. They'll even take you below the building to see the worm bed where organic material from the dining hall is deposited and scarfed up by red wigglers. The inn's philosophy of environmental preservation fits the facilities' namesake, Leonard E. Foote, a biologist, conservationist, and photographer who dedicated his life to protecting Georgia's natural resources.

The Len Foote Hike Inn Trail continues on the northwest side of the inn and goes a little more than a mile to intersect with the Appalachian Approach Trail. To return to the parking area at Amicalola Falls State Park, from the inn retrace your steps to the trailhead.

UTM WAYPOINTS

1. 16S 752895E 3828515N
2. 16S 754352E 3830808N
3. 16S 755170E 3830724N
4. 16S 755948E 3831261N
5. 16S 756028E 3831348N

TRIP 12 Appalachian Approach Trail

Distance	16.2 miles, out-and-back
Hiking Time	8–10 hours
Difficulty	Moderate to strenuous
Elevation Gain/Loss	+4340/-4350 feet
Trail Uses	Leashed dogs and backpacking
Best Times	Year-round
Agency	Amicalola Falls State Park and U.S. Forest Service, Blue Ridge District
Recommended Map	Appalachian Trail Conference *Appalachian Trail* map

HIGHLIGHTS Big decisions are made on this 8.1-mile path that runs from Amicalola Falls State Park to the beginning of the Appalachian Trail (AT) at Springer Mountain. Many people intending to complete the entire AT get their first sobering dose of rugged backpacking on the Approach Trail. It is here that a good number of hikers realize they are not fit enough, have an overloaded pack, or lack the desire to walk all the way to Maine. If you're considering an AT thru-hike, or if you're just seeking a good backcountry trip, the Approach Trail will give you a good taste of the AT.

From the visitors center, the trail climbs gradually through Amicalola Falls State Park, and then traverses the Amicalola Mountain ridgeline. Moderate hiking takes you over a series of knobs and gaps in a mix of hardwoods and pines. There are plenty of ups and downs, with a visit to the summit of Frosty Mountain and a notable steep, rocky descent to Nimblewell Gap. You conclude with switchbacks leading to the summit of Springer Mountain (3782 feet).

DIRECTIONS From Atlanta take Interstate 75 north to Interstate 575. Travel north on I-575 to GA Highway 5/515. Go north on GA 5/515 through East Ellijay, and turn right onto GA Highway 52 to go east. Take GA 52 east 19 miles to the Amicalola Falls State Park entrance on the left. Take the entrance road to the parking area near the visitors center.

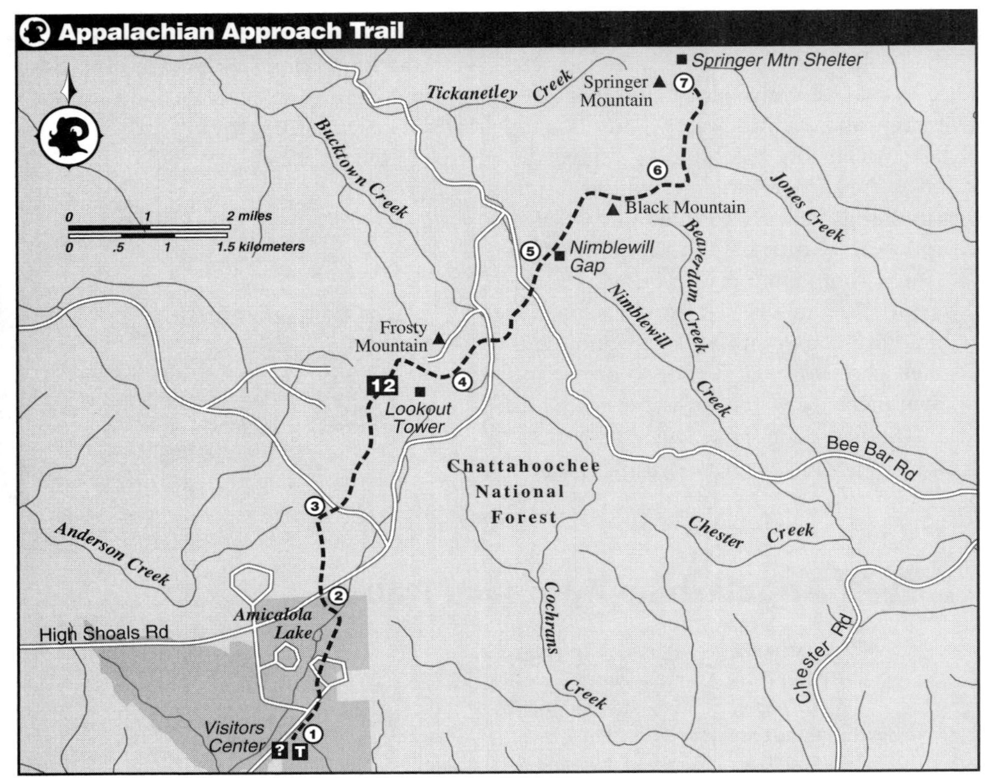

FACILITIES/TRAILHEAD There are restrooms at the visitors center. There is a $3 parking fee for the park. You can purchase an Annual ParkPass for $30 by calling (770) 389-7401. There is no fee to hike or camp. From the end of the Appalachian Approach Trail, walk 0.2 mile on the AT to reach the Springer Mountain Shelter, which has a privy and spring. There are also tent sites.

At the rear (or east side) of the visitors center **(Waypoint 1)**, enter the Appalachian Approach Trail at the stone arch and follow blue blazes. Climb moderately for 0.5 mile, and then take steep switchbacks to an old roadbed. Turn left and travel north to a paved parking area. Here, ascend wood and earth steps on the right and follow blue blazes. The trail then runs north beside Amicalola Lake.

At 1.4 miles **(Waypoint 2)**, take a wood footbridge across Little Amicalola Creek and cross the gravel road. Climb gradually to the crest of a ridge where there are intermittent views to the west of mountains that pile up in endless waves of green. The trail drops from the ridge and then begins a steep climb to High Shoals Road.

At 3.1 miles **(Waypoint 3)** cross High Shoals Road and climb onto a ridge. The trail drops into a gap and then moves up Frosty Mountain's western slopes. At 4.6 miles **(Waypoint 4)** the trail reaches the high point of Frosty Mountain (3382 feet) where a fire tower once stood. You then make a gradual descent from Frosty Mountain, cross a Forest Service road, and climb over Woody Knob.

The path becomes steep and rocky as you move down to Nimblewill Gap (3049 feet) at 5.9 miles **(Waypoint 5)**. As you move through the gap, you will pass the intersection of Forest Service roads 46 and 28, and then climb to a hilltop where there is a small clearing with a fire ring, which is used as a campsite. The trail takes a moderate course, following the western mountain slopes before dropping to Black Gap **(Waypoint 6)** at 7.1 miles. The Black Gap Shelter lies to the left, and a water source is to the right. From the gap the trail runs east and then swings north to climb Springer Mountain.

At 8.1 miles **(Waypoint 7)** the trail reaches the summit of Springer Mountain (3782 feet) and the southern terminus of the AT. The Appalachian Trail begins at an overlook on Springer Mountain, and in spring there is usually plenty of activity at this rock outcrop set in a stand of short, twisted oaks. Preparing to set off on their long journey, thru-hikers gather here to chat, sign the trail register, and take in the view while contemplating what could be a seminal experience in their lives.

The Springer Mountain Shelter lies to the right. Maine's Mount Katahdin is *only* about 2155 miles to the north.

UTM WAYPOINTS

1. 16S 752377E 3827419N
2. 16S 753026E 3828973N
3. 16S 753392E 3830850N
4. 16S 754350E 3831802N
5. 16S 755442E 3833195N
6. 16S 756877E 3834067N
7. 16S 757263E 3835226N

TRIP 13 Benton MacKaye Trail: Wilscot Gap to Shallowford Bridge

Distance	7.6 miles, point-to-point
Hiking Time	4–5 hours
Difficulty	Strenuous
Elevation Gain/Loss	+1885 feet/-2530 feet (one way)
Trail Use	Backpacking
Best Times	Winter, spring, and fall
Agency	Chattahoochee National Forest, Blue Ridge Ranger District. The best information source is the Benton MacKaye Trail Association.
Recommended Map	USGS 7.5-min. *Blue Ridge*

HIGHLIGHTS Traversing the rugged Wilscot Mountain Range, Section 5 of the Benton MacKaye Trail (BMT) begins with a challenging hike through rugged forest and ends with a stroll across the Shallowford Bridge, where the Toccoa River draws tourists in spring and summer. The hike includes a climb to the summit of Tiptop Mountain (3147 feet) and Brawley Mountain (site of the trail's last remaining fire tower).

Due to significant gains and losses in elevation, it's best to do this as a one-way trip, spotting cars at each end or using a shuttle to return to the trailhead. Also, this is a good option for a winter trip, as many of the views along the way are obscured by heavy foliage in spring.

DIRECTIONS There are parking areas at Wilscot Gap and Shallowford Bridge. Note that the parking area at Shallowford Bridge is the lot for the Toccoa Wilderness Outpost, and spots may not be available late May through summer due to heavy tourist traffic. In winter and early spring, you shouldn't have a problem getting a space.

If you wish to use a shuttle for your hike, you can make arrangements with commercial shuttle operators or members of the Benton MacKaye Trail Association. For a list of commercial vendors, or to get contact information for individual volunteers, check out the Hiker Resources link on the BMTA website.

To reach Shallowford Bridge from Atlanta, take GA Highway 400 north to the end of GA 400 at the intersection with GA Highway 60/U.S. Highway 19. Turn left onto GA 60/ U.S. 19 north and travel toward Dahlonega. From Dahlonega take GA 60/U.S. 19 north to where GA 60 and U.S. 19 split at Stonepile Gap. Take GA 60 north 23.8 miles and turn left onto Dial Road (look carefully for this turn as it's difficult to see). Go 5.9 miles and turn left onto Shallowford Bridge Road. Go 1.3 miles and turn left to cross Shallowford Bridge. Once across, turn right onto Aska Road. Parking is immediately on the right.

To reach Wilscot Gap from Atlanta, take GA Highway 400 north to the end of GA 400 at the intersection with GA Highway 60/U.S. Highway 19. Turn left onto GA 60/U.S. 19 north and travel toward Dahlonega. From Dahlonega take GA 60/U.S. 19 north to where GA 60 and U.S. 19 split at Stonepile Gap. Take GA 60 north for 26.5 miles to Wilscot Gap where there is a large clearing on the right side of the road. A green and white sign indicates that the trail crosses the road here.

FACILITIES/TRAILHEAD There are no facilities at the trailhead. The Toccoa Wilderness Outpost at Shallowford Bridge has restrooms, groceries, pizza, burgers, and sandwiches. There are

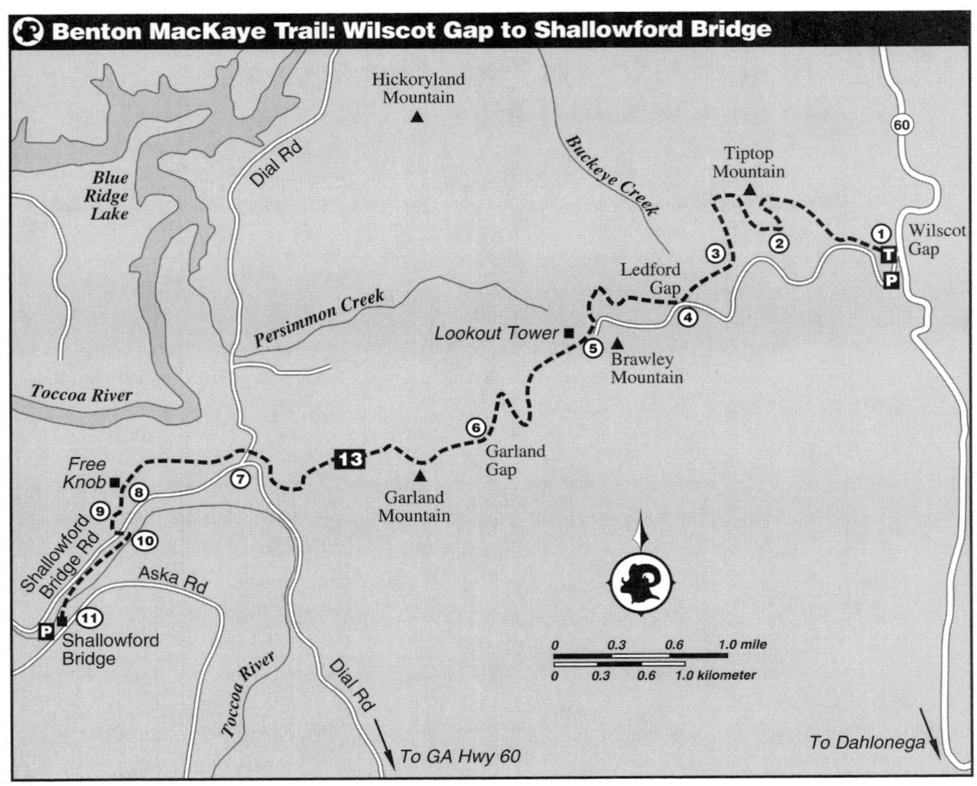

no shelters along the trail, but there are clearings suitable for camping on Tiptop Mountain (water is about a half mile west of the summit); the gap between Tiptop Mountain and Bald Top (with water on the north slope); Brawley Mountain fire tower (no water nearby); and Garland Gap (water is 500 feet north down a side trail).

From the parking area at Wilscot Gap, cross GA 60 and enter the narrow path at the BMT trail marker **(Waypoint 1)**. You'll immediately climb through a mix of white pines and hardwoods. The grades are moderate to steep as the trail winds around a series of draws populated with poplars and oaks, and you'll catch glimpses of distant ridges.

At 1.1 miles **(Waypoint 2)** the trail crosses Tiptop Mountain (3170 feet), which is the high point of this section of the BMT. In spring you'll see plenty of May-apples covering the forest floor. As you curl around the north-facing slopes of the mountain, the scenery to the right is intriguing as low hills and pastures in the foreground are juxtaposed against high peaks on the horizon.

The BMT gradually descends the western slope of Tiptop Mountain, and at 1.9 miles **(Waypoint 3)**, a side trail leads to a large, grassy clearing that serves as grazing land for wildlife. The trail drops quickly to the gap between Tiptop Mountain and Bald Top and then curls around the northwest slope of Bald Top.

You reach Ledford Gap at 2.3 miles **(Waypoint 4)**. Turn right onto Forest Service Road 64, walk west for about 120 feet, and turn right at a trail marker with double white blazes. The climb toward Brawley Mountain begins as a moderate ascent through dense forest, as the trail winds around a knob and a ridge spur. The path becomes steeper and then mellows a bit, finally intersecting a road near the fire tower atop Brawley Mountain at 3030 feet **(Waypoint 5)**. Views here are limited, and it's not possible to climb the fire towers, but you could camp in the wide, flat clearing here. To continue, turn right onto the road, walk about 200 feet, and turn right onto the narrow path that goes southwest.

The trail moves through a saddle, crosses a ridgecrest, and begins moving down the ridge over steep ground. At 3.9 miles, the grade markedly mellows as the

View along the Benton MacKaye Trail

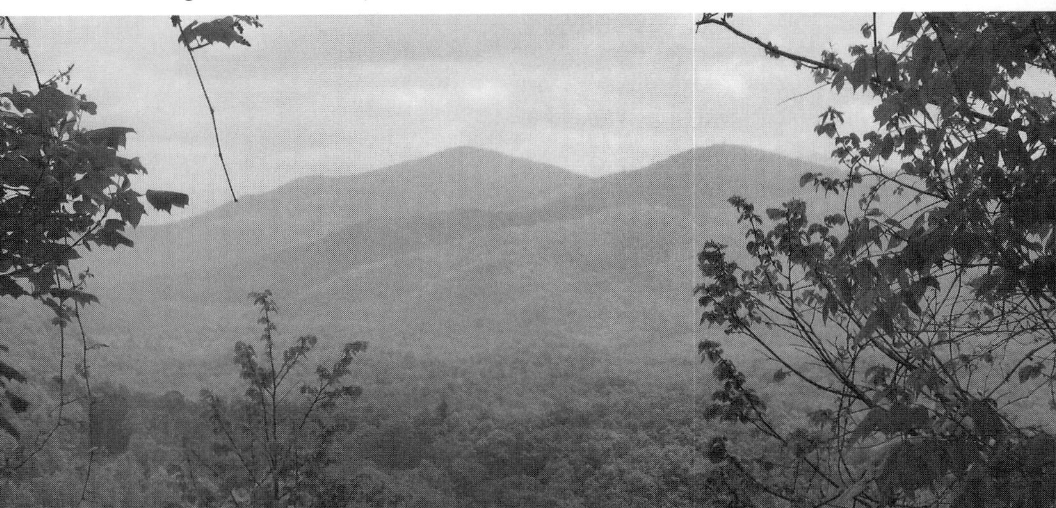

North Central Georgia

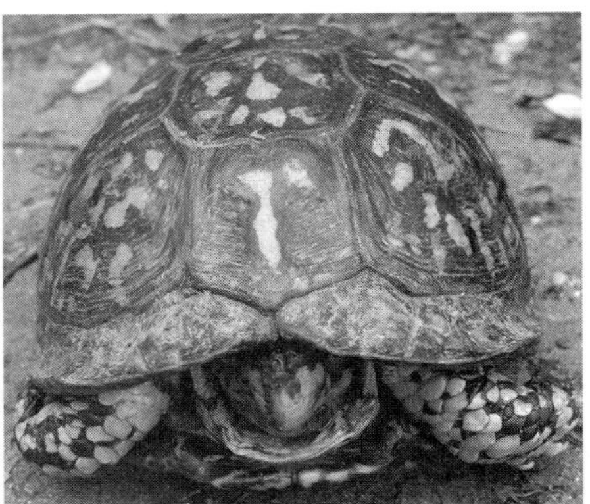
Eastern box turtle

trail swings to the northwest across the easy mountain slope and then takes a horseshoe turn to the south.

At 4.2 miles you enter Garland Gap **(Waypoint 6)** where a campsite sits next to the trail. A narrow path just beyond the campsite leads to water about 500 feet away. From the gap the trail ascends moderately on the northern slope of Garland Mountain where large poplars and oaks dominate the forest. As you approach the top of Garland Mountain, the trail becomes more difficult, but it eases again before reaching the trail's high point on the mountain at 4.7 miles. The descent from the mountain is at times steep and traverses sunny south-facing slopes. As the path takes a right turn to the west, you can peek through the treetops to see a prominent bald peak across the river basin.

A gradual descent takes you into a mix of hickory, oak, white pine, and Virginia pine, and the trail follows an old logging road. At 5.8 miles the trail intersects with the junction of Dial Road and Shallowford Bridge Road **(Waypoint 7)**. Continue straight, walking west across the intersection for 100 feet, and then turn right onto the trail on the right side of Shallowford Bridge Road.

From the gap at Dial Road, the trail rises gradually, alternating between the ridgecrest and southern slopes. It then levels out and crosses a ridge east of Free Knob. At 6.6 miles bear left at a Y junction **(Waypoint 8)** and follow the trail marked with white blazes. The trail slips off the ridge to traverse the southern side of Free Knob on a path covered by a thick bed of leaves. The trail widens as it drops gradually into a lively forest of mountain laurel, poplars, a variety of oaks and flame azalea. The trail becomes narrows, passes through corridors of mountain laurel, and intersects a trail at 7 miles **(Waypoint 9)**. Turn left and descend to the southeast.

The trail intersects with Shallowford Bridge Road at 7.1 miles **(Waypoint 10)**. Turn right and follow the road, which skirts the Toccoa River and passes through a neighborhood of riverside cabins. Walk 0.5 mile and turn left to cross the Shallowford Bridge and reach the parking area on Aska Road **(Waypoint 11)**. The central fixture here is the Toccoa Wilderness Outpost, which serves as a grocery store and grill. While tourist traffic can be heavy in warm months, activity fades in winter and early spring, and it's a welcome end to a challenging hike. Reward yourself with a tasty burger at the Outpost, or simply relax on the riverbank and watch people fly-fishing and wading in the shoals.

UTM WAYPOINTS

1. 16S 757242E 3855384N
2. 16S 756347E 3855534N
3. 16S 755982E 3855288N
4. 16S 755586E 3854963N
5. 16S 754862E 3854662N
6. 16S 754068E 3853892N
7. 16S 752222E 3853803N
8. 16S 751291E 3853626N
9. 16S 751086E 3853127N
10. 16S 751266E 3853108N
11. 16S 750779E 3852462N

TRIP 14 Cooper Creek Yellow Mountain Trail

Distance	6.4 miles, out-and-back
Hiking Time	3 hours
Difficulty	Moderate
Elevation Gain/Loss	+/-1320 feet
Trail Use	None
Best Times	Spring, fall, and winter
Agency	U.S. Forest Service, Blue Ridge District
Recommended Map	USGS 7.5-min. *Mulky Gap*

HIGHLIGHTS Part of the Cooper Creek Scenic Area, the Yellow Mountain Trail follows an old logging road through exceptional forest of old-growth trees, and its high point—just shy of 3000 feet—allow views into the wild heart of the Chattahoochee National Forest. Dropping down through rhododendron thickets, the trail crosses Bryant Creek in a ravine with towering pines and hemlocks. If you can, time your hike to cross this area in late afternoon when sunset bathes the forest floor in an orange glow.

DIRECTIONS From Atlanta take GA Highway 400 north to its end at the intersection with GA Highway 60/U.S. Highway 19. Turn left onto GA 60/U.S. 19 north toward Dahlonega. From Dahlonega take GA 60 north 19 miles, passing through Suches, and turn right onto Cooper Creek Road at the signs for Cavendar Gap and Cooper Creek Recreation Area. Travel 0.8 mile and turn left onto Forest Service Road 236 at the signs for Cooper Creek Wildlife Management Area and Cooper Creek Recreation Area. Travel 2.3 miles to the parking area before the bridge.

FACILITIES/TRAILHEAD There is no fee for day use. There are no facilities at the trailhead, but the Cooper Creek Campground. The campground has 17 campsites and is open March through October.

From the parking area **(Waypoint 1)**, cross the bridge over the creek and walk northwest on the road for 0.1 mile. At **Waypoint 2**, enter the Yellow Mountain Trail on the right side of the road. Follow yellow blazes and ascend through oaks, poplars, hemlocks, and white pines on the southeast slope of Yellow Mountain.

At 1.1 miles **(Waypoint 3)** the blue-blazed Cooper Creek Trail enters on the left. (If you want to loop back to the campground at this point, follow this to

Cooper Creek Yellow Mountain Trail

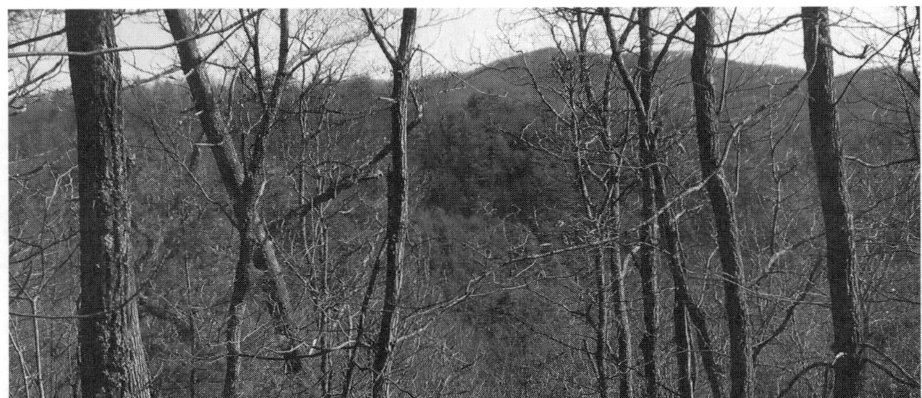

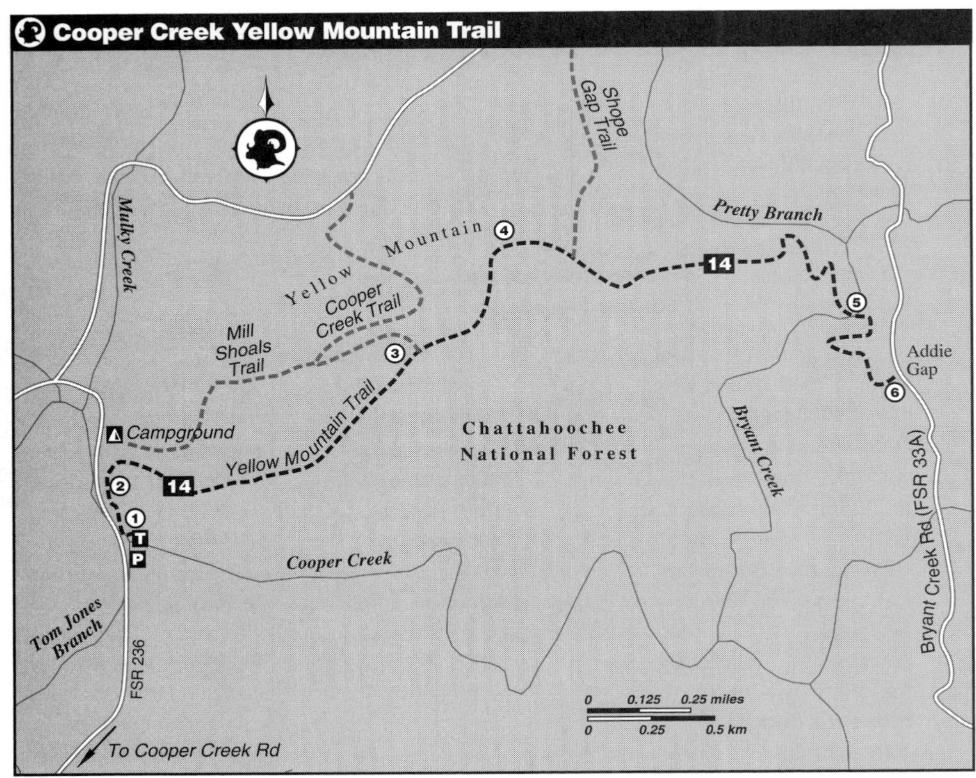

Mill Shoals Trail.) Continue straight, traveling east, to stay on the Yellow Mountain Trail. As you cross a ridge, you will have views (especially in winter) of far ridges to the south.

The trail reaches the summit of Yellow Mountain (2963 feet) at 1.4 miles (**Waypoint 4**), and in winter you can see across forested valleys and high peaks. Continue on the ridge, and at 1.6 miles the Shope Gap Trail enters on the left. (This trail goes 1.8 miles to Mulky Gap.) Continue straight, traveling southeast to cross a hilltop and then descend through tall pines and hemlocks. The trail snakes down the eastern slopes of the mountain where mountain laurel gathers at the base of pines.

The trail drops into the Bryant Creek ravine shaded by massive pines and hemlocks. This can be a glorious place in late afternoon when the fading sunlight casts an orange glow over the tree trunks and rhododendron thickets that surround the cascading stream. At 2.6 miles (**Waypoint 5**), cross Bryant Creek and climb steeply from the ravine.

At 3 miles continue straight at a four-way trail junction. The trail ends at 3.2 miles at Addie Gap, beside Bryant Creek Road, or Forest Service Road 33A (**Waypoint 6**). Retrace your steps to return to the trailhead.

UTM WAYPOINTS

1. 16S 768544E 3850224N
2. 16S 768432E 3850381N
3. 16S 769618E 3850979N
4. 16S 770003E 3851403N
5. 16S 771335E 3851076N
6. 16S 771516E 3850831N

TRIP 15 Vogel State Park: Coosa Backcountry Trail

Distance	12.9 miles, loop
Hiking Time	9 hours
Difficulty	Strenuous
Elevation Gain/Loss	+4210/-4180 feet
Trail Uses	Leashed dogs and backpacking
Best Times	Year-round
Agency	Vogel State Park
Recommended Map	A *Vogel State Park Trail Map* is available in the park office and at www.gastateparks.org/info/vogel.

HIGHLIGHTS The sign at the beginning of the Coosa Backcountry Trail warns that this 12.5-mile loop is "More than a day's hike." I've done it in a day, and consider it a pretty good challenge, but it's much easier on the body to approach this as an overnight excursion. Actually, one of the best aspects of Vogel State Park is that its Coosa Backcountry Trail is perfect for intermediate backpackers who are seeking a trail that is easy to access but still offers a challenge and access to remote backcountry. The trail begins off the side of a main park road, so it's easy to reach, but it runs deep into the backcountry to escape the park crowds and offer plenty of solitude. The loop is difficult, with great gains in elevation, whether you hike it clockwise or counterclockwise.

DIRECTIONS From Atlanta take GA Highway 400 north to the end of GA 400 at the intersection with GA Highway 60/U.S. Highway 19. Turn left onto GA 60/U.S. 19 north toward Dahlonega. Continue 5 miles and turn right at the traffic light to continue on U.S. 19 north (avoiding the highway business route). Continue on U.S. 19 north to U.S. 19/129. Turn left onto U.S. 19/129, travel north 10.5 miles, and turn left onto Vogel State Park Road.

FACILITIES/TRAILHEAD There is a restroom at the park office in the parking area. Pack in plenty of water. There are water sources along the trail, but be sure to treat it. The park charges a $3 parking fee; you can purchase an Annual ParkPass for $30 by calling (770) 389-7401. Before hiking the Coosa Backcountry Trail, you must obtain a permit, and let rangers know whether you plan to camp in the backcountry. Portions of the Coosa Trail lie outside of the state park boundary, so you do not have to camp in designated spots.

From the parking area, go to the right side of the park office and walk west on the park road 1050 feet. Turn right at the sign marked TRAIL ENTRANCE **(Waypoint 1)**. Go up the stone steps, walk to the left side of the vending machine shack, and follow green blazes through a hemlock forest.

At 0.2 mile bear right at the Y intersection and follow orange and yellow blazes as you ascend rocky steps. At 0.4 mile turn right at a four-way trail junction to go west on the approach trail for the Bear Hair Gap and Coosa Backcountry trails. At the next Y junction **(Waypoint 2)**, bear right onto the Coosa Backcountry Trail, which begins as a flat path in poplars and hemlocks.

Mushrooms on the Coosa Backcountry Trail

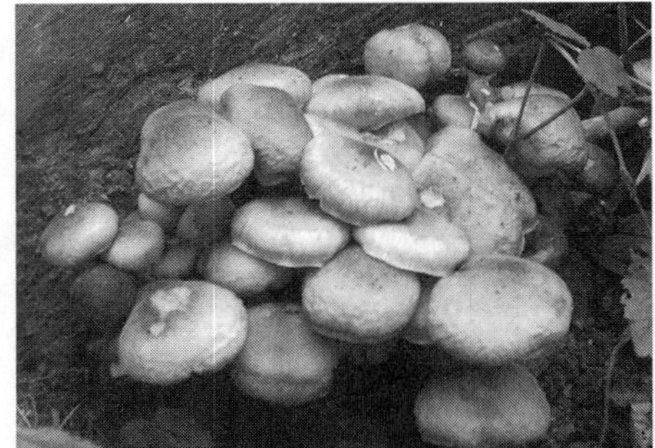

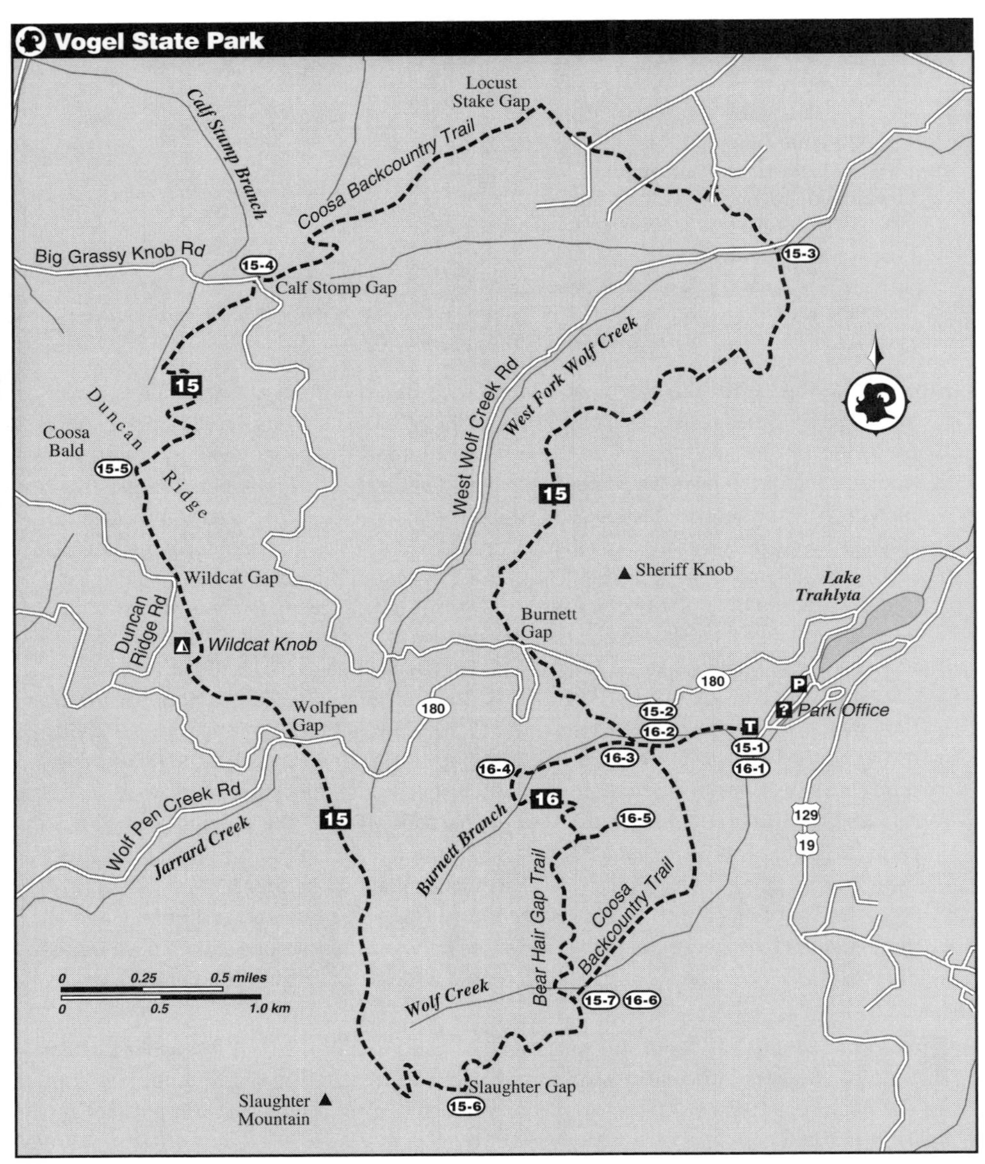

Just past the 1-mile mark the trail crosses GA Highway 180, and then drops gradually over the next 3 miles, following the sides of hills. As you continue down, off your left shoulder you have consistent winter views of the hills to the north. At 3.3 miles a wood footbridge crosses the West Fork of Wolf Creek, and there is a large clearing to the right **(Waypoint 3)**. Cross a gravel road, enter the narrow path marked with yellow blazes, and begin a steep climb through mountain laurel and pines. At 3.6 miles the trail passes a rocky stream while the forest transitions to hemlocks. After dropping into Locust Stake Gap, the steady march upward continues to a ridgetop where the land falls away steeply on each side of the path.

A series of switchbacks and a lengthy stand of mountain laurel lead to Calf Stomp Gap. At 5.9 miles **(Waypoint 4)** to the right is a stand of hemlocks that shade a clearing with room for several tents. Turn left (southwest), and cross the rough road to continue. Galax, moss, and grasses line the narrow, rocky, and rooted trail, which makes a long climb up a draw. The path levels briefly before a final climb to Coosa Bald, one of the highest points on the hike. At 7.1 miles **(Waypoint 5)** turn left at the T intersection to follow the yellow-blazed Coosa Backcountry Trail, which shares a treadway with the Duncan Ridge Trail. A steep descent down a grassy path lined with ferns takes you to Wildcat Gap.

At the gravel road turn left and walk south for 70 feet, enter the trail on the left, and climb to a clearing atop Wildcat Knob where a small patch of ground has a fire ring and room for one tent. The path turns rough and roller coasters to a rock outcrop just beyond the 8-mile mark, where you have winter views to the south. A steep descent down Duncan Ridge brings you to Wolfpen Gap where you cross GA 180 to continue.

The next half mile approaching Slaughter Mountain is the steepest section of the trail. Atop the mountain the trail mercifully levels off and at 9.8 miles begins to move down Slaughter's eastern slope. Poplars, oaks, and hemlocks tower above the fern-covered ground as you drop to Slaughter Gap. At 10.5 miles **(Waypoint 6)**, the Duncan Ridge Trail goes to the right. The Duncan Ridge and Slaughter Creek trails intersect on the right. Continue straight on the Coosa Backcountry Trail, moving downward to the east, as rhododendron and mountain laurel become more prevalent.

At 11.5 miles **(Waypoint 7)** the Bear Hair Gap Trail intersects on the left. Turn right to descend north on the path marked with yellow and orange blazes and cross a stream. The next section is especially attractive as you pass through groves of large hemlocks. The trail stays on a fairly even contour as it runs beside the Wolf Creek Basin and returns you to the four-way trail junction you passed at the beginning of the hike. Continue straight (northeast) following the trail for the PARK TRAILHEAD ENTRANCE.

UTM WAYPOINTS

1. 17S 232141E 3850746N
2. 17S 231535E 3850678N
3. 17S 232358E 3853222N
4. 17S 229727E 3853270N
5. 17S 229064E 3852356N
6. 17S 230561E 3848962N
7. 17S 231086E 3849443N

Hang a right for the Coosa Backcountry Trail

BEAR HAIR GAP TRAIL
3.5 MILES
COOSA BACKCOUNTRY TRAIL
12.5 MILES STRENUOUS
THAN A DAYS HIKE

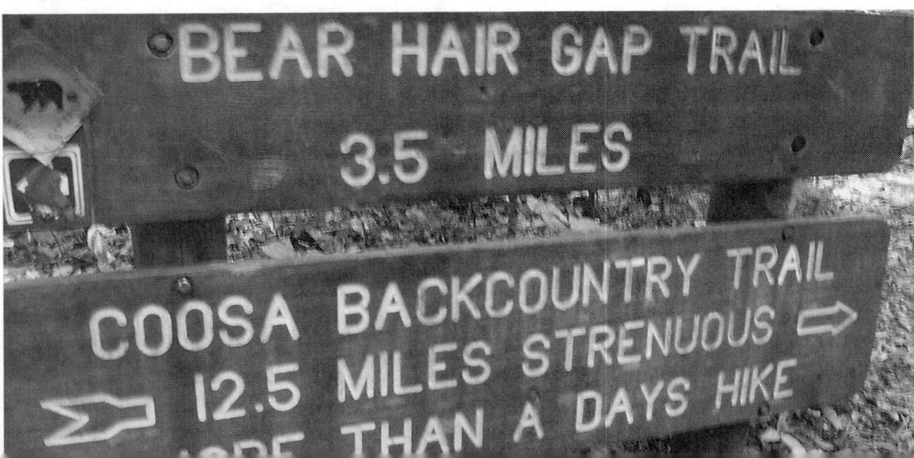

TRIP 16 Vogel State Park: Bear Hair Gap Trail

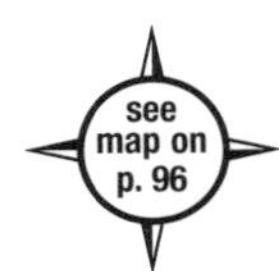

Distance	4.1 miles, semiloop
Hiking Time	2 hours
Difficulty	Moderate
Elevation Gain/Loss	+1335/-1360 feet
Trail Use	Leashed dogs
Best Times	Year-round
Agency	Vogel State Park
Recommended Map	A *Vogel State Park Trail Map* is available in the park office and online at www.gastateparks.org/info/vogel.

HIGHLIGHTS The Bear Hair Gap Trail is the perfect length for a day trip; plus, it's only moderately difficult, so it should suit most hikers visiting the park. The trail alternates between rocky paths and old roadbeds as it climbs a creek ravine adorned with poplars, hemlocks, and mountain laurel. A winding climb brings you to the top of a hill, the most notable spot on the trail, where a wide opening in the trees perfectly frames Lake Trahlyta to the northeast. The lake is named for the Cherokee princess Trahlyta, who is reportedly buried north of Dahlonega in a grave marked by a pile of stones at the junction of GA Highway 60 and U.S. Highway 19. After visiting the overlook, you drop gradually to the junction with the Coosa Backcountry Trail and take that path back to the park trailhead.

DIRECTIONS From Atlanta take GA Highway 400 north to the end of GA 400 at the intersection with GA Highway 60/U.S. Highway 19. Turn left onto GA 60/U.S. 19 north toward Dahlonega. Continue 5 miles and turn right at the traffic light to continue on U.S. 19 north (avoiding the highway business route). Continue on U.S. 19 north to U.S. 19/129. Turn left onto U.S. 19/129, travel north 10.5 miles, and turn left onto Vogel State Park Road.

FACILITIES/TRAILHEAD There is a restroom at the park office in the parking area. The park charges a $3 parking fee; you can purchase an Annual ParkPass for $30 by calling (770) 389-7401. The park has 103 tent, trailer, and RV sites ($25), as well as 18 walk-in campsites ($12).

From the parking area, go to the right side of the park office and walk west on the park road 1050 feet. Turn right at the sign marked TRAIL ENTRANCE (**Waypoint 1**). Go up the stone steps, walk to the left side of the vending machine shack, and follow green blazes through a hemlock forest.

Mountain laurel in bloom

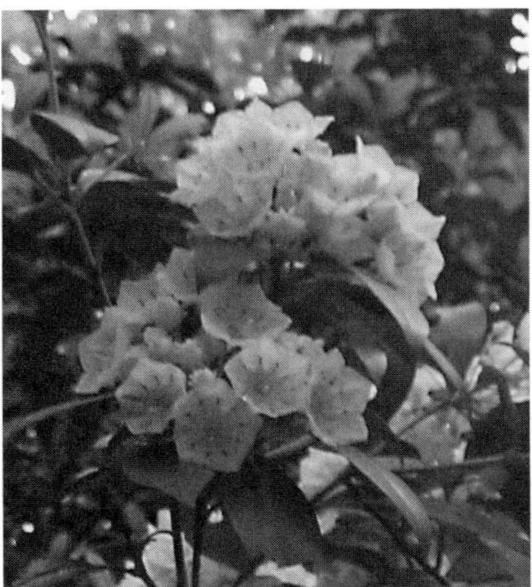

At 0.1 mile bear right at the Y junction and travel northwest following orange and yellow blazes. At the next Y junction (0.2 mile) bear right and travel southwest, again following orange and yellow blazes.

At 0.4 mile you reach a four-way trail junction (**Waypoint 2**). Turn right and travel northwest to take the approach trail for the Bear Hair Gap and Coosa

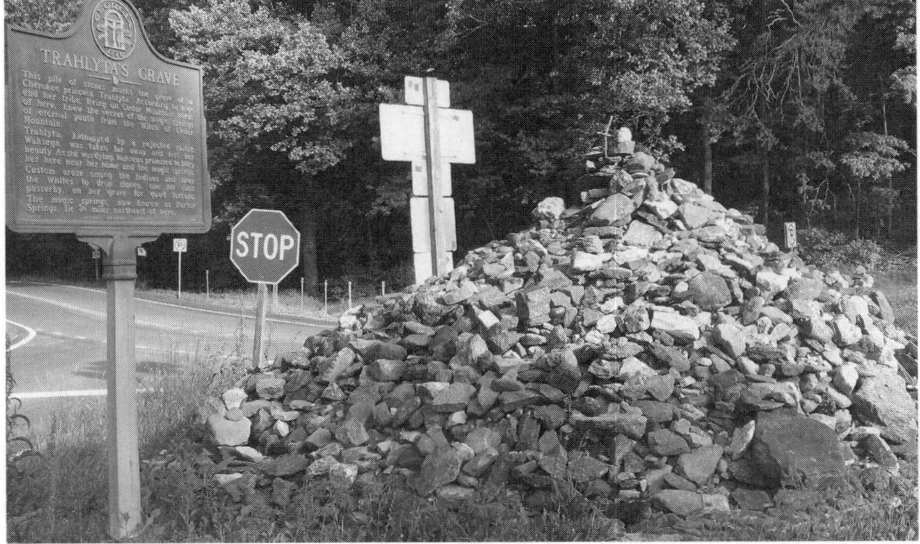

Supposed resting place of Princess Trahlyta at the junction of GA Highway 60 and U.S. Highway 19

Backcountry trails (marked with orange and yellow blazes).

Walk a little more than 200 feet and bear left at the Y intersection **(Waypoint 3)** to take the Bear Hair Gap Trail, ascending to the west (following orange blazes). The rocky trail rises alongside Burnett Branch creek and crosses the stream at 0.9 mile.

Just beyond the 1-mile point the trail ends at an unimproved road **(Waypoint 4)**. Turn sharply left onto the road to travel south and begin a steady climb on a wide, flat dirt path. As you round a bend at 1.4 miles, look left—to the north you can see Sheriff Knob rising on the far side of the creek ravine.

Steep switchbacks lead to a trail junction at 1.6 miles. Turn left and take the trail to Vogel Overlook. At 1.7 miles **(Waypoint 5)** a clearing in the trees provides a lofty view of Lake Trahlyta. According to a historical marker at the junction of GA Highway 60 and U.S. Highway 19, Princess Trahlyta and her tribe lived on Cedar Mountain (north of the grave site) where they discovered springs that offered eternal youth. When the princess rejected a suitor, the man kidnapped her and took her away from the mountain, causing Trahlyta to lose her beauty and begin to die. As she was dying she made a last wish—to be buried near the mountain and its magic springs.

After you circle the hilltop, walk back down to the junction of the main trail and descend to the southwest. The path crosses Wolf Creek at 2.6 miles, and you wind around a moss-covered boulder to enter a lush area of rhododendron and stands of hemlock. Along steep switchbacks the trail becomes rocky and rooted and passes through high boulders in the creek ravine.

At 2.7 miles **(Waypoint 6)** Bear Hair Gap joins the Coosa Backcountry Trail. Turn left and travel northeast following orange and yellow blazes toward Vogel State Park. A great forest of high hemlocks and hardwoods surrounds the path, which rolls easily and takes you back to the four-way intersection at **Waypoint 2**. Go straight (northeast) to return to the trailhead in the park.

UTM WAYPOINTS

1. 17S 231251E 3850753N
2. 17S 231599E 3850695N
3. 17S 231529E 3850714N
4. 17S 230895E 3850629N
5. 17S 231382E 3850316N
6. 17S 231125E 3849425N

TRIP 17 Desoto Falls Recreation Area: Lower & Upper Falls

Distance	2 miles, out-and-back
Hiking Time	1 hour
Difficulty	Easy
Elevation Gain/Loss	+/-180 feet
Trail Uses	Leashed dogs and good for kids
Best Times	Spring, summer, and fall
Agency	U.S. Forest Service, Blue Ridge District
Recommended Map	USGS 7.5-min. *Neels Gap*

HIGHLIGHTS In 1540, the Spanish explorer Hernando de Soto and his army of about 600 men left the area now known as the Florida panhandle and headed northeast through what is now Georgia in search of gold. Supposedly, in the 1880s a plate of Spanish armor was discovered near one of the waterfalls in what is now the Desoto Falls Recreation Area. The validity of the find has been lost to the ages, and the area is now mostly known for two waterfalls accessible by easy to moderate trails. From the parking area, a gradual 0.4-mile ascent to the southwest leads you to Lower Falls, some 35 feet high. The 0.7-mile hike from the trailhead to Middle Falls, a 200-foot-high cascade, is a bit more difficult, but you'll encounter only a few steep hills. (Note that the trail to Upper Falls is closed due to erosion.) The diverse forest, modest trail grades, and waterfalls make this a popular destination for dayhikers.

DIRECTIONS From Atlanta take GA Highway 400 north to the end of GA 400 at the intersection with GA Highway 60/U.S. Highway 19. Turn left onto GA 60/U.S. 19 north toward Dahlonega. Continue 5 miles and turn right onto U.S. 19/GA 60/GA 9. Travel 4.1 miles to the junction where GA 60 and U.S. 19 split at Stonepile Gap. Turn right to take U.S. 19 north. Travel 5.4 miles and turn left onto U.S. 19/129. Travel north on U.S. 19/129 4.1 miles. The entrance to the Desoto Falls Recreation Area is on the left.

FACILITIES/TRAILHEAD There is a restroom at the trailhead (open late April through late November) and a fee for day-use parking. You can hike the trails and camp in Desoto Falls Recreation Area campground year-round. There are 24 campsites, and each has a tent pad, grill, and picnic table.

At the north corner of the parking area, enter the trail between the restroom and kiosk **(Waypoint 1)**. Pass through a picnic area and turn left onto a paved path. Walk to a kiosk with a sign for Upper Falls and Lower Falls. Turn left, cross a wood footbridge, and walk to a T junction **(Waypoint 2)** where a sign relays how Desoto Falls got its name. The path to the left leads to Lower Falls, while the path to the right heads to Middle Falls. From **Waypoint 2**, turn left and travel west on the level path that skirts Frogtown Creek, a lively stream that flows through a nice mix of pines, oaks, poplars, and hickory trees. The trail soon climbs through hemlocks and oaks, and then switchbacks carry you higher into mountain laurel and a jumble of rocks covered in lichen. On the upper slopes above the creek basin, mountain laurel joins the mix of pines and hardwoods.

At 0.4 mile you reach the observation platform that stands before Lower

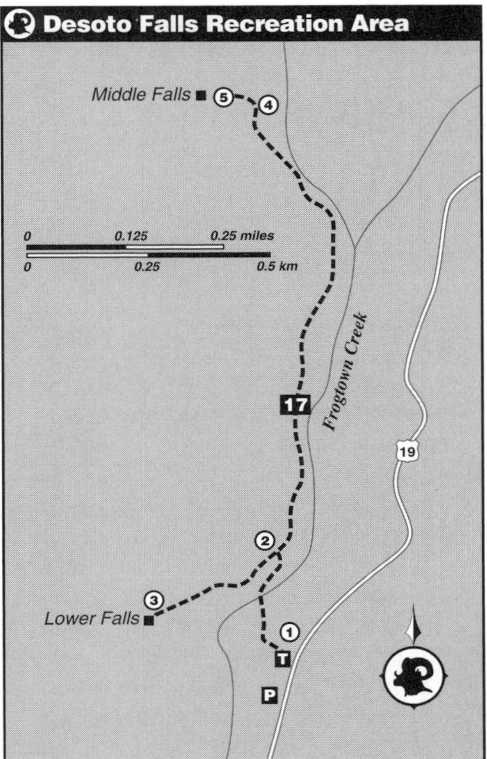

Falls, which is part of a Frogtown Creek tributary **(Waypoint 3)**. Laurel and other greenery form a wreath around the rock face where water pours down the sheer wall to crash on a lower shelf.

From Lower Falls, retrace your steps to **Waypoint 2**, and continue straight, traveling northeast along Frogtown Creek to reach Middle Falls. Weathered logs covered in thick moss lie along the wide trail bordered by deep green leaves of rhododendron. You take a footbridge over a tributary of the creek and walk among widely spaced hardwoods and hemlocks.

At the 1-mile mark of the hike you climb briefly with the creek visible on the right. The trail then steps upward, alternately climbing and leveling off. At 1.3 miles cross a wood footbridge and look left to see Middle Falls on the upper slope. Not far ahead there is a trail junction **(Waypoint 4)**. The trail that continues straight is closed. Turn left and walk 170 feet to the observation platform for Middle Falls **(Waypoint 5)**. From a high ledge, a narrow column of water drops to a wide ledge, widens, spills over a series of rocky platforms, and washes into a pool.

From the falls, retrace your steps to return to **Waypoint 2**, and turn left to reach the parking area.

UTM WAYPOINTS

1. 17S 233001E 3844370N
2. 17S 233024E 3844565N
3. 17S 232770E 3844438N
4. 17S 233043E 3845516N
5. 17S 233003E 3845532N

Middle Falls, Desoto Falls

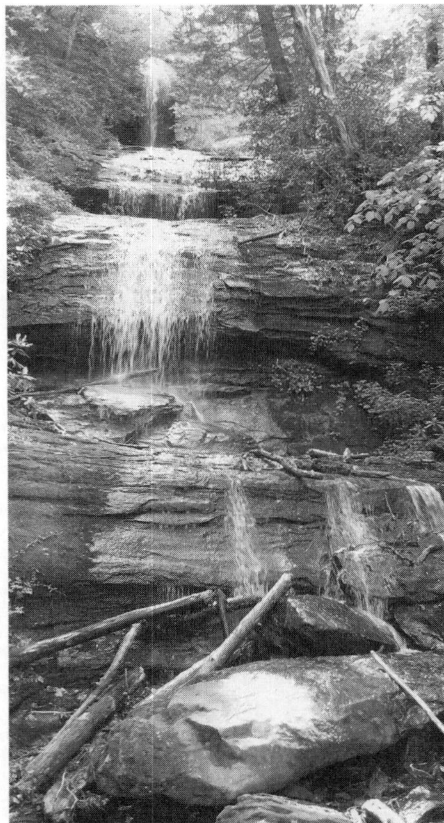

Chapter 3

Northeast Georgia

A journey of 1000 miles begins with a single step, and a journey of 3000 miles begins in northeast Georgia. Each spring, hikers venture to the state's northern mountains to begin their trek to Maine on the Appalachian Trail (AT). While the AT is certainly the crown jewel in the state's trail system, paths in this region also circle the deepest cut in the East, Tallulah Gorge, and carry hikers to the state's high point, Brasstown Bald. Northeast Georgia holds many other treasures as well, such as Smithgall Woods where you can explore the site of an old gold mine and hike along a stream that may have been the birthplace of the Georgia gold rush. From its deep coves with waterfalls and swimming holes, to its lush forests of massive hemlocks, this mountainous corner is truly a hiker's paradise.

Appalachian Trail

In 1921, Benton MacKaye envisioned a trail system that would run "over the full length of the Appalachian skyline" in the eastern U.S. In "An Appalachian Trail: A Project in Regional Planning" published in the *Journal of the American Institute of Architects*, MacKaye said that modern society had robbed people of their leisure time and that a long natural corridor would serve as a place for people to relax and rejuvenate themselves. His vision led to the formation of the Appalachian Trail Conference, which worked with volunteers to complete the AT in 1937. The AT now stretches 2175 miles from Georgia to Maine, and each year 3 million to 4 million people hike some section of it and several hundred "2000-milers" hike its entire length.

About 80 miles of the AT lies within Georgia, a section that is exceptionally beautiful and very popular. Dayhikers benefit from this section's several access points with parking, which allow them to place cars at both ends of a section and do a one-way day trip or to arrange for

AT marker at Unicoi Gap (Trip 5)

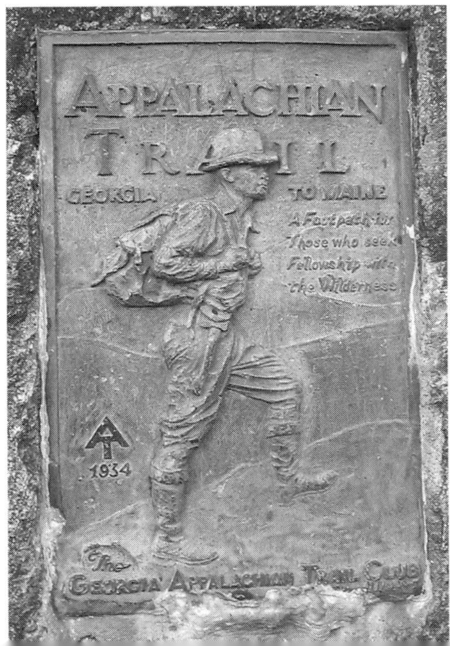

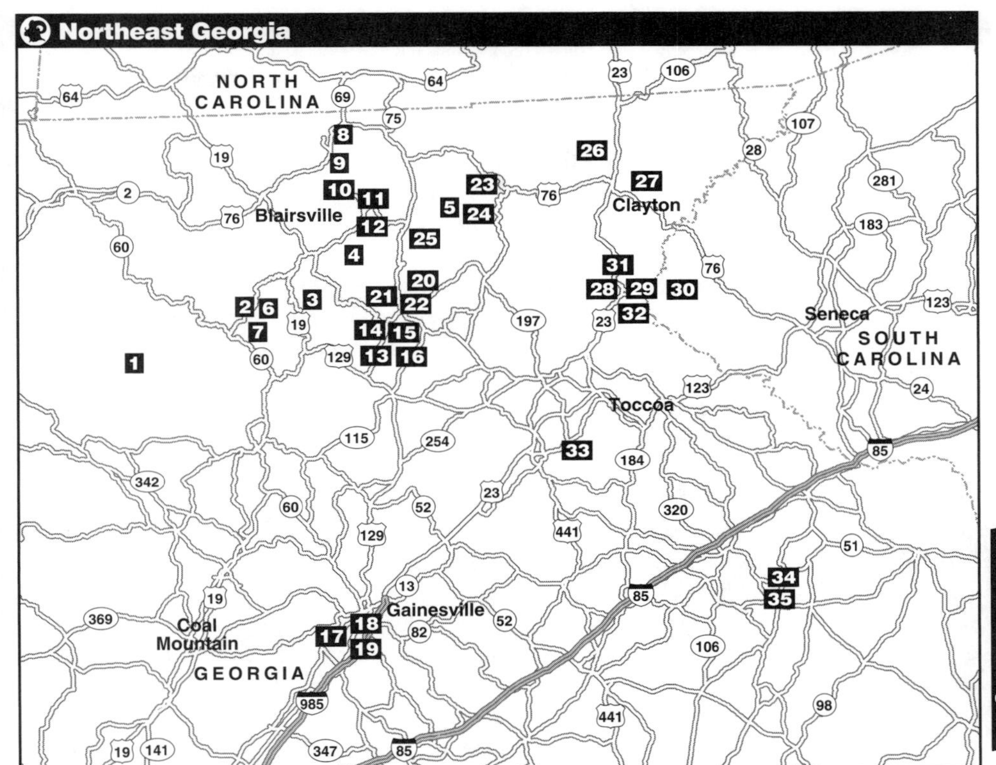

a shuttle. This portion of the AT is also popular with backpackers who link sections for multiday treks.

This book includes selected sections that accommodate full-day, one-way hikes as well as longer trips. Most of these hikes are moderate, with a few strenuous ascents and descents, but keep in mind that the AT in Georgia can be physically demanding, especially if you carry a full backpack. If you are relatively inexperienced, start by doing an out-and-back walk that covers just 2 or 3 miles of a section before attempting an ambitious 10-mile day. You don't have to go very far. The beauty of the Georgia portion of the AT is that, within 30 minutes of leaving the car, you can find yourself in a quiet, remote stretch of woods that will free your mind of your everyday concerns, just as MacKaye intended.

Smithgall Woods Conservation Area

In the 1800s, Dukes Creek and surrounding north Georgia streams attracted miners who panned the waters for gold. As easily accessible deposits grew scarce, people turned to hard-rock mining, digging tunnels to tap gold veins in the hills. By the 1840s, most mining activity had ceased, but there was a resurgence when hydraulic mining was introduced to Georgia in the 1850s. Unfortunately, this practice had devastated much of the landscape by the 1880s. The scene today is dramatically different. In 1994, businessman George Smithgall, Jr. gave the state of Georgia 5555 acres of land now known as Smithgall Woods Conservation Area. Dukes Creek remains the centerpiece of the property, but panning for gold is no longer permitted, and the stream now serves as a major destination for trout fishing. Several trails wind through Smithgall Woods, including a wildlife interpretive trail, a path that explores the former site of a gold mine, and trails that wander the creek and wetlands. It's worth noting that this area was preserved partly to provide environmental education, and each year there are a number of events and programs for the public.

Chicopee Woods Nature Preserve & Elachee Nature Science Center

Set in the 1500-acre Chicopee Woods Nature Preserve, the Elachee Nature Science Center educates tens of thousands of young students each year and runs public programs for adults as well. The center (a nonprofit institution) houses a museum with information on ecology, astronomy, geology, and archaeology. Plus, it has live animal exhibits, including a room with reptiles and an aviary with red-tailed hawks. The center also manages more than 12 miles of trails that cross ridges of hardwoods and pines, explore creeks, and circle Chicopee Lake where you might see an osprey or green heron. There are short, medium, and long trails configured to form several loops, so you can find a hike to suit just about anybody's desires and abilities. A half-mile, paved trail for people with limited mobility winds through the forest just south of the center and stops by a nice overlook.

Unicoi State Park

In autumn a scarlet and gold forest surrounds Unicoi Lake, drawing hikers and bikers, as well as droves of people from the tourist hot spot of Helen. While the fall foliage makes Unicoi one of Georgia's most popular state parks, it has a good mix of trails suitable for families, as well as those seeking a longer trek through remote forest. A 2.5-mile loop is an easy stroll around 53-acre Unicoi Lake, while the 2-mile Bottoms Loop Trail is a slightly more moderate walk through hemlocks, rhododendron, and mountain laurel with a visit to Smith Creek. For a longer walk, take the 3-mile Unicoi to Helen Trail, which passes through hardwood forest and crosses several streams before ending at the alpine village of Helen. One of the best hikes in the area is the Smith Creek

Suspension bridge in Chicopee Woods Nature Preserve (Trip 17)

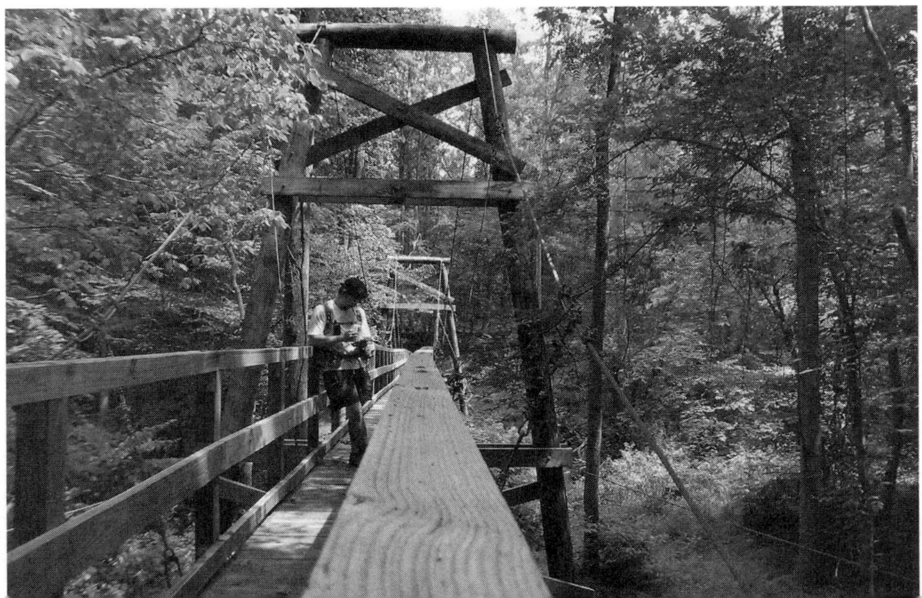

Trail, which does not follow the creek but instead climbs Hickory Nut Ridge and drops to end at Anna Ruby Falls. These dual waterfalls pour into a lush ravine where Smith Creek cascades through a cathedral of hemlocks and hardwoods.

Moccasin Creek State Park

With a wildlife trail, waterfalls, and a stream teeming with trout, Moccasin Creek State Park is a great playground for kids and adults. Located on the shore of Lake Burton in Georgia's Blue Ridge Mountains, the park lies next to the Burton Fish Hatchery, which raises rainbow and brown trout to stock many of Georgia's trout streams. The stretch of Moccasin Creek between the hatchery and Lake Burton is open to fishing for kids 11 and younger. Another kid-friendly option is the 1-mile Non-Game Interpretive Trail, a loop through forest and fields with interpretive signs that highlight local plants and animals. From the observation tower situated along the path you might spy a hawk, turkey, or deer. Nestled in the woods, a small pond holds wood duck boxes, and set high in trees are boxes for bluebirds and bats. The other main attraction is this area is the nearby Hemlock Falls Trail, an easy to moderate path that follows Moccasin Creek through a spectacular forest of hemlocks, rhododendron, and mountain laurel. About a mile in lies the main prize—Hemlock Falls, a 15-foot gush of water that pours into a wide, dark pool.

Tallulah Gorge State Park

Two miles long and almost 1000 feet deep, Tallulah Gorge is one of the most fantastic natural features in the Southeast. It has attracted visitors since the 1800s, when settlers would venture to see its steep granite walls and spectacular waterfalls, one plunging nearly 100 feet.

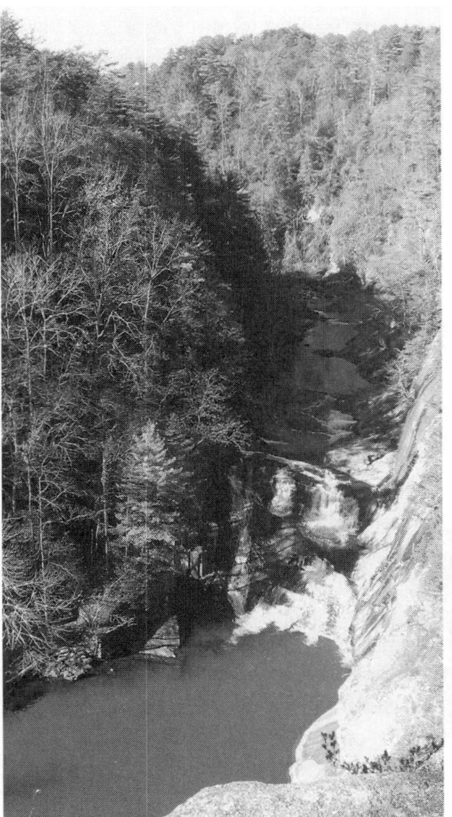

Tallulah Gorge State Park

In 1913, the Georgia Power Company built a dam at the falls and constructed a hydroelectric plant to feed the state's growing power demands. As the dam reduced water flow into the gorge, the tourist business dried up, and the place was largely deserted, save for a few hermits who lived in the canyon in the 1930s and '40s. Though it received less attention over the next several decades, Tallulah Gorge was once again in the spotlight in 1971 when portions of the movie *Deliverance* were filmed in the canyon, and John Voight's character Ed Gentry scaled the granite cliffs. The next significant point in the canyon's history was 1992 when the State of Georgia and the Georgia Power Company partnered to form Tallulah Gorge State Park. Now water from the Tallulah River is released to restore the aesthetics of the gorge, and trails along the rim provide lofty views of the canyon's five waterfalls. Also, the Hurricane Falls Trail includes 600 steps that descend into the gorge. As this book was being completed, the park had begun to offer guided hikes down into the gorge so that hikers could watch kayakers running Bridal Veil Falls.

While it doesn't run along the gorge, the Stoneplace Trail is worth exploring as it takes you to a cove on Tugaloo Lake, which feeds into the Tallulah River. This small, remote inlet surrounded by forested hills can be a wonderful place to swim or simply relax on the pier stretching out over the water. When I scouted this area on a Thanksgiving weekend, I enjoyed a sunny, 70-degree day without another soul in sight. Backcountry camping is also allowed on this trail, and you might consider that option since it's 5 miles one-way.

The park's Jane Hurt Yarn Interpretive Center is also worth a visit. This 16,000-square-foot modern facility has an impressive film about the gorge and excellent displays concerning its history and environment.

Lake Russell Recreation Area

A 100-acre lake is the centerpiece of the Lake Russell Recreation Area, and its easily accessible shoreline makes it a popular place for fishing, canoeing, and swimming. A series of easy and moderate trails hug the shore and wind through the surrounding hills. And no outboard motors are allowed on the lake, so you can walk without the disturbance of loud engines—a good thing for hikers and the healthy population of campers who take advantage of the 42 campsites that overlook the lake. The area is named for Richard Brevard Russell, governor of Georgia from 1931 to 1933 and a U.S. senator from 1933 to 1971. In the 1960s, construction of the Richard B. Russell Dam and Lake was authorized to produce power, control floods, and provide an area for wildlife management and recreation. The lake was filled in the early 1980s and has been a recreation destination ever since.

Victoria Bryant State Park

Established in 1952, Victoria Bryant State Park rests on fertile land that once provided Native Americans with bountiful hunting grounds, croplands, and fresh water from creeks and springs. When settlers arrived, they found swampy regions suitable for growing rice, thus the name for Rice Creek, which flows through the park. Now this is a modern playground with a golf course, places to swim, fishing ponds, and trails that allow hikers to observe wildlife, walk through quiet woods, or relax by a picturesque creek. Its two main hiking paths, the Perimeter Trail and Broad River Loop Trail, are ideal for an easy morning or afternoon hike.

TRIP 1 Appalachian Trail & Benton MacKaye Trail Loop

Distance	5.8 miles, loop
Hiking Time	3 hours
Difficulty	Moderate
Elevation Gain/Loss	+/-1250 feet
Trail Uses	Leashed dogs and backpacking
Best Times	Year-round
Agency	U.S. Forest Service, Blue Ridge District
Recommended Map	Appalachian Trail Conference *Appalachian Trail* map

HIGHLIGHTS This pleasant dayhike gives you a taste of two of the Southeast's long-distance paths, the Appalachian Trail (AT) and the Benton MacKaye Trail (BMT). The hike begins just north of Springer Mountain, which marks the beginning of the AT. Starting on the AT, you begin in hardwoods and pines, and soon the AT and BMT share the same treadway. After descending through thickets of rhododendron and mountain laurel, the trails split and you follow the AT to Stover Creek. The trail then passes eastern hemlock trees that are hundreds of years old. Just south of Three Forks (the confluence of Stover, Chester, and Long creeks) you turn south to take the BMT and begin a gradual climb up Rich Mountain. The BMT finally descends from the mountain, and you rejoin the AT to return to the trailhead.

DIRECTIONS From Atlanta take Interstate 75 north to Interstate 575. Travel north on I-575 to GA Highway 5/515. Go north on GA 5/515 through East Ellijay and turn right onto GA Highway 52 to go east. Take GA 52 east to Cartecay. In Cartecay turn left onto Roy Road (between the Methodist Church and Stanley's Grocery) and travel north 9.7 miles to the end of the road. Turn right and go 2.2 miles to Mt. Pleasant Baptist Church. Turn right onto gravel Forest Service Road 42, and go 6.8 miles to the parking area on the north side of the road.

FACILITIES/TRAILHEAD The trailhead has no facilities, and there is no fee for parking, hiking, or camping. Stover Creek is a reliable water source—be sure to treat any water you take from it.

At the east end of the gravel parking area, enter the white-blazed Appalachian Trail **(Waypoint 1)** and descend through a mix of hardwoods and pines and large beds of ferns. At 0.3 mile **(Waypoint 2)** bear right and travel northeast on the AT. In spring, look for pink ladyslippers growing beside the trail in this area.

Ahead, ferns cover a forest floor shaded by tall oaks and pines. Pass through heavy rhododendron to cross a branch of Davis Creek, and then climb the slopes of Rich Mountain to the junction of the AT and BMT **(Waypoint 3)**. Go straight to travel on the AT, following rectangular white blazes. The path turns to the southwest and drops through dense forest.

Rhododendrons form a hallway, and at 1.6 miles there is a trail junction **(Waypoint 4)**. You can turn left here and walk the short distance to investigate the Stover Creek Shelter, a three-sided structure typical of the shelters located along the AT. Continuing from **Waypoint 4**, take the log bridge across Stover Creek and then turn northwest to parallel the stream, descending gradually. Heavy foliage through here hides the creek from view.

At 2 miles **(Waypoint 5)** you pass by a stand of old-growth hemlocks with

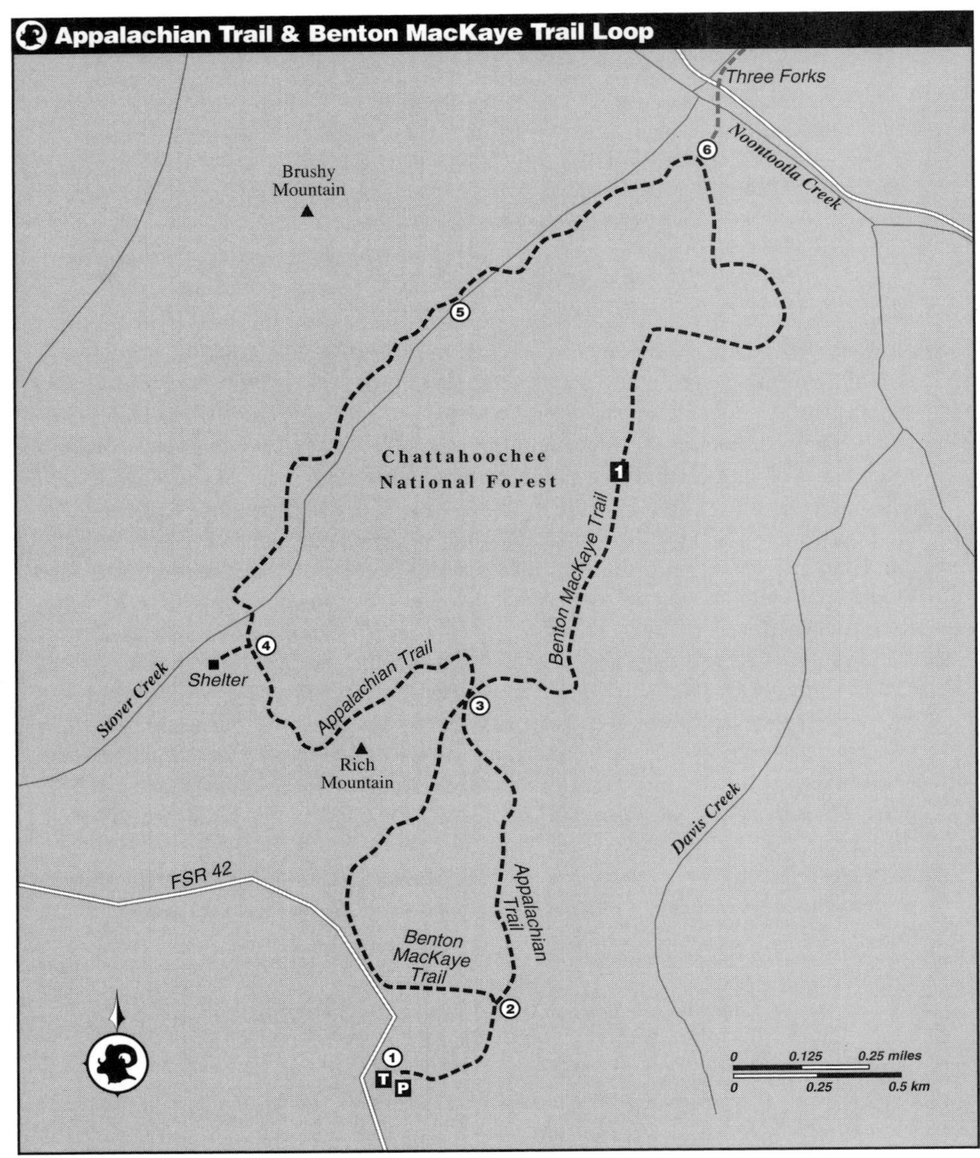

trees more than 200 years old. The AT continues to drop until it intersects with the BMT south of Three Forks (**Waypoint 6**). Travel east and climb to take the BMT, following white diamond blazes. The trail quickly turns to the south and then curls around the eastern slope of a hill. Ferns thrive in a forest of widely spaced hardwoods where the path climbs to the crest of the Rich Mountain ridge. Here, the level path moves through oaks and other hardwoods, then crosses a hill at an elevation of 3357 feet, and turns to the west.

At 4.6 miles you reach **Waypoint 3** once again. Go straight to travel southwest on the BMT, which climbs above 3400 feet in elevation before dropping from the top of Rich Mountain. The path is narrow and loses elevation gradually in classic mixed hardwood forest. When you reach **Waypoint 2** once again, turn right to travel south on the AT and return to the trailhead.

UTM WAYPOINTS

1. 16S 757118E 3836439N
2. 16S 757411E 3836659N
3. 16S 757328E 3837542N
4. 16S 756709E 3837704N
5. 16S 757300E 3838740N
6. 16S 757998E 3839158N

TRIP 2 Appalachian Trail: Woody Gap to Neels Gap

Distance	10.7 miles, point-to-point
Hiking Time	6 hours
Difficulty	Moderate
Elevation Gain/Loss	+3130/-3225 feet
Trail Uses	Leashed dogs and backpacking
Best Times	Year-round
Agency	U.S. Forest Service, Blue Ridge District; Georgia Appalachian Trail Club; and Appalachian Trail Conservancy
Recommended Maps	Appalachian Trail Conference *Appalachian Trail* map, USGS 7.5-min. *Neels Gap*

HIGHLIGHTS A long dayhike or mellow overnight trip, this trek takes you to Blood Mountain, the highest point, at 4461 feet, of the Appalachian Trail (AT) in Georgia. The don't-miss spot on this trip is the Blood Mountain Shelter, a stone building that the Civilian Conservation Corps (CCC) built in the 1930s. From the shelter you can scramble up to a large, flat rock that offers a spectacular view to the south where ridges extend as far as you can see. The hike ends at the unique Mountain Crossings @ Walasi-Yi, a center where the AT actually passes through a store's breezeway. The CCC constructed the building from 1934 to 1937, and it has served as a restaurant and inn. Now, it's a thru-hiker mecca, and many people attempting to complete the AT stop at Mountain Crossings to fine-tune their pack load, purchase gear, and just chill out and mingle with fellow hikers.

DIRECTIONS There are parking areas at Woody Gap and Neels Gap. To reach Woody Gap from Atlanta, take GA Highway 400 north to its end at the intersection with GA Highway 60/ U.S. Highway 19. Turn left onto GA 60/U.S. 19 north toward Dahlonega. From Dahlonega take U.S. 19/GA 60 north to Stonepile Gap where the two roads split. Take GA 60 north 5.5 miles to Woody Gap, and look for the Woody Gap sign on the right side of the road.

To reach Neels Gap from Atlanta, take GA 400 north to its end at the intersection with GA 60/U.S. 19. Turn left onto GA 60/U.S. 19 north toward Dahlonega. Go 5 miles, and at the traffic light turn right to continue on U.S. 19 north (avoiding the highway business route). Continue on U.S. 19 north to U.S. 19/129. Take U.S. 19/129 north 7.7 miles to the Walasi-Yi Center at Neels Gap. The hiker parking lot is a bit farther down U.S. 19/129 on the left.

You can park cars at either end of the hike, or arrange for shuttle service. There is no formal shuttle service, but you can arrange transportation with individuals. For a listing of people who run shuttles, check out the Georgia Appalachian Trail club website: www.georgia-atclub.org/directions.html.

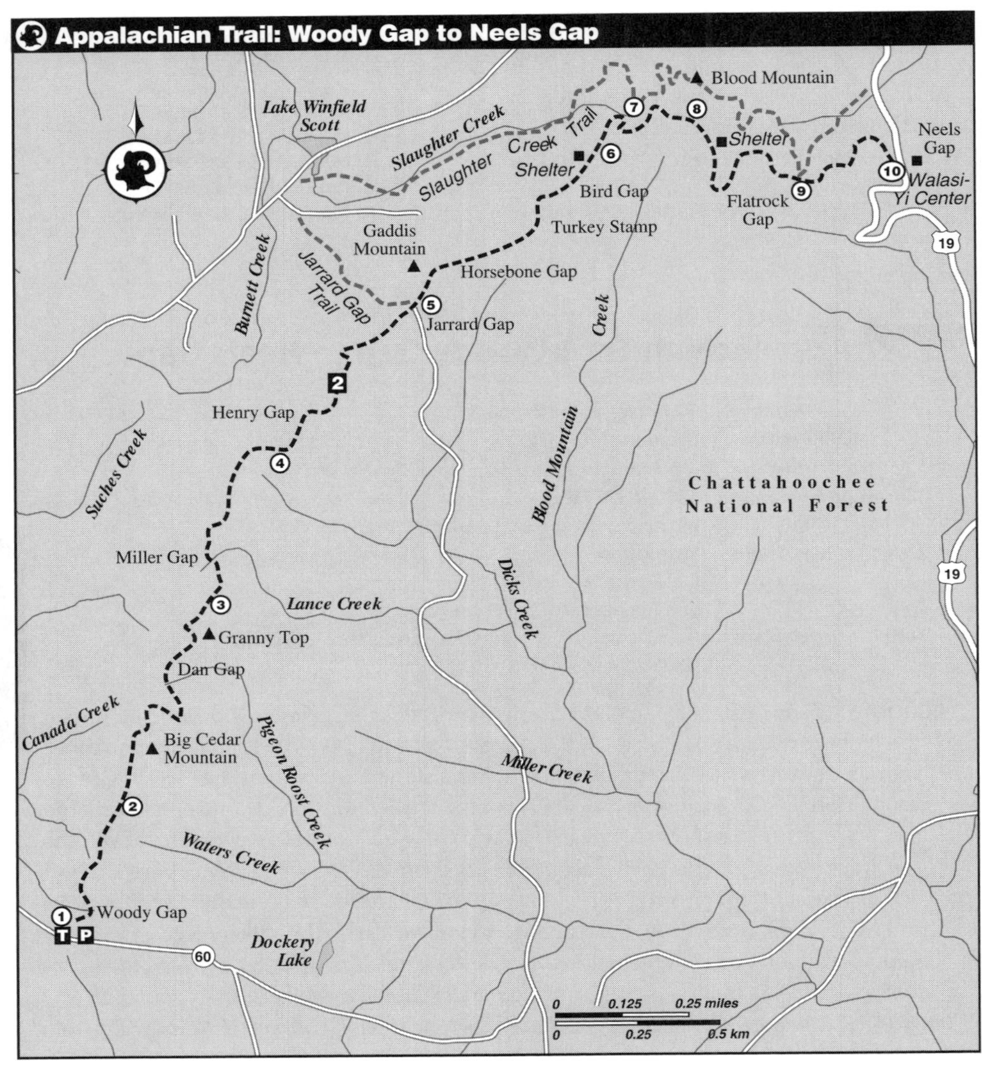

FACILITIES/TRAILHEAD There is a restroom at the Woody Gap Trailhead, as well as one at the Walasi-Yi Center at Neels Gap. There is a $2 parking fee at Woody Gap. While there are some water sources along the trail, they are not always reliable—contact the Georgia Appalachian Trail Club (www.georgia-atclub.org) to get updates on the latest conditions. Side trails leading to water sources are marked with blue blazes.

From the north side of the Woody Gap parking area **(Waypoint 1)**, enter the Appalachian Trail (AT) and travel north, climbing gradually through hardwoods and high mountain laurel. As you continue toward Big Cedar Mountain, you enjoy a good view of distant ridges, and 1 mile in **(Waypoint 2)** a rock outcrop on Big Cedar Mountain looks over layer upon layer of mountains stretching from

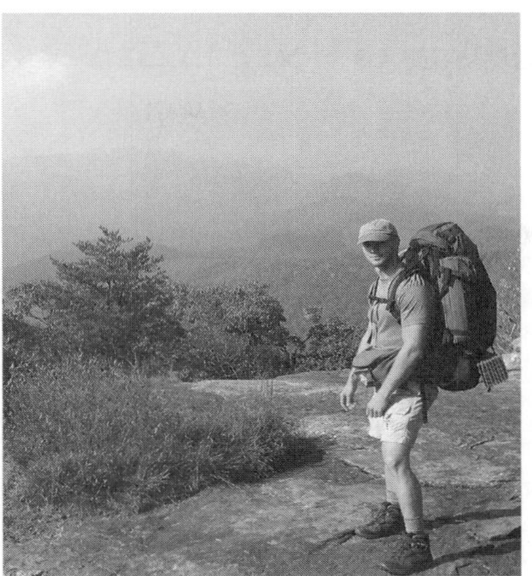

On the AT near Blood Mountain Shelter

southeast to northeast. At mile 1.5 there is a spring on the west side of the trail.

The AT descends gradually, first to Dan Gap, and then to Miller Gap at 2.6 miles **(Waypoint 3)**. As you enter Miller Gap, the blue-blazed Dockery Lake Trail intersects on the right. Continue traveling northeast along the ridge and make a steep climb to Henry Gap. After passing through Henry Gap a break in the foliage at 3.7 miles affords views to the southwest **(Waypoint 4)**. From here, the trail generally climbs as it makes a series of brief ascents and drops.

At 5.2 miles, intermittent springs lie to the east side of the path. At 5.3 miles the AT enters Jarrard Gap **(Waypoint 5)**. To the left is the Jarrard Gap Trail, which proceeds 0.3 mile to a stream and 1 mile to Lake Winfield Scott. Continue straight on the AT to cross a road and take switchbacks to the top of Gaddis Mountain. A relatively brief descent brings you to Horsebone Gap, and then a mellow climb takes you to Bird Gap at 6.8 miles **(Waypoint 6)**. The Woods Hole Shelter sits to the left, and just ahead, the Freeman Trail enters on the right. Continue on the AT, with Slaughter Mountain looming on the left. At 7.1 miles you cross Slaughter Creek, and from this point to Neels Gap campfires are not permitted.

At 7.4 miles **(Waypoint 7)**, pass through Slaughter Gap (3800 feet). The blue-blazed Slaughter Creek Trail intersects to the left and leads to Lake Winfield Scott State Park. As you move through the gap, you'll encounter a large campsite and the intersection of the Duncan Ridge Trail, which connects with the Coosa Backcountry Trail. From the gap, begin the easy to moderate climb up Blood Mountain walking among thick stands of rhododendron and oaks.

At 8.3 miles, you reach the Blood Mountain Shelter **(Waypoint 8)**, where there is no water source. Scramble up the prominent rock formation to the right of the shelter to reach a flat outcrop to gaze over a massive tract of valleys and ridges to the south. Beyond the shelter, the AT crosses exposed rock with hallways of laurel and clear views of mountains to the south.

The path becomes a series of switchbacks that drop to Flatrock Gap at 9.6 miles **(Waypoint 9)**. Here, the Freeman Trail intersects on the right and the Byron Herbert Reece Trail intersects to the left. Continue a gradual descent through thick mountain laurel and large oaks, and finish with an easy walk to Neels Gap and Mountain Crossings @ Walasi-Yi at 10.7 miles **(Waypoint 10)**.

UTM WAYPOINTS

1. 17S 225185E 3841429N
2. 17S 225707E 3842435N
3. 17S 226580E 3844217N
4. 17S 227303E 3845534N
5. 17S 228484E 3846707N
6. 17S 230056E 3847851N
7. 17S 230470E 3848250N
8. 17S 231064E 3848146N
9. 17S 231883E 3847616N
10. 17S 232841E 3847519N

TRIP 3 Appalachian Trail: Neels Gap to Hog Pen Gap

Distance 6.4 miles, point-to-point
Hiking Time 3 hours
Difficulty Moderate to strenuous
Elevation Gain/Loss +2160/-1820 feet
Trail Use Leashed dogs and backpacking
Best Times Year-round
Agency U.S. Forest Service, Blue Ridge District; Georgia Appalachian Trail Club; and Appalachian Trail Conservancy
Recommended Map Appalachian Trail Conference *Appalachian Trail* map, USGS 7.5-min. *Neels Gap*

HIGHLIGHTS This hike serves as a good introduction to the Appalachian Trail (AT), as it passes through the rich Raven Cliff Wilderness and includes mostly moderate hiking. There is one especially challenging ascent from Tesnatee Gap up Wildcat Mountain, so you should be in good physical condition to do this section of the AT. Also, the hike begins at the Mountain Crossings gear store where thru-hikers resupply and get trail information.

The trail reaches altitudes just shy of 4000 feet as it climbs Levelland Mountain and then roller coasters across a series of knobs. Where the trail reaches Wolf Laurel Top there are good views, and then more scenic stops on Cowrock Mountain. Near the end of the hike, the trail intersects with a 1.2-mile side trail that leads to Whitley Gap Shelter. This adds a bit of steep hiking on the climb back up, but there are views of Brasstown Bald, the state's high point, and Cowrock Mountain.

DIRECTIONS There are parking areas at Neels Gap and Hog Pen Gap. To reach Neels Gap from Atlanta, take GA Highway 400 north to the end of GA 400 at the intersection with GA Highway 60/U.S. Highway 19. Turn left onto GA 60/U.S.19 north toward Dahlonega. Go 5 miles, and at the traffic light turn right to continue on U.S. 19 north (avoiding the highway business route). Continue on U.S. 19 north to U.S. 19/129. Take U.S. 19/129 north 7.7 miles to reach the Walasi-Yi Center at Neels Gap. Hikers should not park at the Walasi-Yi Center. Continue 0.5 mile on U.S. 19/129 to the Byron Herbert Reece parking area.

To reach Hog Pen Gap from Neels Gap take U.S. 19/129 north 5.4 miles and turn right onto GA Highway 180, traveling east. Take GA 180 0.9 mile and turn right onto GA Highway 348 (Richard B. Russell Scenic Highway), traveling south. Travel 7 miles on GA 348 to Hog Pen Gap.

You can park cars at either end of the hike or arrange for shuttle service with an individual. For a list of people who run shuttles, check the Georgia Appalachian Trail club website: www.georgia-atclub.org/directions.html.

FACILITIES/TRAILHEAD There are restroom facilities at the Walasi-Yi Center. Snacks, drinks, and water are available at Mountain Crossings. While there are some water sources along the trail, they are not always reliable—contact the Georgia Appalachian Trail Club (www.georgia-atclub.org) to get updates on the latest conditions. Side trails leading to water sources are marked with blue blazes.

Follow the white-blazed Appalachian Trail through the breezeway at the Walasi-Yi Center **(Waypoint 1)** and climb moderately through oaks and mountain laurel. At 1.1 miles you reach Bull Gap, and a trail to the left leads 200 yards to

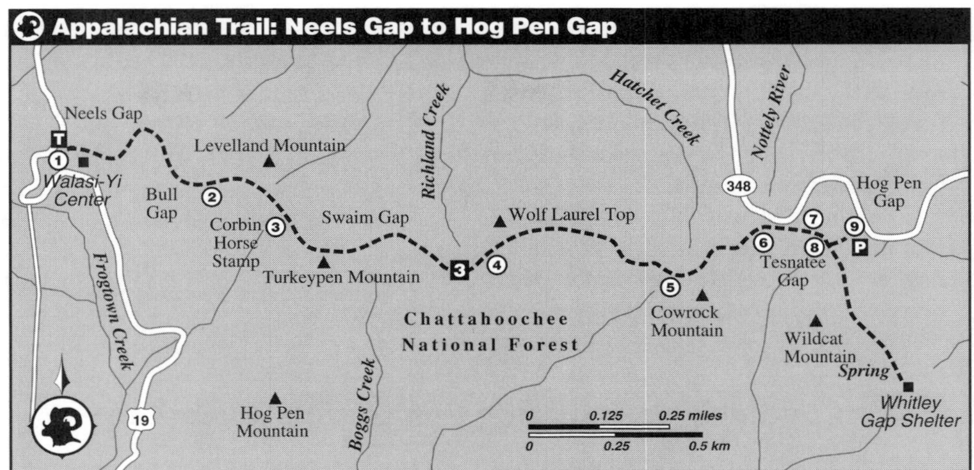

a spring. At 1.5 miles **(Waypoint 2)**, the AT crosses Levelland Mountain in a dense hardwood forest. You soon have good views of Hog Pen Mountain (3421 feet) to the south.

Switchbacks take you down to Swaim Gap **(Waypoint 3)** at 2.1 miles. From the gap, cross a knob and continue along a ridgecrest, walking south of Rock Spring Top and crossing Corbin Horse Stamp. At 2.8 miles, a spring lies to the west of the path. A short climb carries you to Reach Wolf Laurel Top (3766 feet) at 3.4 miles **(Waypoint 4)**. To the right, a trail leads to a cleared area with nice views of three ridges to the southeast. Pass through tall, straight oaks, and you see another clearing used as campsite. Descend gradually and take a level walk to Baggs Creek Gap at 4.2 miles. In the gap, a trail on the left leads to a spring.

The trail remains easy to moderate as you reach the top of Cowrock Mountain at 4.9 miles **(Waypoint 5)**. Then, begin a steep descent over a rocky section of trail to Tesnatee Gap at 5.5 miles **(Waypoint 6)**. At Tesnatee Gap, walk to the northeast side of the parking area, where the AT continues near the right side of GA Highway 348. Begin a very steep climb up Wildcat Mountain, gaining more than 500 feet of elevation in less than a half mile.

At 6.0 miles **(Waypoint 7)** the trail nears the top of Wildcat Mountain, and a rock outcrop offers views to the south of the Town Creek Cove and the Logan Turnpike. Another 0.2 mile ahead **(Waypoint 8)**, a trail on the right descends steeply 1.2

Appalachian Trail between Neels and Hog Pen gaps

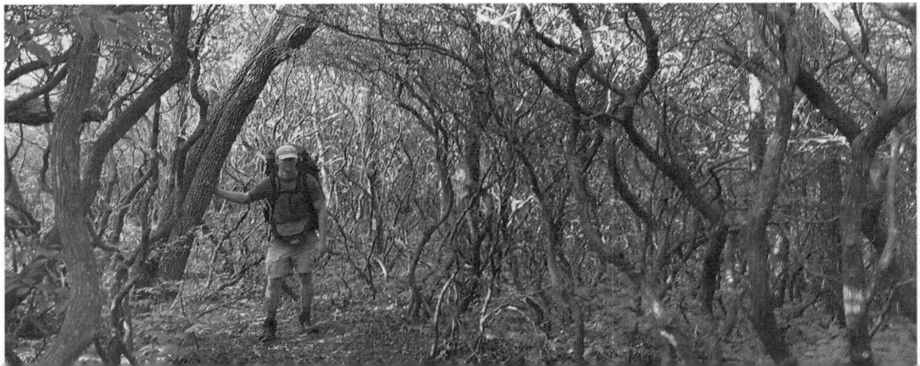

miles to the Whitley Gap Shelter where there is a nearby stream. If you don't wish to go to the shelter, continue northeast on the AT and enjoy a leisurely walk down a series of switchbacks toward Hog Pen Gap. Just before you reach GA 348, a side trail on the right with blue blazes leads to water. At GA 348, bear left to cross the road and reach the parking area for Hog Pen Gap at 6.4 miles **(Waypoint 9)**.

UTM WAYPOINTS

1. 17S 232841E 3847519N
2. 17S 234129E 3847086N
3. 17S 234858E 3846652N
4. 17S 236761E 3846331N
5. 17S 238421E 3845885N
6. 17S 239247E 3846345N
7. 17S 239664E 3846282N
8. 17S 239850E 3846187N
9. 17S 240022E 3846245N

TRIP 4 Appalachian Trail: Hog Pen Gap to Unicoi Gap

Distance	13.6 miles, point-to-point
Hiking Time	7 hours
Difficulty	Moderate
Elevation Gain/Loss	+2805/-3280 feet
Trail Uses	Leashed dogs and backpacking
Best Times	Year-round
Agency	U.S. Forest Service, Blue Ridge District; Georgia Appalachian Trail Club; and Appalachian Trail Conservancy
Recommended Maps	Appalachian Trail Conference *Appalachian Trail* map, USGS 7.5-min. *Neels Gap*

HIGHLIGHTS While this is one of the longer section hikes on the Appalachian Trail (AT) in Georgia, the terrain is mostly moderate, so this serves as a fine dayhike or comfortable overnight backpacking trip. From Hog Pen Gap, the trail undulates as it crosses a series of gaps and reaches the site of the Low Gap Shelter. You then meander through hardwoods along Horsetrough Mountain, and reach a steep section between Cold Springs Gap and Chattahoochee Gap. To the right of Chattahoochee Gap is the headwaters of the Chattahoochee River, which flows 436 miles through Georgia before it forms the Apalachicola River in Florida. From Chattahoochee Gap, the AT is rough and rocky as it cut across the slopes of Spaniards Knob and climbs to the summit of Blue Mountain (4030 feet). The trail then drops, sometimes steeply, from Blue Mountain to Unicoi Gap.

DIRECTIONS There are parking areas at Hog Pen Gap and Unicoi Gap. To reach Hog Pen Gap from Atlanta, take Interstate 85 north to Interstate 985. Take I-985 to Exit 24 for GA Highway 369. Turn left onto GA 369 west, go 0.6 mile, and turn right onto U.S. Highway 129 north. Go 23 miles (passing through Cleveland) and turn right onto GA Highway 75 Alt. Travel 5.9 miles on GA 75 Alt and turn left onto GA Highway 348 (Richard B. Russell Scenic Highway). Travel 10.6 miles on GA 348 to Hog Pen Gap.

To travel from Hog Pen Gap to Unicoi Gap, take GA 348 (Richard B. Russell Scenic Highway) east 10.6 miles to GA 75 Alt. Turn left and travel north on GA 75 Alt to the junction of GA Highway 17/75. Turn left onto GA 17/75 and travel north 7.7 miles to Unicoi Gap.

You can park cars at either end of the hike or arrange for a shuttle service with an individual. For a list of people who run shuttles, check the Georgia Appalachian Trail club website: www.georgia-atclub.org/directions.html.

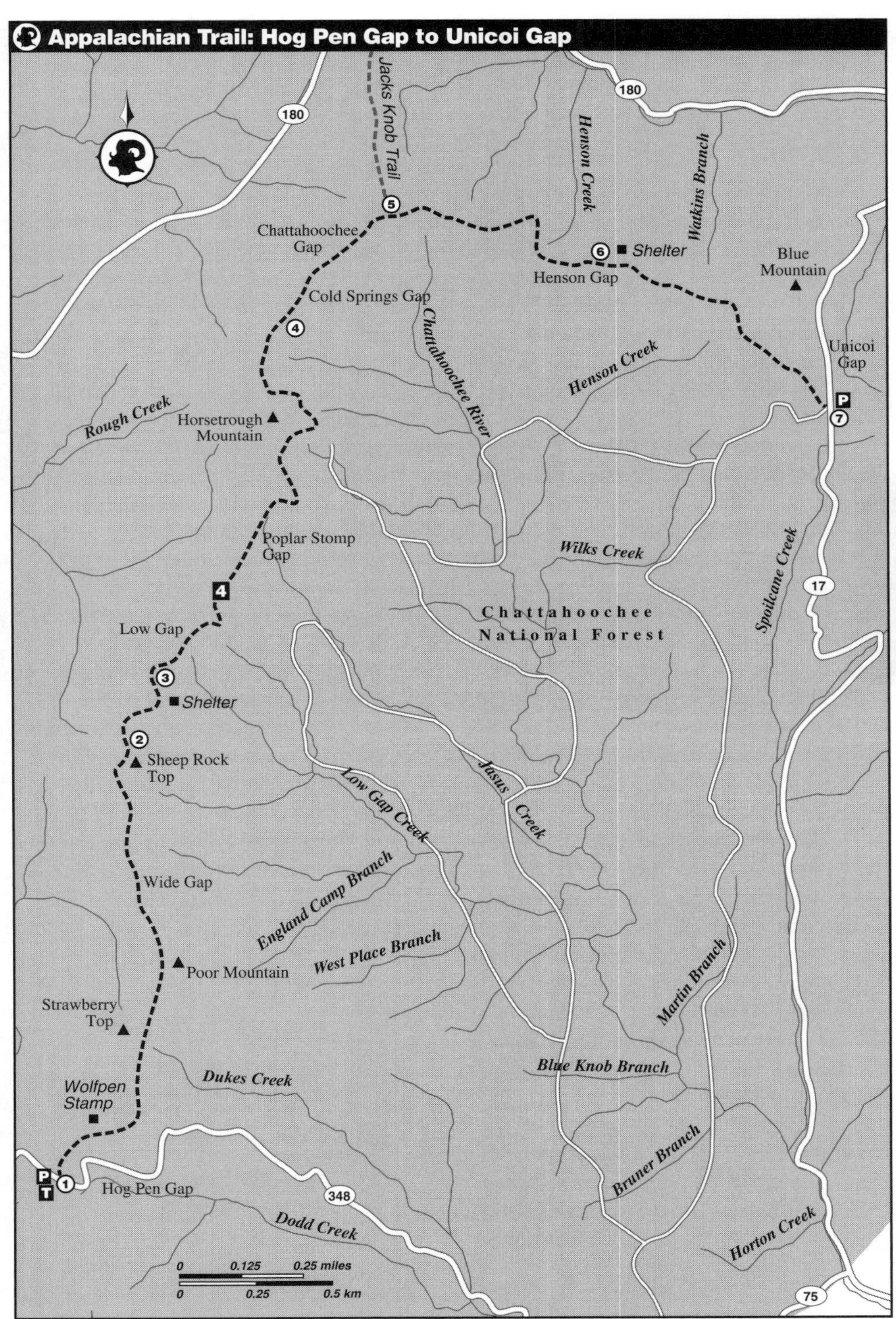
Appalachian Trail: Hog Pen Gap to Unicoi Gap
Jacks Knob Trail
180
Henson Creek
Watkins Branch
Chattahoochee Gap
Shelter
Henson Gap
Blue Mountain
Cold Springs Gap
Chattahoochee River
Unicoi Gap
Henson Creek
Rough Creek
Horsetrough Mountain
Poplar Stomp Gap
Wilks Creek
Spoilcane Creek
17
Low Gap
Chattahoochee National Forest
Shelter
Sheep Rock Top
Jasus Creek
Low Gap Creek
England Camp Branch
Wide Gap
West Place Branch
Poor Mountain
Strawberry Top
Martin Branch
Blue Knob Branch
Dukes Creek
Wolfpen Stamp
Bruner Branch
Hog Pen Gap
348
Dodd Creek
Horton Creek
0 0.125 0.25 miles
0 0.25 0.5 km
75

FACILITIES/TRAILHEAD There are no facilities at the trailhead. AT shelters are located at Low Gap and Blue Mountain. While there are some water sources along the trail, they are not always reliable—contact the Georgia Appalachian Trail Club (www.georgia-atclub.org) to get updates on the latest conditions. Side trails leading to water sources are marked with blue blazes.

From Hog Pen Gap **(Waypoint 1)**, climb gradually to the east of Wolfpen Stamp. You'll make a series of brief, gradual climbs and descents through pines and hardwoods, crossing Strawberry Top and the top of Poor Mountain (3640 feet). You then begin a long descent to Wide Gap.

At 2.5 miles **(Waypoint 2)** the AT crosses Sheep Rock Top (3572 feet), and then moves downward through mixed hardwoods to Low Gap at 4.2 miles. Passing through Low Gap **(Waypoint 3)**, a side trail on the right proceeds 0.1 mile to a cove where the Low Gap Shelter sits near a stream. As you continue on the AT from Low Gap, the walking is fairly easy as the trail follows an old roadbed. The trail rises to Poplar Stomp Gap and then allows an easy stroll across Horsetrough Mountain, with oaks, mountain laurel, and hickory trees keeping you company.

At 8.0 miles cross Cold Springs Gap **(Waypoint 4)**. After a brief climb and a quick descent, there's a strenuous uphill section that, thankfully, becomes less of a strain as you reach the top of a knob. The AT then turns downward to cross Chattahoochee Gap at 9.2 miles **(Waypoint 5)**. While this remote section of forest seems a world away from Atlanta, it actually shares one of the city's landmarks. As you walk through the gap, look for a blue-blazed trail on the right. Walk about 200 yards down this path to reach a spring that is recognized as the headwaters of the Chattahoochee River—from small things big things one day come. In the gap Jacks Knob Trail on the left leads to the summit of Brasstown Bald, Georgia's high point.

From Chattahoochee Gap, the AT drops into Red Clay Gap and becomes much rockier while traversing Spaniards Knob. At 10.8 miles, a spring is located to the west several yards off the trail. At 11 miles you reach Henson Gap and then climb again on a rough, rock-strewn path. At 11.3 miles there is a spring on the left side of the trail.

At 11.4 miles **(Waypoint 6)**, a trail on the left leads to the Blue Mountain Shelter. There are also flat areas here to pitch tents, as well as a relatively new compost toilet (remarkably free of foul odor and a welcome improvement over past privy designs). From the shelter, the trail rises and falls as it proceeds to the top of Blue Mountain (4030 feet). From the summit, a long descent, that is at times steep and rocky, leads you into Unicoi Gap at 13.6 miles **(Waypoint 7)**.

UTM WAYPOINTS

1. 17S 240022E 3846245N
2. 17S 241102E 3851057N
3. 17S 241363E 3851910N
4. 17S 242958E 3855643N
5. 17S 244177E 3856927N
6. 17S 246902E 3856202N
7. 17S 249052E 3854455N

TRIP 5 Appalachian Trail: Unicoi Gap to Dicks Creek Gap

Distance	16.1 miles, point-to-point
Hiking Time	8–10 hours
Difficulty	Moderate to strenuous
Elevation Gain/Loss	+5165/-5390 feet
Trail Uses	Leashed dogs and backpacking
Best Times	Year-round
Agency	U.S. Forest Service, Blue Ridge District; Georgia Appalachian Trail Club; and Appalachian Trail Conservancy
Recommended Maps	Appalachian Trail Conference *Appalachian Trail* map, USGS 7.5-min. *Neels Gap*

HIGHLIGHTS This section of the AT is strenuous only in spots, but it's a long haul, so it's best as a two- or three-day trip. Along the trail there are several clearings where you can camp, or you can spend the night at the Tray Mountain Shelter or Deep Gap Shelter, both of which have nearby water sources. An early climb leads to great views of Yonah Mountain, and the scenery is excellent as you proceed to Indian Grave Gap. The trail climbs to Tray Mountain, the AT's highest point in Georgia at 4430 feet, and then enters the Tray Mountain Wilderness. Here, you'll encounter brief climbs, ridge walks, and several gaps before dropping into Addis Gap, which is another good place to camp. As you approach Powell Mountain, look for a side trail that leads to an excellent overlook. From Powell Mountain the trail drops easily to Dicks Creek.

DIRECTIONS There are parking areas at Unicoi Gap and Dicks Creek Gap. From Atlanta take Interstate 85 north to Interstate 985. Take I-985 to Exit 24 for GA Highway 369. Turn left onto GA 369 west, go 0.6 mile, and turn right onto U.S. Highway 129 north. Take U.S. 129 to Cleveland. From the town square in Cleveland go 0.4 mile and turn right onto GA Highway 75. Take GA 75 to Helen, and from Helen continue on GA 75 about 9 miles to Unicoi Gap.

To reach Dicks Creek from Unicoi Gap, travel north on GA 75 8.9 miles and turn right onto U.S. Highway 76. Continue east on U.S. 76 for 7.7 miles to Dicks Creek Gap.

You can park cars at either end of the hike or arrange for a shuttle service with an individual. For a list of people who run shuttles, check the Georgia Appalachian Trail club website: www.georgia-atclub.org/directions.html.

FACILITIES/TRAILHEAD There are no facilities at the trailhead. While there are some water sources along the trail, they are not always reliable—contact the Georgia Appalachian Trail Club (www.georgia-atclub.org) to get updates on the latest conditions. Side trails leading to water sources are marked with blue blazes.

From the southwest end of the Unicoi Gap parking area **(Waypoint 1)**, ascend stone steps and climb through dense hardwood forest, following white blazes. At 0.6 mile you cross a stream, and then, at the 1-mile mark, reach a Y junction with the Rocky Mountain Trail. Bear right to continue on the AT and cross Rocky Mountain. At 1.5 miles **(Waypoint 2)**, look to the right to see Yonah Mountain rising prominently to the south. The clear views continue on your descent to Indian Grave Gap.

At 2.7 miles, enter Indian Grave Gap **(Waypoint 3)**, cross the gravel road and begin a gradual ascent. At 3.5 miles the

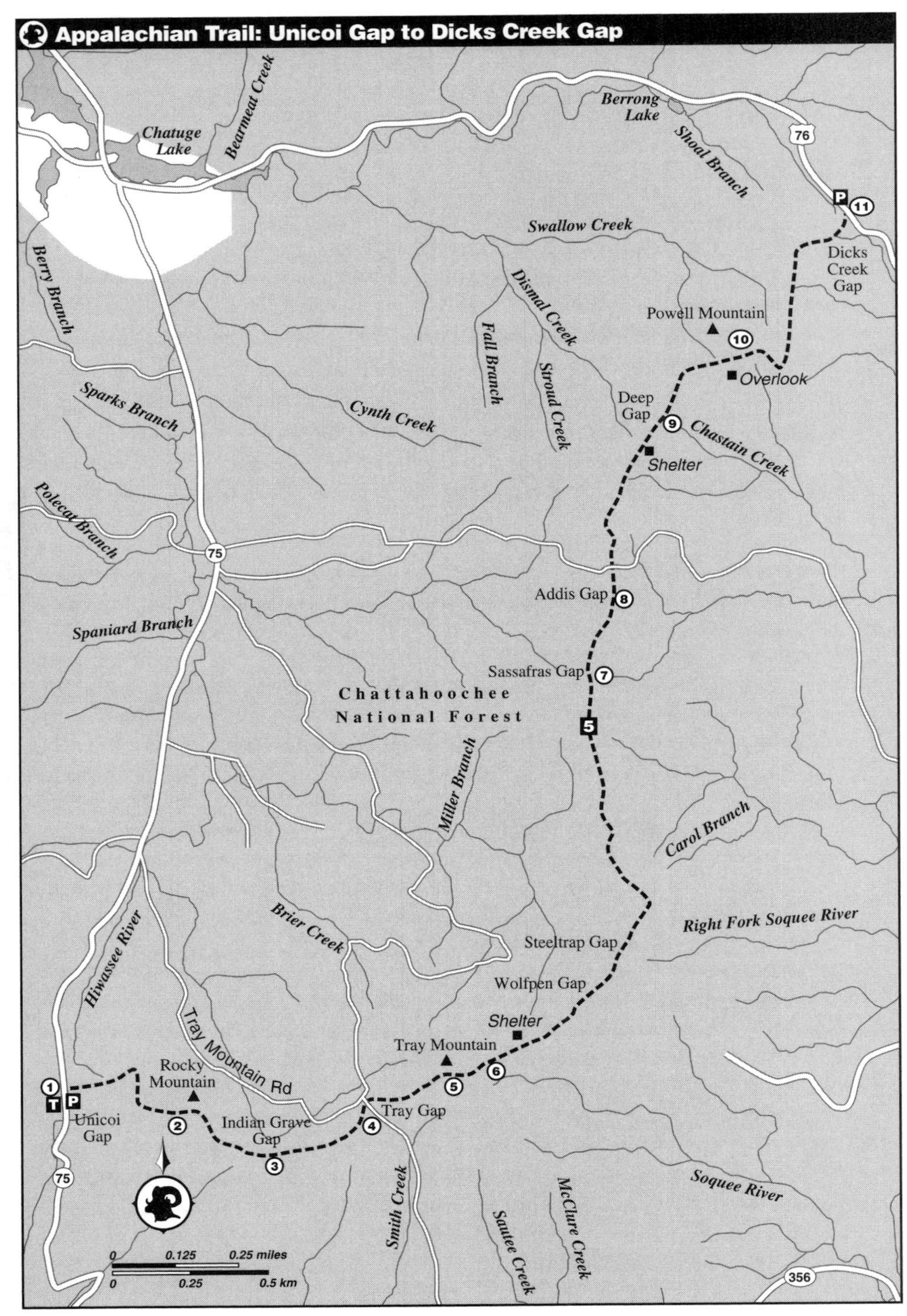
Appalachian Trail: Unicoi Gap to Dicks Creek Gap
Chatuge Lake
Bearmeat Creek
Berrong Lake
Shoal Branch
76
11
Swallow Creek
Dicks Creek Gap
Berry Branch
Dismal Creek
Fall Branch
Powell Mountain
10
Overlook
Stroud Creek
Sparks Branch
Cynth Creek
Deep Gap
9
Chastain Creek
Shelter
Polecat Branch
75
Addis Gap
8
Spaniard Branch
Sassafras Gap
7
Chattahoochee National Forest
5
Miller Branch
Carol Branch
Brier Creek
Hiwassee River
Right Fork Soquee River
Steeltrap Gap
Wolfpen Gap
Shelter
Tray Mountain
Tray Mountain Rd
6
5
Rocky Mountain
1
Unicoi Gap
2
Indian Grave Gap
3
4
Tray Gap
75
Smith Creek
Sautee Creek
McClure Creek
Soquee River
356
0 0.125 0.25 miles
0 0.25 0.5 km

AT crosses Tray Mountain Road, and a large clearing ahead marks the former site of an old goat cheese factory. Tray Mountain Road and a spring lie about 50 yards to the west. From the clearing, the AT snakes its way up onto a ridge, and then flattens in an odd grove of short and twisted oaks. At 4.4 miles you reach Tray Gap **(Waypoint 4)** where Forest Service Road 79 and Forest Service Road 698 intersect. Cross to the northeast side of the gravel area and climb rocky switchbacks to the top of Tray Mountain.

At 5.2 miles **(Waypoint 5)** you reach the exposed top of Tray Mountain, which rises to 4340 feet of elevation. From here you can look across pastureland to the north and see the observation tower at Brasstown Bald, while Yonah Mountain and a distant ridgeline rise in the southern sky. Walk another 0.3 mile, and a trail to the left **(Waypoint 6)** leads to the Tray Mountain Shelter and a spring. From this junction, make an overall descent, passing through Wolfpen Gap and Steeltrap Gap.

The AT enters Sassafrass Gap at 10.1 miles **(Waypoint 7)**, an option for camping if you are too tired to go farther. There is a small clearing, and a water source lies about 0.2 mile east of the gap. At 10.8 miles you reach Addis Gap **(Waypoint 8)** where there is a campsite clearing as well as a stream another 0.5 mile down an old road. From the gap, you begin a long push upward toward Kelly Knob. After traversing the east slope of Kelly Knob, the AT takes a downhill run to Deep Gap.

At 12.6 miles **(Waypoint 9)**, a trail to the right goes 0.3 mile to the Deep Gap Shelter, which sits next to a spring. From Deep Gap, you climb for about 0.4 mile to reach the east flank of Wolfstake Knob. The path then slumps briefly before moving up again toward Powell Mountain. At 13.5 miles **(Waypoint 10)**, a side trail leads to an overlook with a wide-open view of low ridges and a creek basin. From the overlook, return to the AT and make the final short push to the top of Powell Mountain. The trail then loses elevation gradually, leaving the mountain on its way to Dicks Creek Gap. The final descent is a delight, with long corridors of mountain laurel and ribbons of water flowing through hardwood coves. At 16.1 miles, the AT finally reaches Dicks Creek Gap **(Waypoint 11)**.

UTM WAYPOINTS

1. 17S 249052E 3854455N
2. 17S 250580E 3854010N
3. 17S 251651E 3853424N
4. 17S 253825E 3854080N
5. 17S 254460E 3854302N
6. 17S 254960E 3854450N
7. 17S 256767E 3860007N
8. 17S 257192E 3861072N
9. 17S 258008E 3863537N
10. 17S 259096E 3864311N
11. 17S 260750E 3865644N

A hazy view of Yonah Mountain from the Appalachian Trail

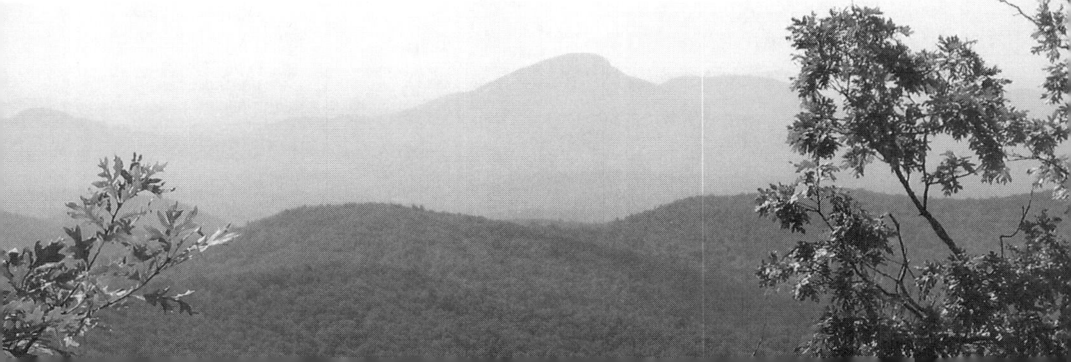

TRIP 6 Lake Winfield Scott Recreation Area: Slaughter Creek Trail, Appalachian Trail, & Jarrard Gap Loop

Distance	5.7 miles, loop
Hiking Time	2–3 hours
Difficulty	Moderate
Elevation Gain/Loss	+1355/-1390 feet
Trail Uses	Leashed dogs and backpacking
Best Times	Year-round
Agency	U.S. Forest Service, Blue Ridge District
Recommended Map	USGS 7.5-min. *Neels Gap*

HIGHLIGHTS Sitting high in the Chattahoochee National Forest, 18-acre Lake Winfield Scott is the launch point for the Slaughter Creek and Jarrard Gap trails. These two paths follow the same treadway for 0.2 mile and then split. Slaughter Creek ascends northeast through a watershed to Slaughter Gap, while Jarrard Gap runs south along Lance Branch before climbing to a gap and intersection with the Appalachian Trail (AT). For a good dayhike you can walk a loop that begins on the Slaughter Creek Trail and then takes the AT southwest to meet the Jarrard Gap Trail. The climbing is mostly moderate as you pass through stands on mountain laurel and rhododendrons as well as hardwood forests of mostly oak.

DIRECTIONS From Atlanta take GA Highway 400 north to its end at the intersection with GA Highway 60/U.S. Highway 19. Turn left onto GA 60/U.S. 19 north toward Dahlonega. From Dahlonega take GA 60 north to the GA 60/U.S. 19 split. Go left to take GA 60 northwest. In Suches turn right onto GA Highway 180 east, go almost 4.5 miles, and turn right onto Forest Service Road 37/Lake Winfield Scott Road. Continue to the southeast end of the lake to reach the hiking parking area.

FACILITIES/TRAILHEAD There are no facilities at the trailhead, but the Lake Winfield Scott Campground has restrooms. There is a $5 vehicle fee. There are 36 campsites, with the 18 sites in the northern loop remaining open all year ($6–$24, depending on camp size and season).

From the parking area **(Waypoint 1)** walk on the gravel path that goes beneath a power line and travel south. You will soon reach a sign for the Slaughter Creek and Jarrard Gap trails. Turn left and travel east into hardwoods, hemlock, and rhododendron.

At 0.2 mile **(Waypoint 2)** continue straight across a gravel road to take the Slaughter Creek Trail east, following blue blazes. Here mountain laurel with thick trunks hangs just overhead, and the trail is rooted and rocky.

White trillium

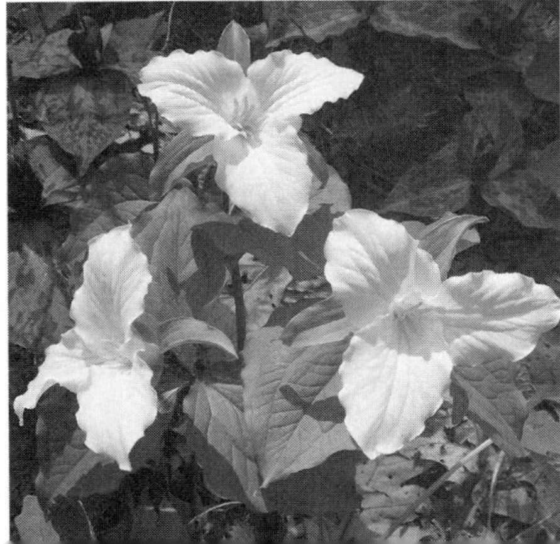

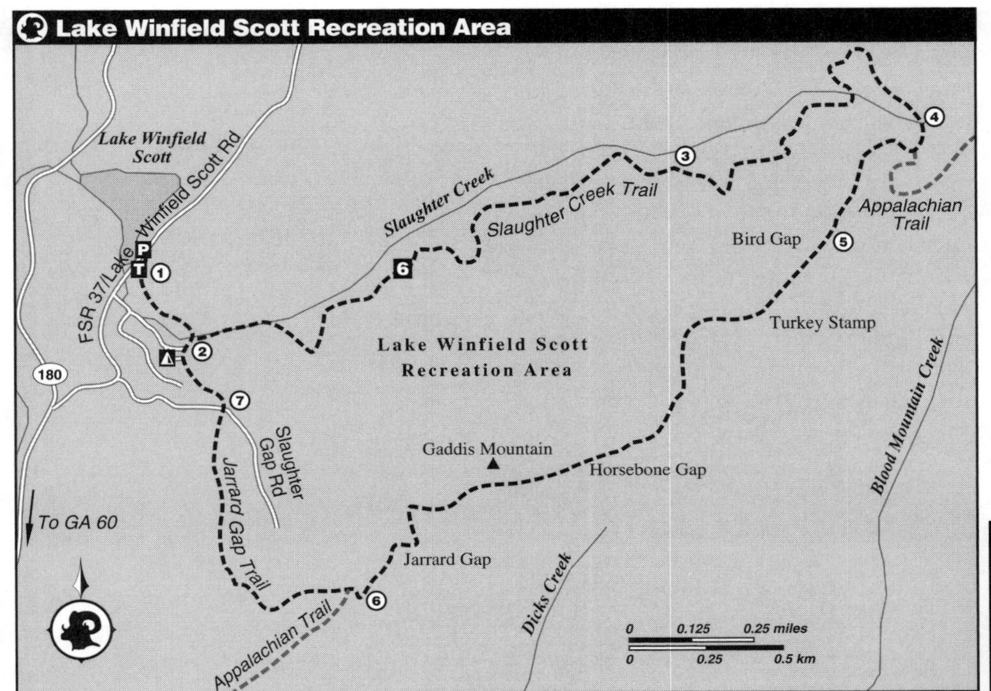

You continue climbing through thick foliage with Slaughter Creek whispering on your left. The trail generally parallels the creek, which is mostly hidden from view, and crosses small feeder streams. At about 1 mile you begin to roll easily through a drier forest of oak, poplars, mountain laurel, and pine. You then moderately ascend where stones on the narrow trail form crude steps, while Slaughter Mountain comes into view to the northeast. The path soon levels as it cuts across a slope.

A side trail enters on the left at 1.7 miles **(Waypoint 3)**. Continue straight, traveling northeast and ascend. The path crosses a tributary of Slaughter Creek at 2.3 miles, and just past the stream a flat rock makes a good bench to sit and enjoy the open forest.

A steady, gradual climb ends at the junction with the Appalachian Trail at 2.7 miles **(Waypoint 4)**. To the left, the AT rises and eventually turns to the east to climb Blood Mountain. (From **Waypoint 4**, about 500 feet down this section of the AT there are several cleared plots of ground for camping.) To continue the hike from **Waypoint 4**, do not turn left, but continue straight and travel northwest on the AT.

The AT runs through Bird Gap, and at 3.2 miles the Freeman Trail enters on the left **(Waypoint 5)**. Continue straight, traveling southwest through attractive forest dominated by tall poplars. The hiking remains easy as you pass through Horsebone Gap and then cross over Gaddis Mountain with views of distant ridges on the left.

At 4.6 miles you reach Jarrard Gap **(Waypoint 6)** and the junction of the AT and Jarrard Gap Trail. At the trail signs in the wide clearing, turn right onto the wide gravel path, traveling north. After a brief walk, turn left onto the blue-blazed Jarrard Gap Trail and descend to the west on the narrow path. You first enter dense forest, but at 4.9 miles the scenery is much better as you move down through hemlocks and cross small streams.

At 5.4 miles the Jarrard Gap Trail intersects with a gravel road **(Waypoint 7)**. Turn right onto the road and walk to the intersection with Slaughter Creek Road. Turn left onto Slaughter Creek Road and walk northwest. (Blazes on the power line poles indicate that the Jarrard Gap Trail follows the road.) Stay on the road until you reach **Waypoint 2** at 5.6 miles. Turn left and travel northwest to return to the trailhead.

UTM WAYPOINTS

1. 17S 227816E 3847954N
2. 17S 227963E 3847672N
3. 17S 229627E 3848212N
4. 17S 230449E 3848249N
5. 17S 230086E 3847878N
6. 17S 228501E 3846708N
7. 17S 228042E 3847419N

TRIP 7 Dockery Lake Trail

Distance	7.3 miles, out-and-back
Hiking Time	4 hours
Difficulty	Moderate to strenuous
Elevation Gain/Loss	+/-2400 feet
Trail Use	Leashed dogs
Best Times	Spring, summer, and fall
Agency	U.S. Forest Service, Blue Ridge District
Recommended Map	USGS 7.5-min. *Neels Gap*, Appalachian Trail Conference *Appalachian Trail* map

HIGHLIGHTS Fed by a cold, clear tributary of Waters Creek, Dockery Lake lies deep within the Chattahoochee National Forest and is known for its rainbow trout. From the water's shore, the Dockery Lake Trail climbs through rich forest, crosses remote streams, and offers lofty views of forested valleys. The trail surpasses 3000 feet of elevation to end at Miller Gap where it meets the Appalachian Trail.

DIRECTIONS From Atlanta take GA Highway 400 north to its end at the intersection with GA Highway 60/U.S. Highway 19. Turn left onto GA 60/U.S. 19 north toward Dahlonega. From Dahlonega take GA 60 north for 12 miles, and turn right onto Forest Service Road 654 at the Dockery Lake sign. Take FSR 654 about 1 mile and turn left at a fork where there is a sign for the picnicking, fishing, and hiking area.

FACILITIES/TRAILHEAD There is a restroom at the Dockery Lake Campground, which is open mid-April through October and has 11 campsites with tent pads and picnic tables.

At the northeast side of the parking lot, enter the path to the right of the bulletin board marked DOCKERY LAKE TRAIL/APPALACHIAN TRAIL 3.7 **(Waypoint 1)**. Walk through the picnic area, and turn left at the lakeshore. Travel along the west side of the lake to the dam with a bridge. Bear left and travel north on the Dockery Lake Trail.

Ascend gradually on a rocky, narrow path, and at 0.3 mile look right for a good view of distant rolling ridges. As the trail

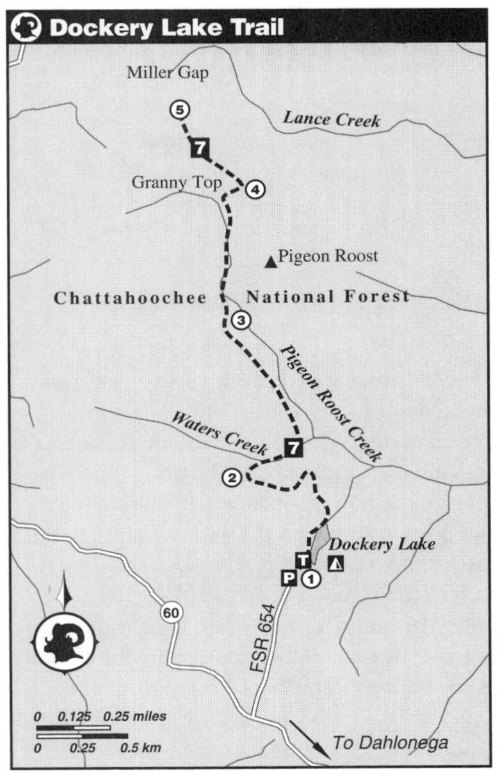

turns to the southwest, you can see high hills looming just opposite a deep valley. The walking is easy as you pass through oak trees, sourwood trees, and stands of tall mountain laurel.

At the 1-mile mark **(Waypoint 2)**, you cross a narrow stream set in a grove of rhododendron and soon bend to the east. The forest is primarily oak and hemlock trees as you descend and make several easy stream crossings. Once you reach Pigeon Roost Creek, you begin a long ascent on a wide, rocky path.

At 2.2 miles **(Waypoint 3)** pause during your ascent to look right and gaze over a sloping mountain shoulder to see a succession of hills and saddles. At 2.3 miles, the trail enters a stand of small hemlocks and nears the shaded creek where the water slides over a dark tongue of rock.

The trail rises steeply from the creek basin in a mixed hardwood forest and reaches a high point at 3.2 miles **(Waypoint 4)**. You might want to pause here for a moment and look to the northeast where the dramatic relief of the forest makes quite a display.

The trail then makes its final, gradual climb to Miller Gap and the junction with the Appalachian Trail **(Waypoint 5)**. In winter, from this spot you can look east down a long valley bordered by waves of hills and saddles. Retrace your steps to return to the trailhead.

UTM WAYPOINTS

1. 17S 227234E 3840847N
2. 17S 226883E 3841521N
3. 17S 226851E 3842748N
4. 17S 227031E 3843634N
5. 17S 226592E 3844222N

Crossing a stream on the Dockery Lake Trail

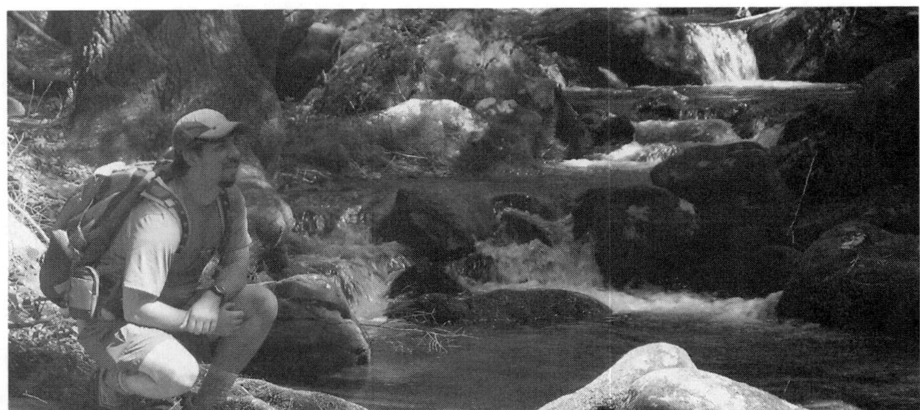

TRIP 8 Brasstown Valley Resort: Miller Trek Trail

Distance	6.1 miles, semiloop
Hiking Time	3 hours
Difficulty	Easy to moderate
Elevation Gain/Loss	+1575/-1590 feet
Trail Use	Leashed dogs
Best Times	Year-round
Agency	Brasstown Valley Resort
Recommended Map	A rough trail map is available at the Brasstown Valley Resort reception counter.

HIGHLIGHTS When the Brasstown Valley Resort was constructed in the mid-1990s, great care was taken to disturb the surrounding natural habitat as little as possible. The resort lies within the Brasstown watershed, which includes Brasstown Creek, a primary trout stream that holds 23 species of fish. The site also has cultural significance as it held prehistoric and historic archaeological sites that were preserved during construction. Preservation efforts have allowed the land to flourish, supporting hardwood forest, wetlands, and diverse animal species from migratory birds to turkeys, deer, and even black bears.

Whether or not you're staying at the resort, it's worth visiting the area's Miller Trek Trail, named after Zell Miller, a former mayor of Young Harris and former U.S. senator. The path rolls through the Chattahoochee National Forest near the resort, passing interpretive signs that call out notable animals and plants. The path is rarely steep, though it does take you above 3300 feet of elevation.

DIRECTIONS From Atlanta take GA Highway 400 north to its end at the intersection with GA Highway 60/U.S. Highway 19. Turn left onto GA 60/U.S. 19 north toward Dahlonega. Go 5 miles, and at the traffic light turn right to continue on U.S. 19 north (avoiding the highway business route). Continue on U.S. 19 north to U.S. 19/129. Take U.S. 19/129 north to Blairsville. At the intersection of U.S. 19 and U.S. Highway 76 in Blairsville, turn right onto U.S. 76 east, continue 10 miles, and turn right at the sign for the Brasstown Valley Resort. To reach the trailhead go 1.3 miles and turn left onto the road toward signed GOLF PARKING. Go 0.2 mile to the hiking parking lot on the left.

FACILITIES/TRAILHEAD The resort lobby has restroom facilities, but the trailhead does not. Plan to pack all the water you'll need for the day.

At the trailhead parking area (**Waypoint 1**), enter the chipped wood path and travel northeast to skirt the road and follow the power line break. At **Waypoint 2**, walk through the elaborate log and stone archway with a sign marked MILLER TREK and follow orange blazes. At 0.2 mile, the blue-blazed Keys Branch Loop Trail intersects on the left. Continue straight to follow the Miller Trek Trail through hardwood bottomland forest. You climb gradually to a watershed and a creek whose clear, cold water allows trout to spawn.

At 0.6 mile bear right at the Y intersection (**Waypoint 3**) and go northeast to begin the Miller Trek loop. Rising out of the bottomland, you move into a hardwood forest of oaks, poplars, red maples, and black locusts. At 1.2 miles, a connector trail intersects on the left. If you wanted to take a shorter, 2.5-mile loop

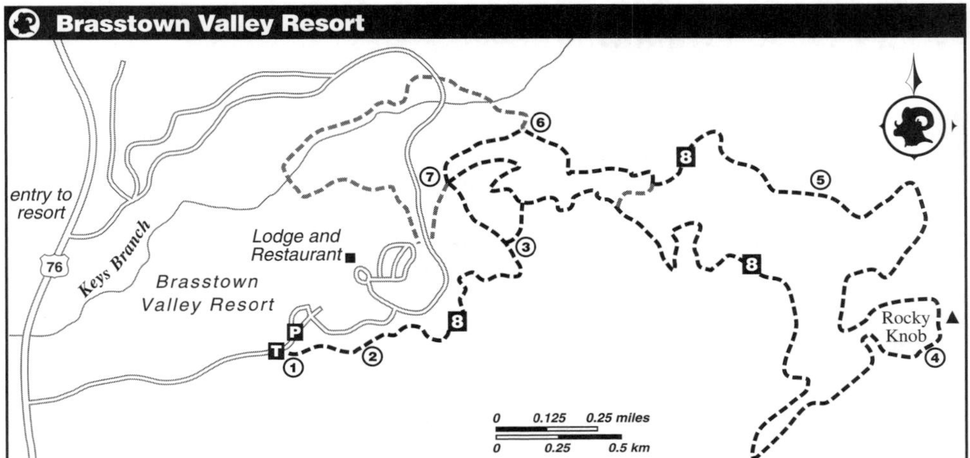

on the Miller Trek Trail, you can turn left here. Go straight to continue the trip as described. A little less than 2 miles into the hike, there are wide winter views of broad pastureland below and, beyond the valley, layers of distant, forested ridges.

At 2.7 miles **(Waypoint 4)** on the western slop of Rocky Knob, a high bluff offers a sweeping view of the valley and ridges to the west. The trail turns southeast, curls around the knob and drops quickly as Long Bullet Creek appears on the right. A walk through clear hardwoods brings you to a long footbridge **(Waypoint 5)** built to protect a watershed. Stretching 230 feet, this may be the longest footbridge in the Chattahoochee National Forest. During construction, 15 tons of lumber were brought in by helicopter and hand to prevent damage to the area.

A moderate descent takes you to the connector trail at 4.6 miles. The trail then drops into Walnut Cove, and at 5.2 miles there is a T junction **(Waypoint 6)** with the Long Bullett Branch. Take the trail on the left marked with orange and blue blazes and travel southwest.

At 5.3 miles there is a Y junction **(Waypoint 7)**. Going left allows you to climb to a high point with 360-degree views. There is also an interpretive sign explaining that migratory songbirds, such as the red-eyed vireo and oriole, summer in this area and in winter move on to Central and South America.

From **Waypoint 7**, bear right to continue on the Miller Trek Trail. At the next Y junction, bear right and follow orange and blue blazes toward the Miller Trek trailhead. At 5.5 miles you reach the end of the Miller Trek loop **(Waypoint 3)** where you bear right and travel south to return to the trailhead. After you hike, take some time to visit the archaeology display in the resort. When the resort was constructed, some sites with artifacts had to be disturbed, so the Georgia Department of Natural Resources worked with the Eastern Band of Cherokees to conduct the state's largest ever archaeological survey.

UTM WAYPOINTS

1. 17S 240484E 3871261N
2. 17S 240667E 3871315N
3. 17S 241261E 3871561N
4. 17S 242534E 3871027N
5. 17S 242436E 3871545N
6. 17S 241276E 3871856N
7. 17S 241122E 3871714N

TRIP 9 Wagon Train Trail

Distance	6.6 miles, point-to-point (13.1 miles, out-and-back)
Hiking Time	3–4 hours one-way
Difficulty	Moderate
Elevation Gain/Loss	+/- 2350 feet
Trail Use	Leashed dogs
Best Times	Year-round, with best views in winter
Agency	U.S. Forest Service, Blue Ridge District
Recommended Map	USGS 7.5-min. *Hiawassee*

HIGHLIGHTS The Wagon Train Trail rises above 4000 feet of elevation and traverses ridge tops to offer plenty of dramatic views, particularly in winter. The grade is primarily moderate, with only brief steep climbs, and unusually wide in places. In the 1930s, prisoners constructed the path, which served as a roadbed for GA Highway 66, linking Young Harris with Brasstown Bald and GA Highway 180. Beginning at Young Harris, the climb up is a steady push, but the rewards are many as breaks in the tall oaks allow you to peer out across the broad valley where Young Harris sits, examine deep coves, and gaze upon distant ridges. The trail ends at the Brasstown Bald parking lot, and from there you can opt to take the Summit Trail to the observation tower, which is the highest point in the state of Georgia at 4784 feet.

DIRECTIONS There are two access points for the Wagon Train Trail, one in Young Harris and another at the summit of Brasstown Bald. You can spot one car at each trailhead or do a long out-and-back trip. The hike detailed below begins at Young Harris.

To start in Young Harris: From Atlanta take GA Highway 400 north to its end at the intersection with GA Highway 60/U.S. Highway 19. Turn left onto GA 60/U.S. 19 north toward Dahlonega. Go 5 miles, and at the traffic light turn right to continue on U.S. 19 north (avoiding the highway business route). Continue on U.S. 19 north to U.S. 19/129. Take U.S. 19/129 north to Blairsville. At the intersection of U.S. 19 and U.S. Highway 76 in Blairsville turn right onto U.S. 76 east and travel 8.5 miles. Turn right onto Bald Mountain Road (just before you reach the Sharp Memorial United Methodist Church). Travel 0.2 mile, and bear right at a split in the road. Continue to the gate, which is usually closed. *This is not a designated parking area, and you may want to park at the church.*

To start at Brasstown Bald: From Atlanta take GA Highway 400 north to its end at the intersection with GA Highway 60/U.S. 19. Turn left onto GA 60/U.S. 19 north toward Dahlonega. Go 5 miles, and at the traffic light turn right to continue on U.S. 19 north (avoiding the highway business route). Continue on U.S. 19 north to U.S. 19/129. Take U.S. 19/129 north to GA Highway 180 east. Turn right onto GA 180 east, and travel 7.5 miles to the GA 180 spur on the left. Take the GA 180 spur to the parking lot at the summit. Near the concession building take the Summit Trail for 400 feet and turn right to begin the Wagon Train Trail.

FACILITIES/TRAILHEAD There are no facilities at the Young Harris Trailhead. There are restrooms and concessions at the Brasstown Bald summit area, which is open daily from Memorial Day through October and weekends in early spring and late fall. There are streams along the trail, but they may not be reliable water sources—be sure to pack plenty of water for your hike.

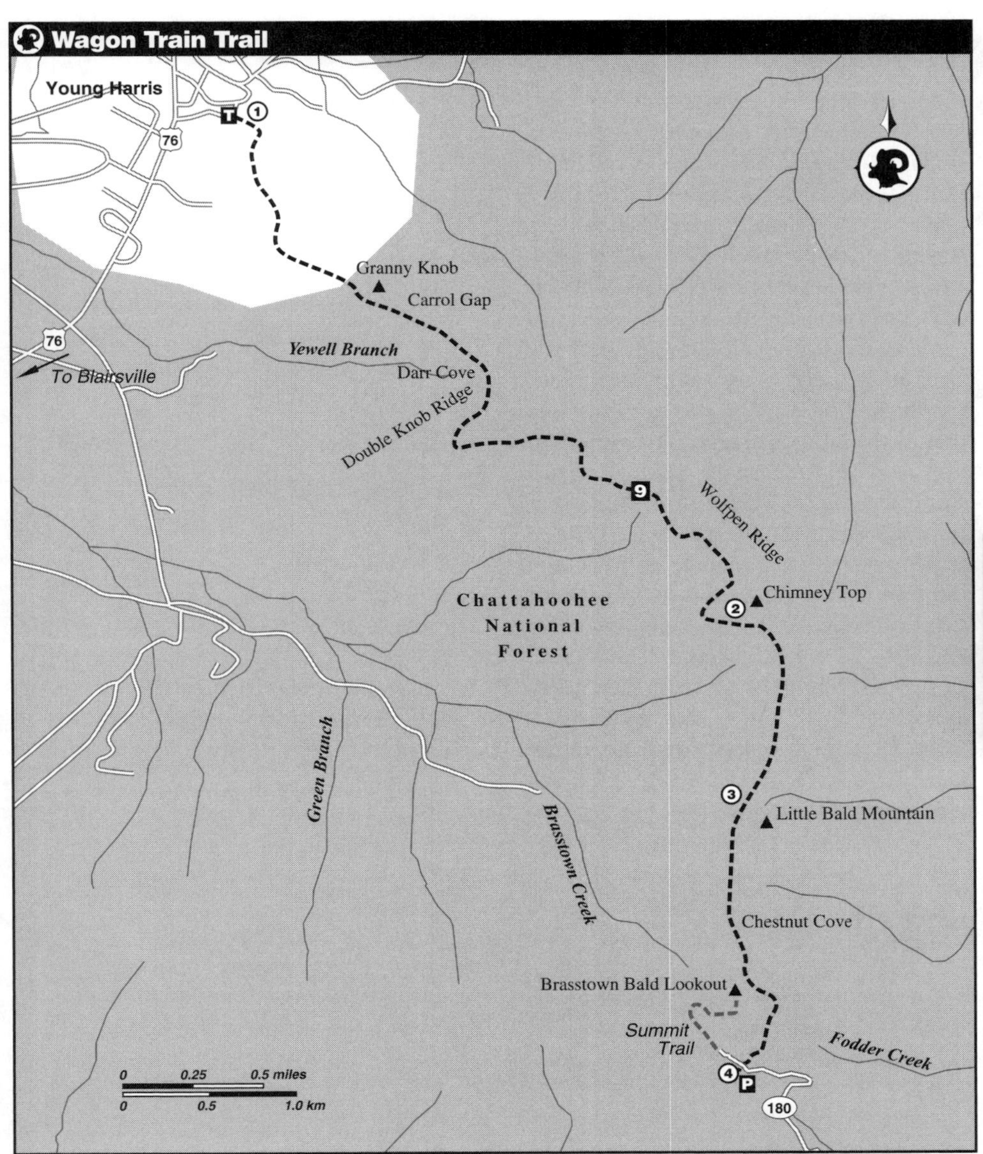

This hike starts at the Young Harris Trailhead **(Waypoint 1)**. Although parking space is limited, don't park in front of the gate. To begin, walk past the gate and ascend a rough roadbed. The pine and oak forest is dense and not very attractive for the first two- to three-tenths of a mile, but you soon pass a draw to the right thick with oaks, poplars, and other hardwoods. In this area I have encountered bears, one of which was so busy digging into a stump for brunch that it took me a few minutes to shoo the animal away. At 0.6 mile you have winter views to the west and northwest of farmland in the Young Harris Valley. A thousand feet ahead, intermittent breaks in the pines reveal prominent peaks far off to the southwest.

The trail circles around Granny Knob, and at 1.8 miles look to the right to see the steep slopes of Darr Cove. As you pass over Double Knob Ridge, at 2.1 miles a small window in the foliage gives a clear look at three layers of distant ridges and a higher hooked peak. The trail turns east, staying in the neighborhood of 3200 feet, while thick stands of mountain laurel and oaks wall the right side of the trail. As you circle to the southwest flank of Chimney Top, at 4.2 miles there is great view of the Brasstown Bald observation tower to the southwest **(Waypoint 2)**. The path then surpasses 4000 feet of elevation as it runs south across a long ridge covered in ferns, rhododendron, and hemlocks.

One of the best vantage points along the trail is at 5.2 miles on the northwest side of Little Bald Mountain **(Waypoint 3)**. To the immediate west are Little Bald Cove and Big Bald Cove, which form great cuts that run to the wide valley splayed out before you. Completing the scene, a stretch of towering hills and saddles rules the landscape.

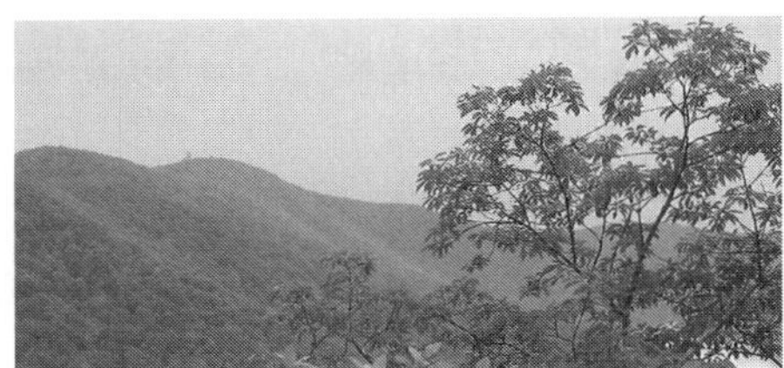

Above 4000 feet on the Wagon Train Trail

Almost due east of Brasstown Bald the path narrows, and an extremely dense forest of rhododendron, magnolias, and beeches close in on the trail to form a tunnel. At 6.2 miles, continue past the metal gate following a wide, grassy path. You soon reach the intersection with the paved Summit Trail. Turn right to walk to the observation tower, or turn left and walk 400 feet to the parking area **(Waypoint 4)**.

UTM WAYPOINTS

1. 17S 240109E 3869130N
2. 17S 243312E 3865317N
3. 17S 243235E 3864029N
4. 17S 243147E 3862293N

TRIP 10 Arkaquah Trail

Distance	5.4 miles, point-to-point (10.8 miles, out-and-back)
Hiking Time	5 hours
Difficulty	Strenuous
Elevation Gain/Loss	+3485/-1050 feet
Trail Use	Leashed dogs
Best Times	Year-round
Agency	U.S. Forest Service, Blue Ridge District
Recommended Map	USGS 7.5-min. *Jacks Gap, Hiawassee, Blairsville*

HIGHLIGHTS The Native Americans dubbed the land near this trail "Arkaquah," which is the Cherokee word for a crooked creek. But the Native American presence here predates the Cherokee, stretching perhaps back to Archaic period (8000 to 1000 BCE). Petroglyphs on boulders near the parking area are evidence of early habitation. It's worth it to take a moment and examine this artwork before starting your trek on the Arkaquah Trail, which runs between Trackrock Gap Road and Brasstown Bald, Georgia's highest point.

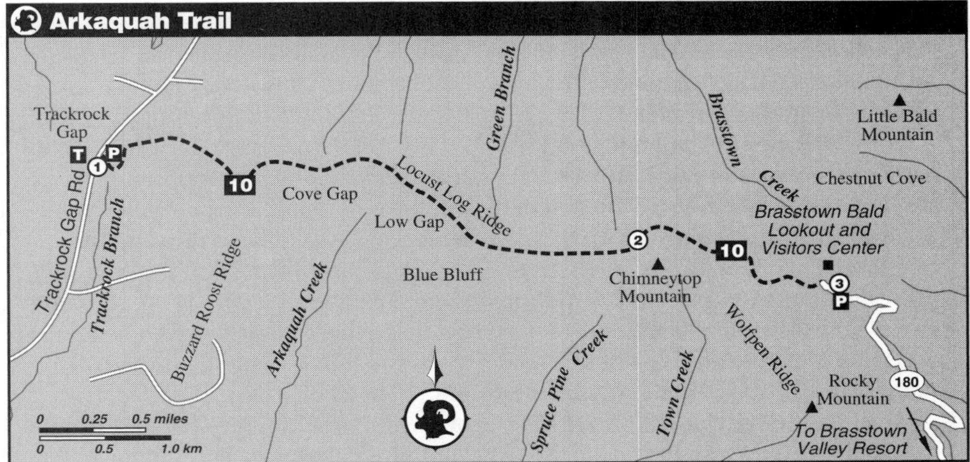

The easiest way to do this trail is to spot cars at each end and begin at Brasstown, hiking down. If you instead begin at Trackrop Gap, as described here, you enjoy a heart-pumping journey that gains more than 2400 feet of elevation in steep ascents. Your efforts are rewarded with great views, especially at 4.1 miles where Chimneytop Mountain overlooks the town of Young Harris to the north and prominent hilltops rise in the south.

DIRECTIONS The Arkaquah Trail can be accessed from Trackrock Gap Road and from Brasstown Bald. The hike detailed below begins in Trackrock Gap. From Atlanta take GA Highway 400 north to its end at the intersection with GA Highway 60/U.S. 19. Turn left onto GA 60/U.S. 19 north toward Dahlonega. Go 5 miles, and at the traffic light turn right to continue on U.S. 19 north (avoiding the highway business route). Continue on U.S. 19 north to U.S. 19/129. Take U.S. 19/129 north to GA Highway 180 east. Turn right onto GA 180 east, travel 2.5 miles, and turn left onto Town Creek School Road. Go 5.3 miles and turn right onto Trackrock Gap Road (across from a church). Go 3.8 miles to the parking area on the left.

To start at Brasstown Bald: From Atlanta take GA Highway 400 north to its end at the intersection with GA Highway 60/U.S. 19. Turn left onto GA 60/U.S. 19 north toward Dahlonega. Go 5 miles, and at the traffic light turn right to continue on U.S. 19 north (avoiding the highway business route). Continue on U.S. 19 north to U.S. 19/129. Take U.S. 19/129 north to GA Highway 180 east. Turn right onto GA 180 east, and travel 7.5 miles to the GA 180 spur on the left. Take the GA 180 spur to the Brasstown Bald parking lot.

FACILITIES/TRAILHEAD There are no facilities at the trailhead off of GA 180, and there is no parking fee. The Brasstown Bald summit has restrooms and concessions and is open daily from Memorial Day through October and weekends in early spring and late fall. Be sure to pack plenty of water for several hours of vigorous hiking.

From the north side of the parking area, a brief trail walk leads to a group of soapstone boulders that have petroglyphs of footprints, bird tracks, and other designs. To reach the Arkaquah Trail from the parking area, cross Trackrock Gap Road, turn left and look for the trailhead on the right **(Waypoint 1)**. Follow red blazes as the narrow path moves through hardwoods. You soon ascend along the side of a hill and begin a steady, steep climb up Buzzard Roost Ridge. The path moves over stony ground with winter views to your left and right.

The trail drops to Cove Gap and then moves up onto Locust Log Ridge, becoming steep once again near the top. A series of hills and saddles along this ridge take you through diverse forest of not only pine and oak but also rhododendron, mountain laurel, and hemlock.

At 2.7 miles the trail goes through Low Gap and then begins a long, gradual rise to the Blue Bluff Overlook at 3.1 miles. The path drops from the ridge along the north slope of the hill, and the environment is noticeably more moist, cool, and shaded. You'll scramble up through moss-covered boulders and stands of rhododendron, and then return to the ridgetop. If you need a breather, at 3.6 miles a gathering of hemlocks form a natural pavilion, and when I passed though here a large log made for a good resting bench.

The path runs level along a ridge before climbing Chimneytop Mountain. At 4.1 miles you can look to the north from a rocky outcrop **(Waypoint 2)** to see the town of Young Harris, while prominent peaks are visible to the southwest.

Continuing your hike, the trail dips then rises above 4200 feet of elevation before leaving Chimneytop. At the 5-mile mark you take a steady, gradual grade up to Brasstown Bald **(Waypoint 3)**. At the end of the trail, you can turn left to reach the Summit Trail, which climbs to the observation tower for one of the most stellar views in Georgia.

UTM WAYPOINTS

1. 17S 237034E 3863796N
2. 17S 241514E 3862753N
3. 17S 243076E 3862287N

TRIP 11 Jacks Knob Trail: North to Brasstown Bald

Distance	4.6 miles, out-and-back
Hiking Time	3 hours
Difficulty	Moderate
Elevation Gain/Loss	+/-1805 feet
Trail Use	Leashed dogs
Best Times	Year-round
Agency	U.S. Forest Service, Blue Ridge District
Recommended Map	USGS 7.5-min. *Jacks Gap*

HIGHLIGHTS The Jacks Knob Trail stretches 4.5 miles from Brasstown Bald to a junction with the Appalachian Trail. At its midpoint, the trail crosses GA Highway 180. If you were to begin at Brasstown Bald and do the entire trail as an out-and-back hike, it would make for a challenging day trip. Another good option is to split the trail into two separate, moderate dayhikes, each beginning at the parking area at the intersection of GA Highway 180 and the GA 180 spur road. To explore the northern half of the trail, begin at the GA 180 parking area, at about 2900 feet of elevation, and climb moderately to the Brasstown Bald parking area, which lies at just over 4500 feet of elevation. This trip takes you up slopes of oaks and pines with an understory of mountain laurel, and just past the 2-mile mark an opening offers an inspiring view of mountain ranges to the east.

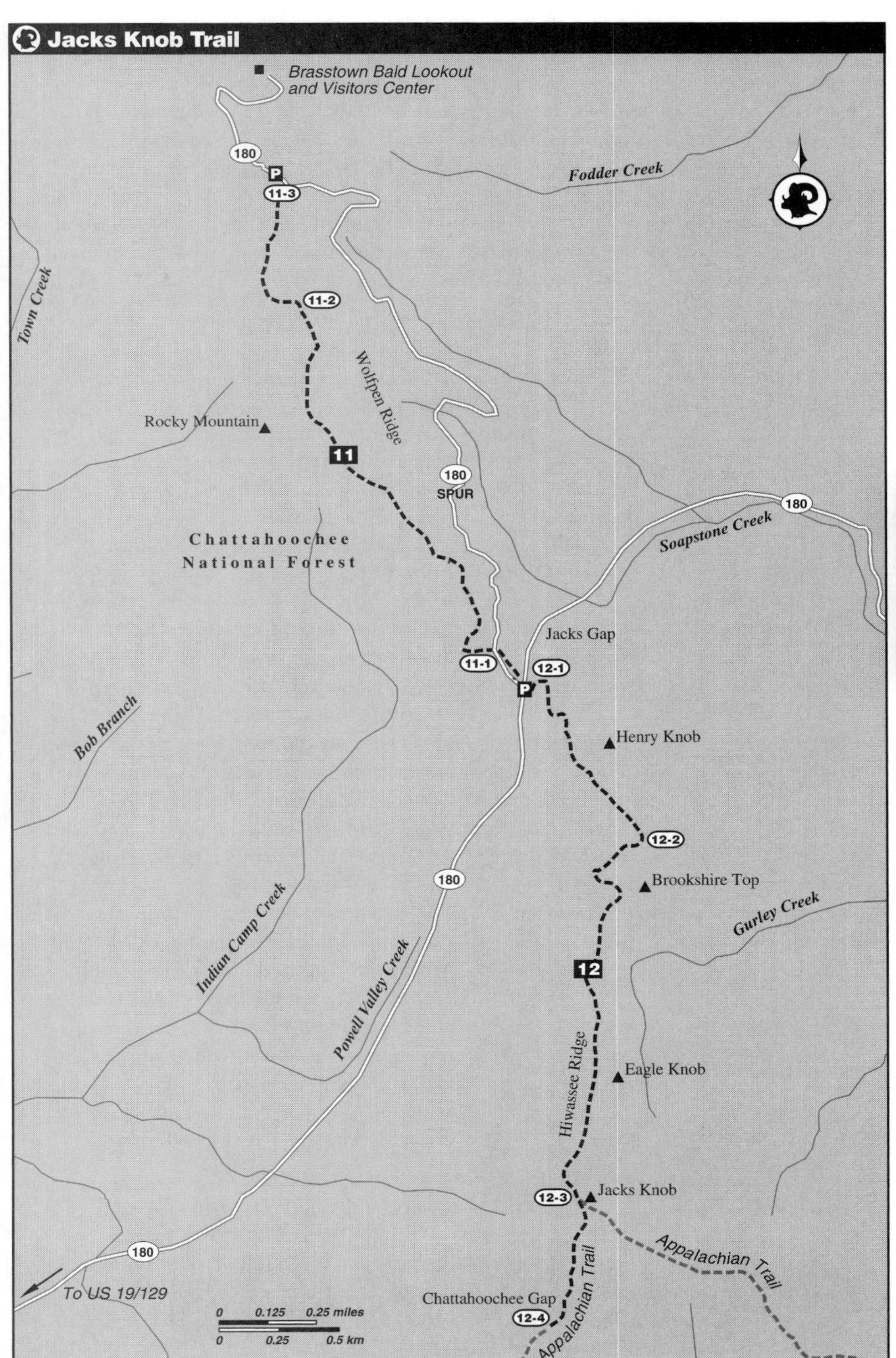

Jacks Knob Trail
Brasstown Bald Lookout and Visitors Center
180
P
11-3
Fodder Creek
Town Creek
11-2
Wolfpen Ridge
Rocky Mountain
11
180
SPUR
180
Soapstone Creek
Chattahoochee National Forest
Jacks Gap
11-1
12-1
P
Bob Branch
Henry Knob
12-2
Brookshire Top
180
Gurley Creek
Indian Camp Creek
12
Powell Valley Creek
Hiwassee Ridge
Eagle Knob
12-3
Jacks Knob
Appalachian Trail
Appalachian Trail
180
To US 19/129
Chattahoochee Gap
12-4
Appalachian Trail
0 0.125 0.25 miles
0 0.25 0.5 km

DIRECTIONS From Atlanta take GA Highway 400 north to its end at the intersection with GA Highway 60/U.S. Highway 19. Turn left onto GA 60/U.S. 19 north toward Dahlonega. Go 5 miles, and at the traffic light turn right to continue on U.S. 19 north (avoiding the highway business route). Continue on U.S. 19 north to U.S. 19/129. Take U.S. 19/129 north to GA Highway 180 east. Turn right onto GA 180 east and travel 7.5 miles. The parking area is on the left shoulder of the road just before you reach the junction with the GA 180 spur.

FACILITIES/TRAILHEAD There are no facilities at the GA 180 trailhead, and there is no parking fee. Brasstown Bald summit has restrooms and concession and charges $3 for parking. The Brasstown Bald summit area is open daily from Memorial Day through October and weekends in early spring and late fall. Pack water for your hike, and keep in mind you'll be ascending quite a bit.

At the northwest (uphill) end of the parking area, enter the path at the HIKER TRAIL sign attached to a poplar **(Waypoint 1)**. Follow blue blazes, ascending moderately through the shade of overhead mountain laurel. As you head toward Wolfpen Ridge, the trail actually runs along the border of Towns County (to the east) and Union County (to the west). The narrow path is mostly surrounded by heavy foliage, but there are occasional views to the east. At the 1-mile mark, the heavy odor of galax hangs in the air.

There is an especially large stand of mountain laurel at 1.2 miles, and the crooked limbs form a strange corridor whose walls are a wavy curtain. Ahead, their trunks grow quite thick and the hallway dims, but you then exit into a forest of pines and hardwoods bright with sunshine.

Brasstown Bald Lookout and Visitors Center

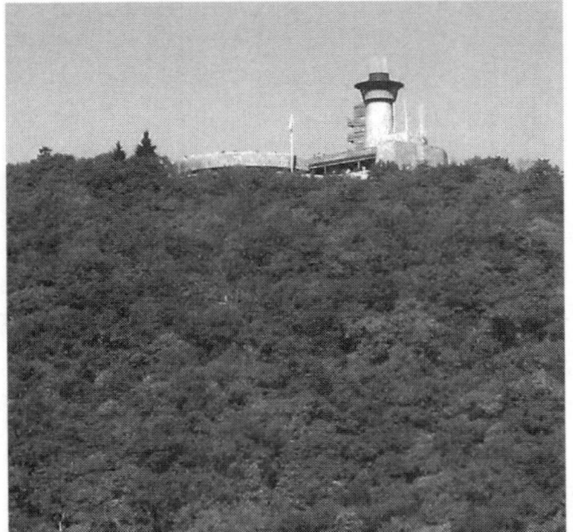

At 1.7 miles the path levels as you reach the upper portion of Wolfpen Ridge. High laurel once again lines the trail at 1.9 miles, and you scramble down boulders where a bed of moss and leaves blanket the ground.

When the trail reaches a hilltop at 2 miles **(Waypoint 2)**, look for a short path to the right that leads to an opening in the trees at the edge of a bluff. Before you lies a broad valley and waves of mountain ridges extending to the horizon. After returning to the main trail, descend, traveling west on the southwest slope where laurel leans hard downhill. The trail dives into a rich stand of rhododendron and passes through boulders before reaching its end at the parking area **(Waypoint 3)**. To the left and right are picnic benches, and you can cross the parking area to reach a restroom. On the far side of the parking lot, the trailhead for the Summit Trail lies between the concession building and the gift shop. This path takes you to the observation tower, which sits at 4784 feet, the highest point in Georgia. From **Waypoint 3**, retrace your steps back down to the parking area at GA 180.

UTM WAYPOINTS

1. 17S 244073E 3859808N
2. 17S 243172E 3861682N
3. 17S 243087E 3862005N

TRIP 12 Jacks Knob Trail: South to Chattahoochee Gap

Distance	4.4 miles, out-and-back
Hiking Time	2 hours
Difficulty	Moderate
Elevation Gain/Loss	+945/-1865 feet
Trail Uses	Leashed dogs and backpacking
Best Times	Year-round
Agency	U.S. Forest Service, Blue Ridge District
Recommended Map	USGS 7.5-min. *Jacks Gap*

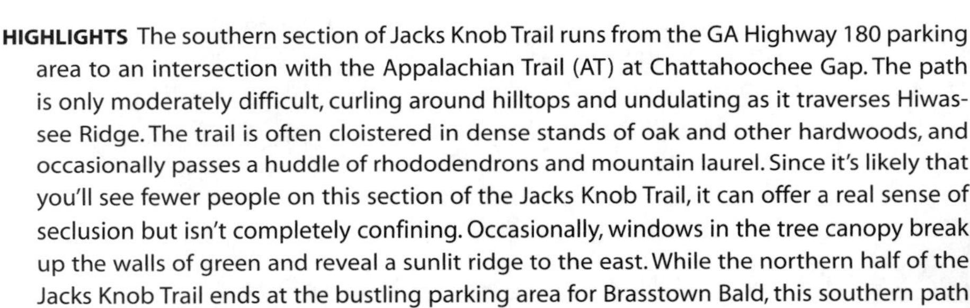

HIGHLIGHTS The southern section of Jacks Knob Trail runs from the GA Highway 180 parking area to an intersection with the Appalachian Trail (AT) at Chattahoochee Gap. The path is only moderately difficult, curling around hilltops and undulating as it traverses Hiwassee Ridge. The trail is often cloistered in dense stands of oak and other hardwoods, and occasionally passes a huddle of rhododendrons and mountain laurel. Since it's likely that you'll see fewer people on this section of the Jacks Knob Trail, it can offer a real sense of seclusion but isn't completely confining. Occasionally, windows in the tree canopy break up the walls of green and reveal a sunlit ridge to the east. While the northern half of the Jacks Knob Trail ends at the bustling parking area for Brasstown Bald, this southern path leads to a gap tucked away deep in the forest.

DIRECTIONS From Atlanta take GA Highway 400 north to its end at the intersection with GA Highway 60/U.S. Highway 19. Turn left onto GA 60/U.S. 19 north toward Dahlonega. Go 5 miles, and at the traffic light turn right to continue on U.S. 19 north (avoiding the highway business route). Continue on U.S. 19 north to U.S. 19/129. Take U.S. 19/129 north to GA Highway 180 east. Turn right onto GA 180 east and travel 7.5 miles. The parking area is on the left shoulder of the road just before you reach the junction with the GA 180 spur.

FACILITIES/TRAILHEAD There are no facilities and no parking fee at the trailhead. The nearest facilities (including restrooms) lie at the Brasstown Bald summit parking area, which charges a $3 parking fee. To reach the area from GA 180, turn left onto the GA 180 spur and drive 3 miles.

From the parking area on GA 180, cross the road, turn left (north) and walk 180 feet to the sign for JACKS KNOB TRAIL on the right **(Waypoint 1)**. Following blue blazes, climb moderately to steeply into hardwoods. As you skirt around Henry Knob, the slopes to your right fall away steeply and Hiwassee Ridge rises prominently in the southwest. The path roller coasters on the flank of the hill, and then at 0.6 mile passes a saddle. To the left, about 30 feet off the trail, there is a small clearing with a fire ring and room for a couple of small tents **(Waypoint 2)**.

After a steep ascent you reach an elevation of about 3460 feet east of the summit of Brookshire Top. The path then gradually moves down a south-facing slope and to your left you have intermittent views of a close ridge to the south. The forest closes in around you again as a steep descent takes you into a saddle. From this low-slung land you climb steeply to Eagle Knob, topping out at about 4560 feet. Here you have views in winter to the east and west, and as the roller coaster trail makes another drop, ridges to the east should be in view when the leaves have fallen.

At 1.9 miles you find yourself on the western flanks of the slopes below Jacks Knob. In fall this hickory-covered hillside is bright with scattered golden leaves. Look right for a small opening in the tree canopy **(Waypoint 3)**. Immediately below is a saddle whose deep-green forest contrasts with the misty blue mountain range that rises high in the distance.

After rounding Jacks Knob and ascending past 4600 feet of elevation, you make the final descent to Chattahoochee Gap **(Waypoint 4)**. On sunny days this small clearing is bathed in light, and it's a great place to relax and eat before the return trek. In the gap there is a side trail and sign marked WATER SOURCE 0.5 MILE; the spring it leads to is the headwaters for the Chattahoochee River. Across the gap clearing, on the south side, is the junction with the AT and a small, cleared space with a fire ring and room for a single tent.

From the gap, retrace your steps and take the Jacks Knob Trail back to GA 180.

UTM WAYPOINTS

1. 17S 244134E 3859808N
2. 17S 244623E 3858960N
3. 17S 244223E 3857265N
4. 17S 244179E 3856916N

TRIP 13 Smithgall Woods: Laurel Ridge Trail

Distance	1.6 miles, loop
Hiking Time	1 hour
Difficulty	Moderate
Elevation Gain/Loss	+/-290 feet
Trail Uses	Leashed dogs and good for kids
Best Times	Year-round
Agency	Smithgall Woods Conservation Area
Recommended Map	A trail map is available at the visitors center and online at www.gastateparks.org.

HIGHLIGHTS This interpretive trail takes you through numerous habitats, from a mountain cove to a ridgetop to wetlands. There are 25 interpretive markers along the trail, all called out in a handy pamphlet that you should pick up at the visitors center. This is a great hike for families, especially kids who can keep their eyes peeled for squirrels, spotted salamanders, and a variety of animal tracks.

DIRECTIONS From Atlanta take Interstate 85 north to Interstate 985. Take I-985 to Exit 24 for GA Highway 369. Turn left onto GA 369 west, go 0.6 mile, and turn right onto U.S. 129 north. Go 23 miles (passing through Cleveland), and turn right onto GA Highway 75 Alt. Go 5.7 miles, and turn right onto Tsalaki Trail at the conservation area entrance.

FACILITIES/TRAILHEAD The visitors center has restrooms. There is a $3 parking fee; you can purchase an Annual ParkPass for $30 by calling (770) 389-7401. Everyone should register at the visitors center. Accommodations include the Lodge at Smithgall Woods and a group campground (for youth groups only).

At the east side of the paved parking area, enter the woodchip path at the wood fence marked with the Laurel Ridge Trail sign **(Waypoint 1)**. You soon cross a small stream that serves as habitat for trout. The first interpretive sign explains

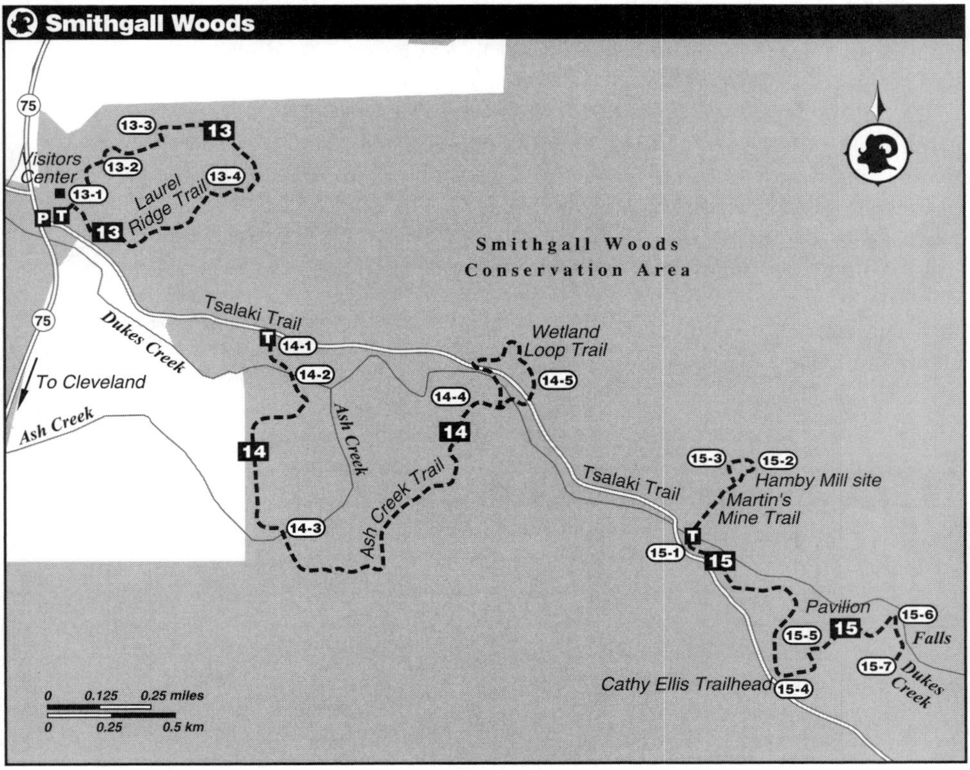
Smithgall Woods
75
13-3
13
Visitors Center
13-2
13-4
Laurel Ridge Trail
13-1
P T
13
Smithgall Woods Conservation Area
Tsalaki Trail
75
Dukes Creek
T
14-1
Wetland Loop Trail
14-2
14-5
To Cleveland
14-4
Ash Creek
Ash Creek
14
14
Ash Creek Trail
15-3
15-2
Tsalaki Trail
Hamby Mill site
Martin's Mine Trail
14-3
T
15-1
15
Pavilion
15-6
15-5
15
Falls
15-7
Dukes Creek
Cathy Ellis Trailhead
15-4
0 0.125 0.25 miles
0 0.25 0.5 km

that a dam was placed here to create a pool to hold the fish. From the stream, the trail turns northwest as you climb through the mountain cove (home of the spotted salamander) and pass through sourwood trees, maples, and white pines. Farther on, the forest includes a mix of hemlocks and rhododendron.

After crossing an intermittent stream, you pass through the lower slope forest where ferns and mosses lie in the shade of pines and hardwoods. Ahead is a spring-fed stream **(Waypoint 2)**; an interpretive sign indicates that this is a feeding ground for ruffed grouse whose diet includes such delicious things as snails and spiders. Not far ahead, after crossing a footbridge, search the sides of the path for resurrection ferns, which curl up in hot, dry weather and then, following a rain, open up and seemingly return to life.

At 0.4 mile **(Waypoint 3)** an opening marks the former site of an old sawmill that operated in the 1930s or 1940s. Actually, there's hardly any trace of it now as second-growth forest has hidden the evidence.

The rhododendron fades as the trail then climbs through a dry area with Virginia pines, hickory trees, and oaks. At 0.7

Holly lining a Smithgall trail

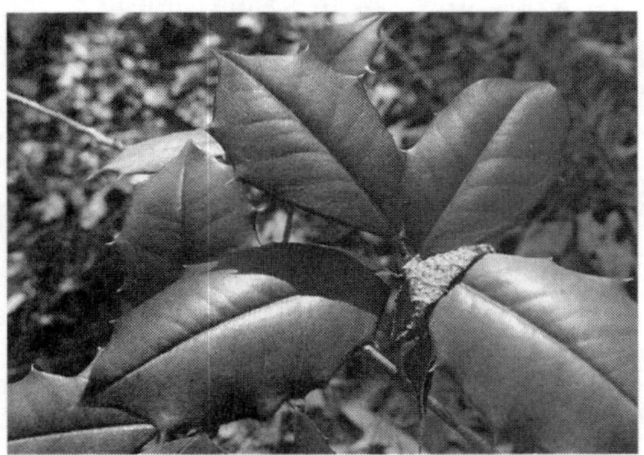

mile you enter forest that is recovering from damage inflicted by a blizzard that hit in 1993.

Traversing Laurel Ridge, at 0.8 mile a break in the trees reveals Yonah Mountain which lords over the landscape, surpassing 3000 feet of elevation. At 0.9 mile **(Waypoint 4)** you reach the top of Laurel Ridge where pines and oaks can withstand the strong winds that sweep across this high feature. As you continue, keep an eye out for soaring hawks.

The path then drops back down into lush vegetation, and a wood footbridge takes you over the creek. At the junction of the Laurel Ridge Loop and trail for the Dukes Creek Loop, go right and travel north back to the parking area.

UTM WAYPOINTS

1. 17S 246432E 3842367N
2. 17S 246531E 3842494N
3. 17S 246769E 3842587N
4. 17S 247049E 3842403N

TRIP 14 Smithgall Woods: Ash Creek Trail & Wetland Loop

Distance	2.2 miles, loop
Hiking Time	1 hour
Difficulty	Moderate
Elevation Gain/Loss	+165/-215 feet
Trail Use	Leashed dogs
Best Times	Year-round
Agency	Smithgall Woods Conservation Area
Recommended Map	A trail map is available at the visitors center and online at www.gastateparks.org.

see map on p. 135

HIGHLIGHTS On a warm day, this is the perfect hike for cooling off. The Ash Creek Trail includes two knee-deep stream crossings and a climb to a ridgetop with a view of Yonah Mountain. After completing the Ash Creek Trail, you can cross Tsalaki Trail to take the short Wetland Loop. This passes a beaver pond and serves as a good spot for birding and identifying frogs. Before you set out on your walk, pick up "The Frogs of Smithgall Woods" brochure at the visitors center.

DIRECTIONS From Atlanta take Interstate 85 north to Interstate 985. Take I-985 to Exit 24 for GA Highway 369. Turn left onto GA 369 west, go 0.6 mile, and turn right onto U.S. Highway 129 north. Go 23 miles (passing through Cleveland), and turn right onto GA Highway 75 Alt. Go 5.7 miles, and turn right onto Tsalaki Trail at the conservation area entrance.

FACILITIES/TRAILHEAD The visitors center has restrooms. There is a $3 parking fee, or you can purchase an Annual ParkPass for $30 by calling (770) 389-7401. All visitors should register at the visitors center. Accommodations include the Lodge at Smithgall Woods and a group campground (for youth groups only).

Ash Creek Trail

To reach the trailhead from the parking area, walk about 0.6 mile down Tsalaki Trail to a sign on the right marked FISHING ACCESS **(Waypoint 1)**. Turn right onto a wide dirt path and travel south for 500 feet to the Ash Creek Trailhead **(Waypoint 2)**. Walk southeast through dense pines

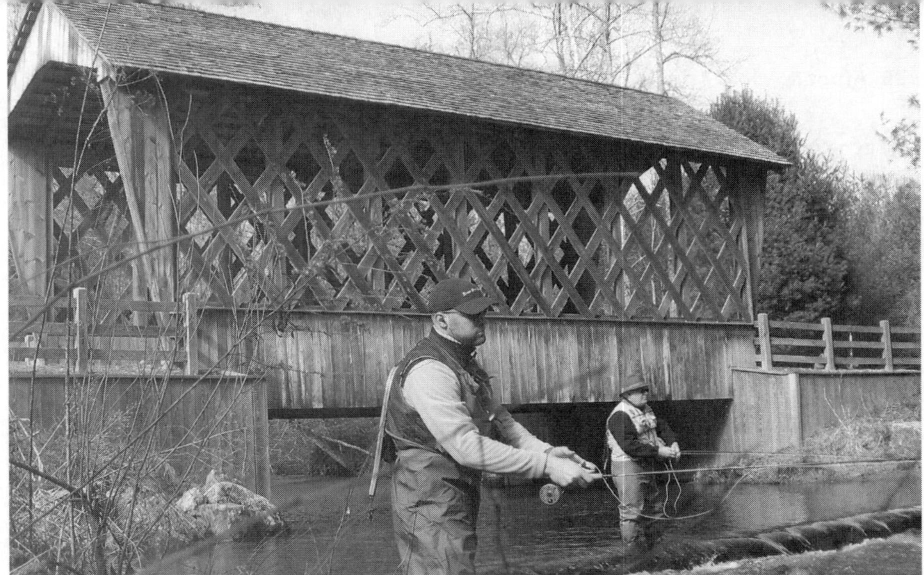

Smithgall Woods is a popular fly-fishing destination in north Georgia.

and hardwoods for another 200 feet and cross Ash Creek where the water is knee deep and about 20 feet wide.

The trail continues through very attractive forest with hemlocks and tall oaks. At 0.2 mile the trail climbs moderately and winds around a hill before dropping again through young pines in forest that feels very secluded.

Towering oaks dominate the forest ahead, and at 0.7 mile **(Waypoint 3)** you cross the stream again, this time about shin deep. Farther on, moss appears at the base of hemlocks, and high rhododendron lines the trail. At 1.1 miles the trail tops a ridge, where you can look north to the distant hills and ridges.

At 1.2 miles pass a large clover field and look southeast to see Yonah Mountain. After walking another 0.3 mile the trail starts to descend from the ridge into dense forest of hemlocks and hardwoods.

The trail Ts into the gravel road at 1.6 miles **(Waypoint 4)**. This is also the location of the Bear Ridge campsite. Turn right (northeast) to continue to the intersection with the paved road. Turn left and go through the covered bridge to reach the Wetlands Loop Trailhead **(Waypoint 5)**.

Wetland Loop

At **Waypoint 5** enter the gravel and dirt path and pass a pond formed by a beaver dam. You can also see wood duck boxes dotting the area. An interpretive sign goes into some detail about the ecology of this type of wetland. Along the loop, a boardwalk allows you to cross wet areas, and an observation platform is ideal for birding. The trail leads to an interpretive sign for "softmast" vegetation, such as dogwood and holly, which provide plenty of nutrition for wildlife. As you proceed, you can watch for a variety of birds, including pileated woodpeckers, cardinals, and towhees. The path drops to a creek and then turns back southeast along the road, returning to the trailhead.

From the trailhead turn right and take Tsalaki Trail northwest back to the parking area.

UTM WAYPOINTS

1. 17S 247256E 3841787N
2. 17S 247262E 3841653N
3. 17S 247240E 3840898N
4. 17S 248005E 3841397N
5. 17S 248198E 3841446N

TRIP 15 Smithgall Woods: Martin's Mine & Cathy Ellis Memorial Trails

Distance	6.8 miles, out-and-back
Hiking Time	3–4 hours
Difficulty	Moderate
Elevation Gain/Loss	+/-440 feet
Trail Use	Leashed dogs
Best Times	Year-round
Agency	Smithgall Woods Conservation Area
Recommended Map	A trail map is available at the visitors center or online at www.gastateparks.org.

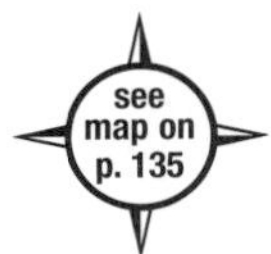

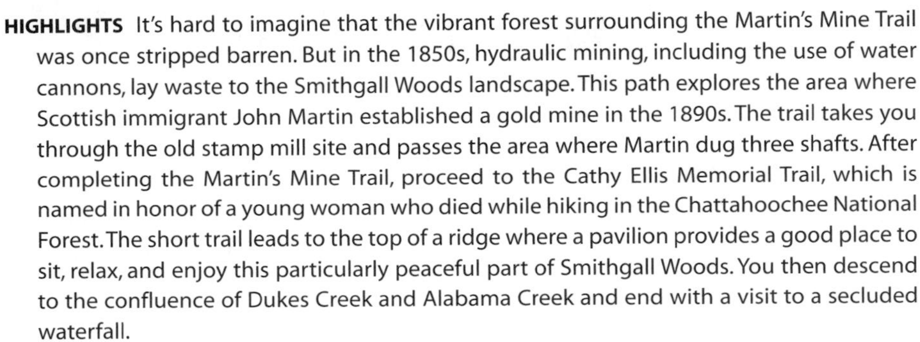

HIGHLIGHTS It's hard to imagine that the vibrant forest surrounding the Martin's Mine Trail was once stripped barren. But in the 1850s, hydraulic mining, including the use of water cannons, lay waste to the Smithgall Woods landscape. This path explores the area where Scottish immigrant John Martin established a gold mine in the 1890s. The trail takes you through the old stamp mill site and passes the area where Martin dug three shafts. After completing the Martin's Mine Trail, proceed to the Cathy Ellis Memorial Trail, which is named in honor of a young woman who died while hiking in the Chattahoochee National Forest. The short trail leads to the top of a ridge where a pavilion provides a good place to sit, relax, and enjoy this particularly peaceful part of Smithgall Woods. You then descend to the confluence of Dukes Creek and Alabama Creek and end with a visit to a secluded waterfall.

DIRECTIONS From Atlanta take Interstate 85 north to Interstate 985. Take I-985 to Exit 24 for GA Highway 369. Turn left onto GA 369 west, go 0.6 mile, and turn right onto U.S. Highway 129 north. Go 23 miles (passing through Cleveland), and turn right onto GA Highway 75 Alt. Go 5.7 miles and turn right onto Tsalaki Trail at the conservation area entrance.

FACILITIES/TRAILHEAD The visitors center has restrooms. There is a $3 parking fee, or you can purchase an Annual ParkPass for $30 by calling (770) 389-7401. All visitors should register at the visitors center. Accommodations include the Lodge at Smithgall Woods and a group campground (for youth groups only).

From the parking area, walk southeast down the Tsalaki Trail about 1.2 miles to the Martin's Mine Trailhead on the left **(Waypoint 1)**. You cross a wood bridge set in hemlocks and take the rolling, rocky path through rhododendron. At 0.1 mile you reach wood platform and an interpretive sign that goes into detail about the mine operation here. To extract gold, miners dug shafts, constructed tunnels, and harnessed the flow of Dukes Creek to run a stamp mill where ore was crushed, washed, and boiled to separate out the gold.

The falls near Martin's Mine

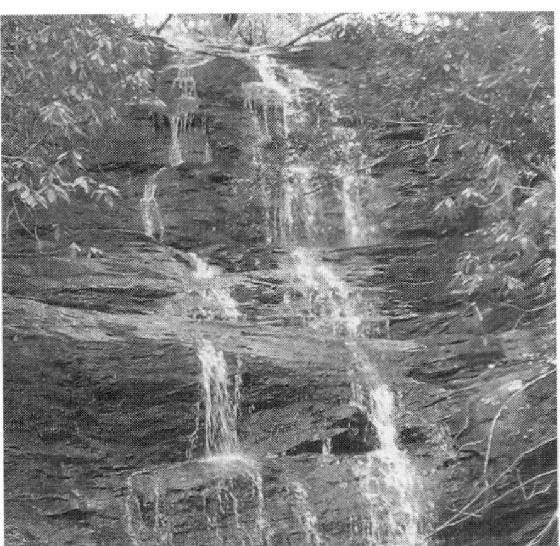

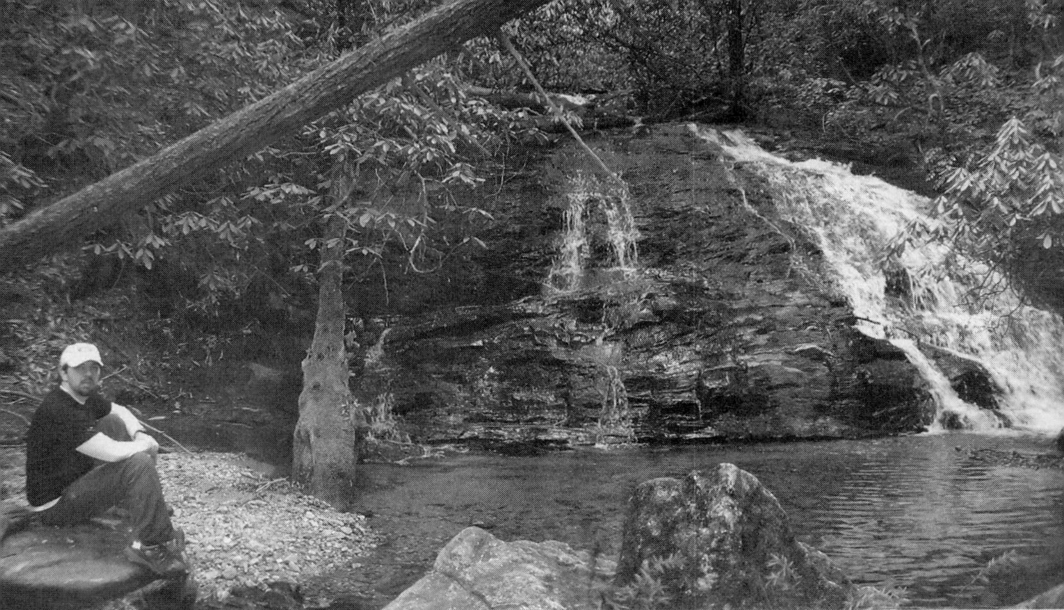
Secluded falls on Dukes Creek

At 0.2 mile the trail passes the Hamby Mill site **(Waypoint 2)** where water flumes delivered ore that was crushed into sand and washed to extract gold. From here, bear right to the northeast and then climb steeply aided by wooden steps and bridges. You encounter a high waterfall at 0.4 mile **(Waypoint 3)**, and then take a sharp turn to descend stone steps and pass through the area where Martin dug mine shafts.

When you've returned to the trailhead at **Waypoint 1**, turn left and walk down Tsalaki Trail 0.6 mile to the Cathy Ellis Trailhead on the left **(Waypoint 4)**. The path climbs to a ridgetop with the Dog Wood Shelter **(Waypoint 5)**, a small pavilion with a picnic table that makes a great place to enjoy a bite to eat while surrounded by quiet woods.

The path then drops off the ridge and passes through oaks and mountain laurel. The terrain to your left drops away steeply as the forest transitions to rhododendron. Pines become prevalent before joining more hardwoods and hemlocks.

After walking about 0.4 mile on the trail you'll reach the bank where Alabama Branch meets Dukes Creek **(Waypoint 6)**. This cool, shaded basin feels very remote as you pass beneath tall hemlocks and low boughs of rhododendron. It was in this area that gold was discovered in 1828, which helped spark the Georgia gold rush. You continue along the creek, and the hike ends on a high note with a visit to a waterfall with streams sliding down sloped rock into a shallow pool **(Waypoint 7)**.

From the falls, retrace your steps to Tsalaki Trail. The walk from the Cathy Ellis Trailhead to the parking area is about 2.7 miles.

UTM WAYPOINTS

1. 17S 248910E 3840770N
2. 17S 249132E 3841062N
3. 17S 249060E 3841101N
4. 17S 249328E 3840194N
5. 17S 249354E 3840291N
6. 17S 249727E 3840333N
7. 17S 249711E 3840257N

TRIP 16 Yonah Mountain

Distance	4.2 miles, out-and-back
Hiking Time	2 hours
Difficulty	Moderate
Elevation Gain/Loss	+/-1545 feet
Trail Uses	Climbing and backpacking
Best Times	Spring, fall, and winter
Agency	Chattahoochee-Oconee national forests
Recommended Map	USGS 7.5-min. *Helen*
Note	To avoid hiking or climbing during ranger training, call the U.S. Army Ranger 5th Battalion at Camp Frank D. Merrill at (706) 864-3367.

HIGHLIGHTS Near the center of White Country lies massive Yonah Mountain, a 3156-foot peak with a great brow of exposed granite stretching across its upper face. That sea of granite has made climbing the primary activity on Yonah, though improved access has attracted more hikers. A new, gravel access road leads to a well-constructed parking area.

A unique aspect of Yonah is that it serves as a training site for the U.S. Army Ranger 5th Battalion. The Mountain Phase of Ranger School includes climbing instruction, so the rangers have established bolted routes that are ideal for beginner or intermediate climbers and are open to the public when not in use by the school. Less than a mile in, a grassy clearing offers views of a placid valley, and higher on the mountain, exposed granite faces make a great perch to look out over rolling forested ridges and the lowlands to the south.

DIRECTIONS From Atlanta take Interstate 85 north to Interstate 985. Take I-985 to Exit 24 for GA Highway 369. Turn left onto GA 369 west, go 0.6 mile, and turn right onto U.S. Highway 129 north. Take U.S. 129 to Cleveland. From the town square in Cleveland go 0.4 mile and turn right onto GA Highway 75. Travel 3.6 miles on GA 75 and turn right on Tom Bell Road. Go 0.1 mile on Tom Bell Road and turn left onto Chambers Road. Travel 0.8 mile on Chambers Road and turn left onto a gravel road. Travel 0.4 mile to the parking area.

FACILITIES/TRAILHEAD There is a privy at the trailhead, and at the clearing at 1.5 miles. There is no fee for parking or camping. There are no water sources, so carry all the water you will need.

At the northeast side of the gravel parking area **(Waypoint 1)**, enter the narrow dirt path that cuts through high grass. You soon walk a shaded trail that rises gradually through mixed hardwoods, pines, and mountain laurel. The path winds among large boulders scattered throughout a modest slope and takes a winding route up the mountain's southwestern flank.

Climb two sets of stone steps, and then walk downhill briefly. At 0.9 mile you scramble over large rocks and pass between two boulders that are about 20 feet high. Another gradual walk uphill brings you to a grassy clearing at 1.1 miles **(Waypoint 2)**. To the left is a wide break in the trees where you can see for miles, with lowlands extending to the western horizon. A trail to the right marked LOWERS leads to the lower climbing crag. Go straight toward the upper climbing area, traveling north across the field to continue up the mountain and begin a steep ascent on an old roadbed of red earth.

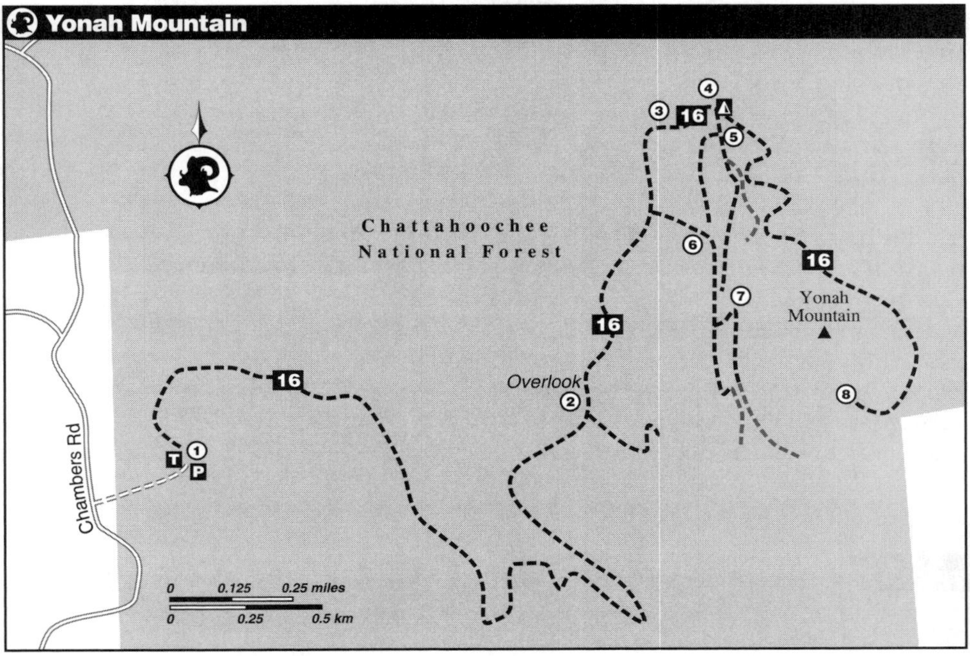

Yonah Mountain

Chattahoochee National Forest
Chambers Rd
Overlook
Yonah Mountain
16
0 0.125 0.25 miles
0 0.25 0.5 km

At 1.4 miles a narrow trail on the right provides alternate access to the upper cliff faces. Continue straight, traveling north. At 1.5 miles **(Waypoint 3)** turn right onto a gravel road and travel east to ascend. You soon reach a wide clearing that rangers use as a staging area and where camping is allowed for those who wish to spend the night on the mountain **(Waypoint 4)**.

To the right are two trails. Of these two trails, the path to the right provides the more direct access to the cliff face, while the one to the left takes you on a nice walk toward the mountain summit. To reach one of the best views on the mountain, take the trail to the right and proceed to **Waypoint 5**. Turn right to follow the trail toward the Boulder, traveling west. At **Waypoint 6**, continue straight toward the Main Face, traveling south on a narrow, rocky path that leads to its base. Turn left and walk north to reach a rock

Climbing the high granite flank of Yonah Mountain

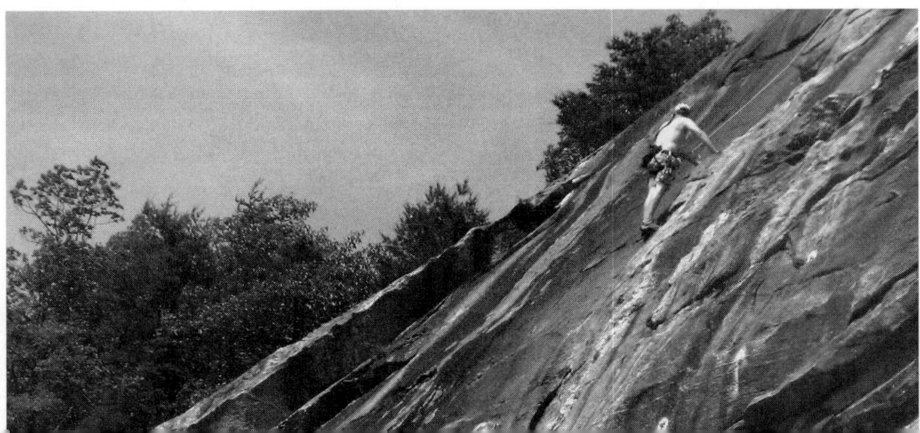

outcrop (**Waypoint 7**). From the base of this large granite face you enjoy an impressive view of a long run of rolling, forested hills in the Chattahoochee National Forest, as well as a broad expanse of farm- and pastureland.

From the clearing at **Waypoint 4**, if you take the trail to the left, you will reach the intersection of several trails at **Waypoint 8.** Take the leftmost path, which is gravel, and climb gradually to the east. Hike for another half mile, crossing beds of exposed granite, to reach the large, circular clearing at the mountain summit. This grassy opening is ringed with trees, so there are no clear views. But, on a blue-sky day it's a good place to rest and enjoy some sunshine. Retrace your step to walk back down the mountain.

UTM WAYPOINTS

1. 17S 250206E 3836205N
2. 17S 250857E 3836212N
3. 17S 251010E 3836674N
4. 17S 251091E 3836706N
5. 17S 251098E 3836660N
6. 17S 251072E 3836498N
7. 17S 251100E 3836377N
8. 17S 251282E 3836210N

TRIP 17 Chicopee Woods: West Lake & East Lake Trails

Distance	4.6 miles, loop
Hiking Time	2–3 hours
Difficulty	Moderate
Elevation Gain/Loss	+480/-505 feet
Trail Use	Leashed dogs (except Monday–Friday 9 AM–3 PM)
Best Times	Year-round
Agency	Elachee Nature Science Center
Recommended Map	A trail map is available at the visitors center and online at www.elachee.org.

HIGHLIGHTS The West Lake Trail begins in open hardwoods and drops to bottomland forest in the Walnut Creek Valley. You'll pass an impressive 150-foot suspension bridge that crosses Walnut Creek, and traverse more hilly terrain to reach Chicopee Lake. Formed in 1973, the lake has a good overlook and detailed interpretive information on the wetland ecology and is prime birding territory. The center even runs an educational program for students called "Birds of a Feather." From the edge of the lake, you'll circle the Chicopee Aquatic Studies Center, which has a long boardwalk used for educating people about lake wildlife. Then, you pick up the East Lake Trail, which winds through hills of pines and hardwoods, descends into bottomland woods, and finally climbs through oaks to meet the Mathis Loop Trail.

DIRECTIONS From Atlanta take Interstate 85 north to Interstate 985. Take Exit 16 for Oakwood and then turn right off the ramp onto GA Highway 53. Go to the second traffic light and turn left onto Atlanta Highway/GA Highway 13. Continue north on Atlanta Highway, pass the Chicopee Woods Golf Course, and then turn right onto Elachee Drive. Cross I-985 and, at the road split, bear right to continue to the trailhead parking loop, or bear left to go to the science center.

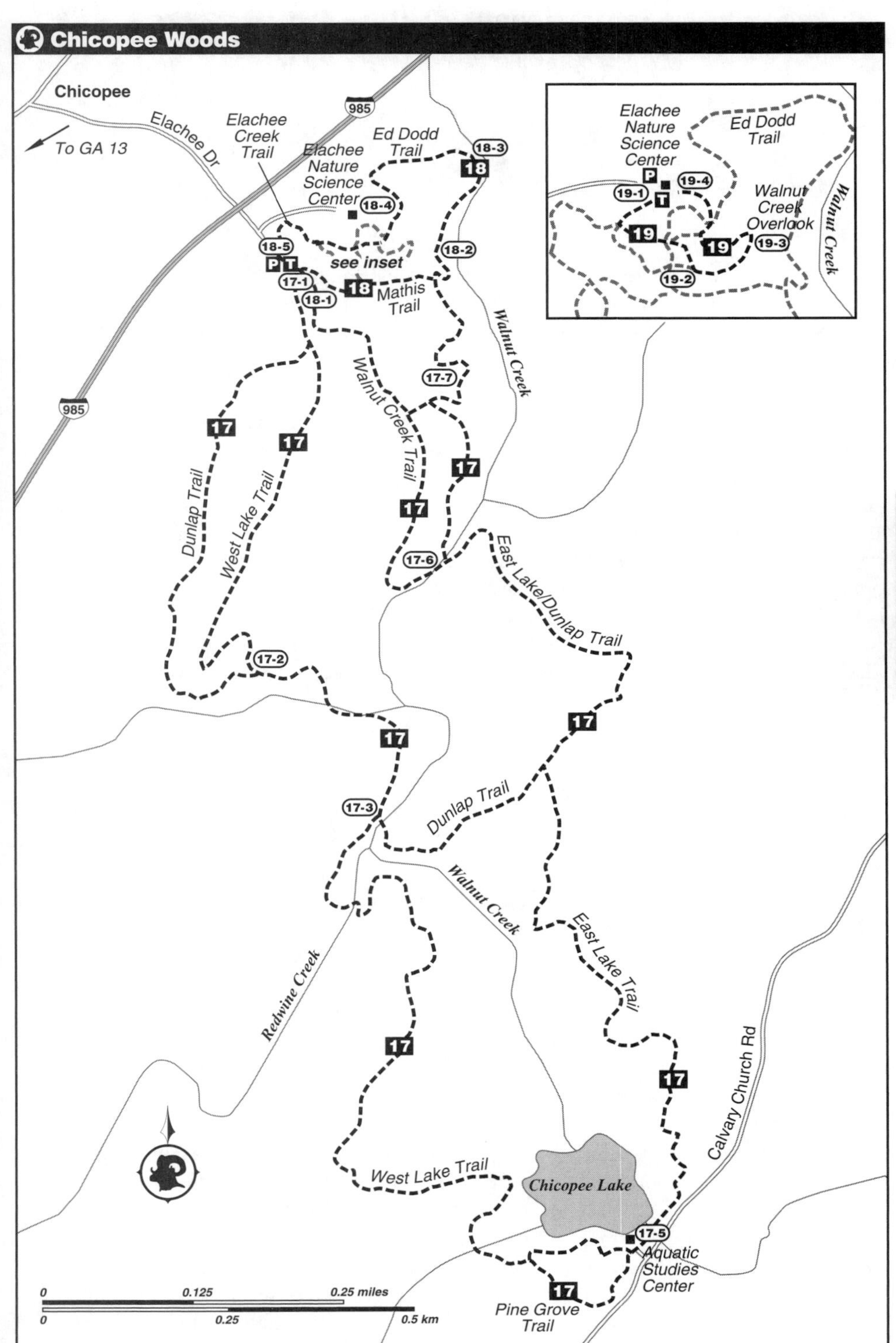
Chicopee Woods
Chicopee
985
Elachee Dr
To GA 13
Elachee Creek Trail
Elachee Nature Science Center
Ed Dodd Trail
18-3
18
18-4
18-5
P
T
17-1
18-1
see inset
18
Mathis Trail
18-2
Walnut Creek
17-7
Walnut Creek Trail
985
17
17
17
17
Dunlap Trail
West Lake Trail
17-6
East Lake/Dunlap Trail
17-2
17
17
17-3
Dunlap Trail
Walnut Creek
East Lake Trail
Redwine Creek
17
17
Calvary Church Rd
West Lake Trail
Chicopee Lake
17-5
Aquatic Studies Center
17
Pine Grove Trail
0
0.125
0.25 miles
0
0.25
0.5 km
Elachee Nature Science Center
Ed Dodd Trail
P
19-4
19-1
T
Walnut Creek Overlook
Walnut Creek
19
19
19-3
19-2

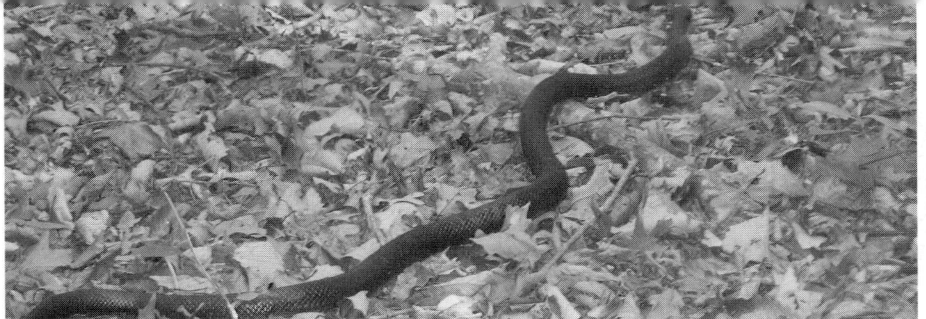

Rat snake slithering beside the Mathis Loop Trail

FACILITIES/TRAILHEAD There are no facilities at the trailhead (the nearest restrooms are at the science center), and you should plan to pack in water for longer hikes. There is no fee to park at the trailhead, though you are encouraged to make a donation to support trail maintenance.

At the south end of the circular parking area enter the West Lake Trail **(Waypoint 1)** and travel southeast through an airy forest of oak and hickory. After 100 feet, the Dunlap Trail enters on the right, but continue southeast following orange blazes to continue on the West Lake Trail.

At 326 feet, to the left is the Lake Loop Mathis Connector Trail. Bear right and keep going southwest on the West Lake Trail. For the next half mile you take an easy walk through more open forest of oaks, hickory trees, maples, and pines. At 0.6 mile the path drops to Vulture Rock Creek **(Waypoint 2)** where the Dunlap Trail joins the West Lake Trail. Turn left and walk east following red and orange blazes. With fern beds covering the forest floor and a heavy tree canopy blocking sunlight, this bottomland forest is more like a jungle. You pass a sign marked NEOTROPICAL BIRD MONITORING STATION. This habitat attracts birds that breed in the U.S. or Canada during summer, and then fly to Mexico, Central America, South America, or the Caribbean during winter. (The science center provides information on why their populations are decreasing.)

Just past the 1-mile point in your hike **(Waypoint 3)** a hefty 150-foot suspension bridge is to your left. (The Dunlap Trail continues across the bridge and connects to the East Lake Trail on the opposite side.) To continue on the West Lake Trail, at **Waypoint 3** turn right and ascend the earth steps. You climb and then level out on a ridge before descending to the overlook on the west side of Chicopee Lake **(Waypoint 4)**.

At 2.3 miles you can bear right at a Y junction to take the short Pine Grove Trail, but I recommend that you continue straight on the West Lake Trail. The path drops to a point just above lake level where an opening in the brush nicely frames the still lake and deep green forest encircling it. An OPEN WATER sign highlights a few of the birds you may spy on the lake, and interpretive signs in this stretch offer good detail on the wetland habitat.

The West Lake Trail ends at the Aquatic Studies Center. Circle around it, and on the northwest side of the parking area enter the East Lake Trail **(Waypoint 5)**. Cross Boulder Creek to reach a trail junction where the Dunlap Trail joins the East Lake Trail. Turn right and travel east to climb briefly through woods with a good mix of sun and shade before dropping steeply back down toward the creek.

At **Waypoint 6** you cross a wood footbridge, and the combination East Lake/Dunlap Trail intersects with the Walnut Creek Trail. Turn right and travel northeast to continue on the East Lake/Dunlap Trail. The path rises gradually to an intersection with the Mathis Loop **(Waypoint 7)**. Turn left onto the blue-blazed Mathis Loop Trail, traveling southwest. Walk 140 feet and turn right at the next trail junction (with the Walnut Creek Trail) to take the Mathis Loop Trail to the parking area. Keep your eyes peeled as you round the next hill—I once came upon a 5-foot rat snake which, according to a local hiker, is a regular around here. This fairly mellow snake, with an impressively thick body, paid me little attention and scooted off into the trees slowly as I approached.

UTM WAYPOINTS

1. 17S 239077E 3792828N
2. 17S 238946E 3792069N
3. 17S 239171E 3791743N
4. 17S 239400E 3790906N
5. 17S 239431E 3790732N
6. 17S 239341E 3792294N
7. 17S 239316E 3792672N

TRIP 18 Chicopee Woods: Mathis Trail, Ed Dodd Trail, & Elachee Creek Loop

see map on p. 143

Distance	1.5–1.8 miles, loop
Hiking Time	1 hour
Difficulty	Moderate
Elevation Gain/Loss	+/-455 feet
Trail Uses	Leashed dogs (except Monday–Friday 9 AM–3 PM) and good for kids
Best Times	Year-round
Agency	Elachee Nature Science Center
Recommended Map	A trail map is available at the visitors center or online at www.elachee.org.

HIGHLIGHTS The Elachee nature trails include several short loops that explore the creeks and rolling hardwood forest areas south and east of the Elachee Nature Science Center. The Ed Dodd Trail (0.75 mile) follows Walnut Creek, passing an interesting stream restoration project. Fern beds surround the Elachee Creek Trail (0.5 mile), which follows the stream and climbs the wooded slopes overlooking the creek valley. The Mathis Trail (0.7 mile) includes some brief, steep climbing as it makes a southern loop, but it then turns north and takes an easy grade to cross Elachee Creek and meet the Ed Dodd Trail. The paved Geiger Trail (also a braille-signed interpretive path) is a 0.5-mile loop that takes you to the Walnut Creek Overlook, which sits at treetop level for a bird's-eye view of the creek valley. The current hike combines several of these trails in a not-so-difficult 1.5-mile loop.

DIRECTIONS From Atlanta take Interstate 85 north to Interstate 985. Take Exit 16 for Oakwood and then turn right off the ramp onto GA Highway 53. Go to the second traffic light and turn left onto Atlanta Highway/GA Highway 13. Continue north on Atlanta Highway, pass the Chicopee Woods Golf Course, and then turn right onto Elachee Drive. Cross I-985 and, at the road split, bear right to continue to the trailhead parking loop, or bear left to go to the science center.

FACILITIES/TRAILHEAD There are no facilities at the trailhead (the nearest restrooms are at the science center), and you should plan to pack in water for longer hikes. There is no fee to park at the trailhead, though you are encouraged to make a donation to support trail maintenance.

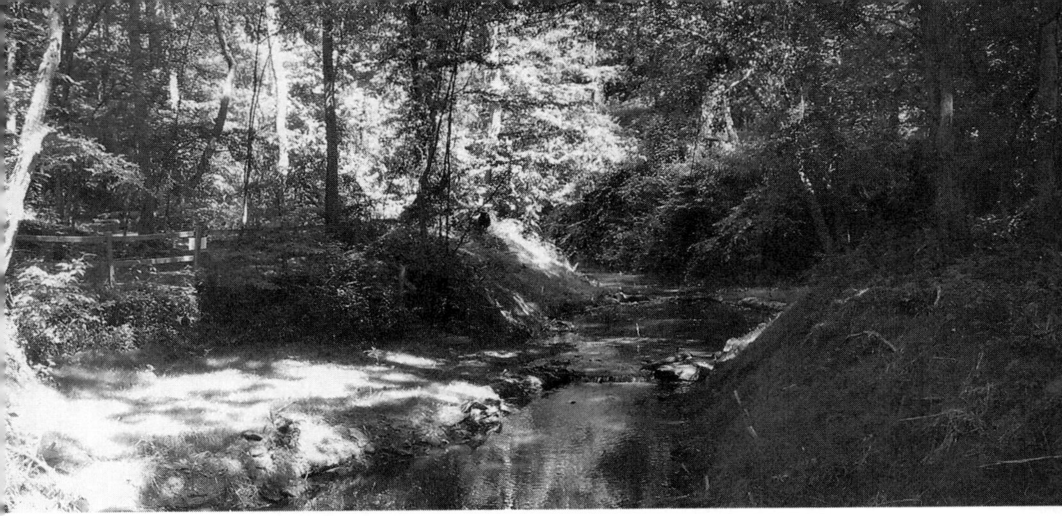

Rehabilitated stretch of Walnut Creek

From the north side of the parking area, enter the trail just beyond the bulletin board **(Waypoint 1)**. You descend immediately to a trail junction. Turn right to travel south on the blue-blazed Mathis Loop Trail. The path climbs through oak-dominated woods and then drops to the junction with the Walnut Creek Trail at 0.3 mile. Turn left to travel northeast and continue your descent. After walking less than a tenth of a mile, you turn sharply to the west to quickly gain 130 feet of elevation before heading down the east side of the slope.

At 0.7 mile the Mathis Trail meets the Ed Dodd Trail at a T junction **(Waypoint 2)**. (If you turn left, the Ed Dodd Trail leads to the Elachee Creek Trail and a spot where benches overlook the stream.) To continue a longer loop, turn right at **Waypoint 2** and descend steps to the bank of Walnut Creek set in hickory trees as well as tall poplars and oaks.

Perhaps the best section of the trail is at 0.8 mile **(Waypoint 3)** where Walnut Creek has been restored to stop bank erosion and improve the water quality. An interpretive sign has dramatic before and after photos of the stream, and you can see that its grassy banks were once crumbling dirt. Flowing through a nice mix of sun and shade, the stream slides over small steps and collects in clear pools.

At 0.9 mile, bear left to turn away from the creek and ascend to the west. The trail ends at the northeast side of the science center (1.1 miles). Take the concrete walkway around the center to rejoin the Ed Dodd Loop at **Waypoint 4**. Walk another 540 feet to the junction of the Ed Dodd and the Elachee Creek trails.

Turn right onto the Elachee Trail and ascend to the picnic area, which sits in the shade of surrounding forest. From the picnic area, turn left onto the paved Geiger Trail to circle around the picnic area and rejoin the Elachee Trail. Traveling northwest, you gain ground in clear forest and bend around a draw. The trail then descends to a junction with the Mathis Trail **(Waypoint 5)**. From here you can bear left to stay on the Elachee Trail and walk down to the creek. Or, bear right onto the Mathis Trail, walk a short distance, and turn right at a trail junction to return to the parking area.

UTM WAYPOINTS

1. 17S 239061E 3792903N
2. 17S 239369E 3792931N
3. 17S 239468E 3793154N
4. 17S 239203E 3793051N
5. 17S 239067E 3792976N

TRIP 19 Chicopee Woods: Geiger Trail

Distance	1.0 mile, out-and-back
Hiking Time	30 minutes to 1 hour
Difficulty	Easy
Elevation Gain/Loss	+90/-80 feet
Trail Uses	Accessible for people with disabilities or limited mobility and good for kids
Best Times	Year-round
Agency	Elachee Nature Science Center
Recommended Map	A trail map is available at the visitors center and online at www.elachee.org.

see map on p. 143

HIGHLIGHTS Designed for people with limited mobility or disabilities, the paved Geiger Trail winds easily along the slopes above the Walnut Creek Valley. It is not only wheelchair accessible, but also has braille interpretive signs. Well-shaded in hardwood forest, the path runs by the Walnut Creek Overlook, which sits among the treetops and provides a good view of the forested creek valley.

DIRECTIONS From Atlanta take Interstate 85 north to Interstate 985. Take Exit 16 for Oakwood and then turn right off the ramp onto GA Highway 53. Go to the second traffic light and turn left onto Atlanta Highway/GA Highway 13. Continue north on Atlanta Highway, pass the Chicopee Woods Golf Course, and then turn right onto Elachee Drive. Cross I-985 and, at the road split, bear right to continue to the trailhead parking loop, or bear left to go to the science center.

FACILITIES/TRAILHEAD There are no facilities at the trailhead (the nearest restrooms are at the science center), and you should plan to pack in water for longer hikes. There is no fee to park at the trailhead, though you are encouraged to make a donation to support trail maintenance.

The trail can be accessed at the picnic area **(Waypoint 1)** or the rear of the science center. From the picnic area, the path goes northwest to a junction with the Elachee Creek Trail. Continue to follow the paved trail, which turns southeast to circle around the picnic area.

You cross the Ed Dodd Trail and then descend gradually to a trail junction **(Waypoint 2)**. The path to the right leads to the Ed Dodd Trail. To continue on the Geiger Trail, turn left and walk east another 360 feet to the Walnut Creek Overlook on the right **(Waypoint 3)**. At this wood platform there is an interpretive sign (including braille) that provides an overview of the plants and animals that thrive in the Walnut Creek Valley.

From the overlook, the trail moves up the slope and hooks to the southeast, arriving at the side of the science center where there are benches and a podium for outdoor education. This is effectively the end of the attractive portion of the Geiger Trail. If you bear right, you can continue circling the east side of the center until the trail ends at the building **(Waypoint 4)**. Retrace your route on the Geiger Trail to return to the picnic area.

UTM WAYPOINTS

1. 17S 239130E 3793043N
2. 17S 239230E 3792956N
3. 17S 239320E 3793003N
4. 17S 239241E 3793120N

TRIP 20 Unicoi State Park: Smith Creek Trail

Distance	8.7 miles, out-and-back
Hiking Time	4 hours
Difficulty	Moderate
Elevation Gain/Loss	+/-1915 feet
Trail Use	Leashed dogs
Best Times	Year-round
Agency	Unicoi State Park
Recommended Map	A *Unicoi State Lodge Park Trail Map* is available at the visitors center and online at www.gastateparks.org.

HIGHLIGHTS The well-marked Smith Creek Trail is not difficult, but its rewards are great. The trail's name is actually deceiving, as it follows another stream (not Smith Creek) briefly before it climbs through open hardwood forest, crosses several streams, and ventures into wild coves of thick rhododendron. The path tops Hickorynut Ridge and then descends a west-facing slope with good winter views. The trail then circles around Smith Mountain and reaches the Anna Ruby Falls Scenic Area where separate falls—one 153 feet tall and another 50 feet tall—plunge into a lush cove.

DIRECTIONS From Atlanta take Interstate 85 north to Interstate 985. Take I-985 to Exit 24 for GA Highway 369. Turn left onto GA 369 west, go 0.6 mile, and turn right onto U.S. Highway 129 north. Take U.S. 129 to Cleveland. From the town square in Cleveland, go 0.4 mile and turn right onto GA Highway 75. Travel east on GA 75 9.7 miles, passing through Helen, and turn right onto GA Highway 356. Go 1.8 miles on GA 356 and turn right at the sign for the Unicoi Lodge and Conference Center. To reach the trailhead from the Unicoi Lodge and Conference Center, turn left onto GA 356, and then take the next right turn onto S. Unicoi Campground Drive. Go 0.6 mile and park at the gray A-frame building on the left. The trailhead is across S. Unicoi Campground Rd.

As described here, the Smith Creek Trail hike begins at Unicoi State Park, but it can also be accessed from the Anna Ruby Falls Scenic Area. To reach this from Atlanta, take I-85 north to I-985. Take I-985 to Exit 24 for GA 369. Turn left onto GA 369 west, go 0.6 mile, and turn right onto U.S. 129 north. Take U.S. 129 to Cleveland. From the town square in Cleveland, go 0.4 mile and turn right onto GA 75. Travel east on GA 75 9.7 miles, passing through Helen, and turn right onto GA 356. Travel 1.3 miles, turn left onto Smith Creek Road, and follow signs for the Anna Ruby Falls parking area.

FACILITIES/TRAILHEAD There are no facilities at the trailhead, but there is a restroom at the parking area for the Anna Ruby Falls Recreation Trail. Pack enough water for several hours of walking. There is a $3 parking fee. You can purchase an Annual ParkPass for $30 by calling (770) 389-7401. The park has 82 tent, trailer, and RV sites ($22–$24), 34 walk-in campsites ($14 per person), and 30 cottages ($99–$139).

On the east side of South Unicoi Campground Drive, enter the marked trail **(Waypoint 1)** and follow blue blazes to climb through hardwoods and high mountain laurel. The path parallels the road for 0.4 mile and then moves away from it and drops into heavy cover of hemlocks. At 0.5 mile, descend wood steps and take a footbridge across the creek.

The trail then moves from moody, shaded areas with multiple layers of tree canopy to stretches where the sun breaks

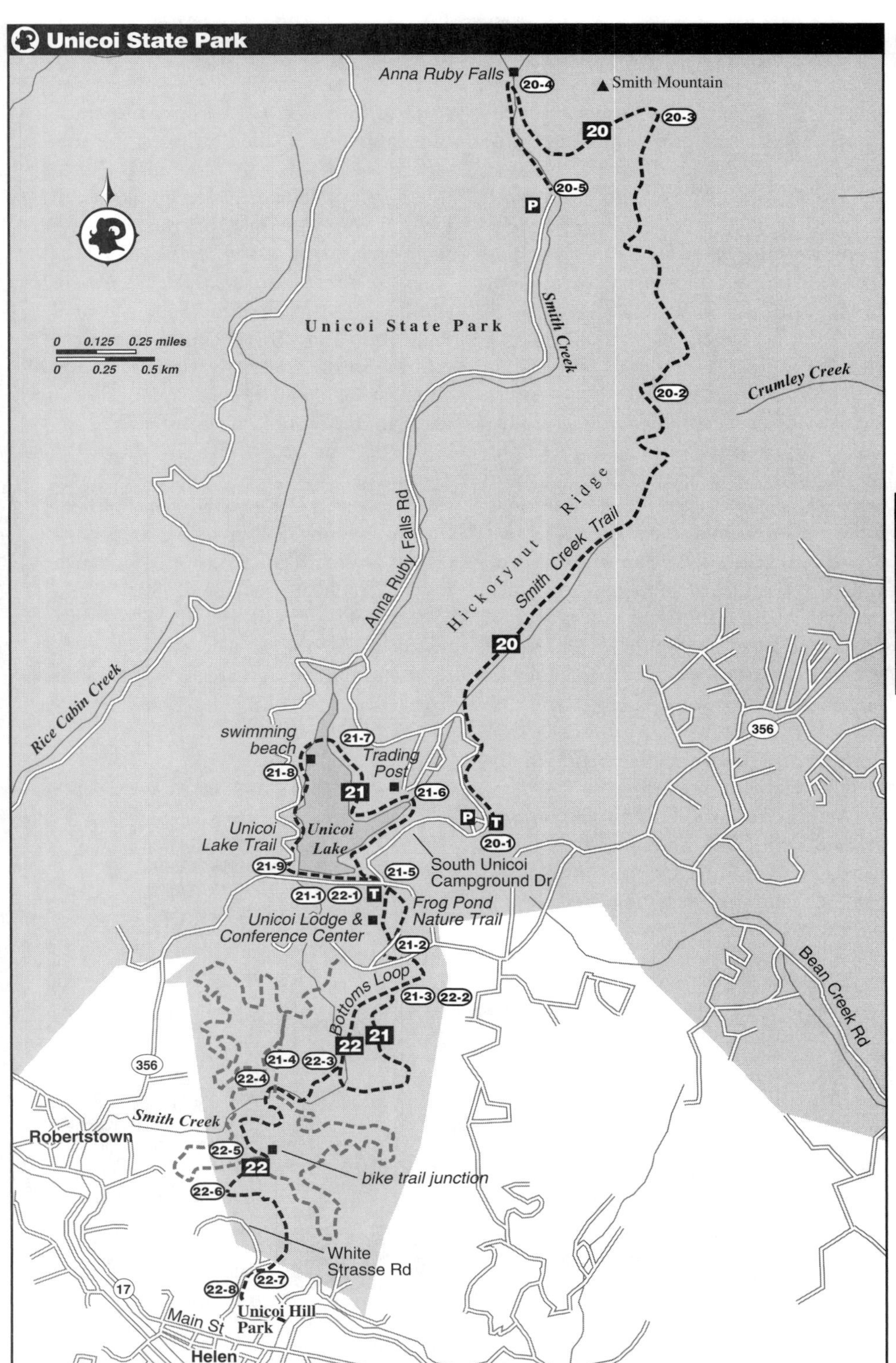
Unicoi State Park
Anna Ruby Falls
20-4
Smith Mountain
20-3
20
20-5
P
Smith Creek
Unicoi State Park
0 0.125 0.25 miles
0 0.25 0.5 km
Crumley Creek
20-2
Hickorynut Ridge
Smith Creek Trail
Anna Ruby Falls Rd
20
Rice Cabin Creek
356
swimming beach
21-7
Trading Post
21-8
21
21-6
P
T
Unicoi Lake Trail
Unicoi Lake
20-1
South Unicoi Campground Dr
21-9
21-5
21-1
22-1
T
Frog Pond Nature Trail
Unicoi Lodge & Conference Center
21-2
Bottoms Loop
21-3
22-2
Bean Creek Rd
22
21
356
21-4
22-3
22-4
Smith Creek
Robertstown
22-5
22
bike trail junction
22-6
White Strasse Rd
17
22-8
22-7
Unicoi Hill Park
Main St
Helen

through the treetops. As you continue along the narrow, shallow creek, the forest opens and fern beds sprawl across its floor. On each side of the trail, the ravine slopes rise steeply, and the path crosses the stream again. You ascend Hickorynut Ridge and at 2 miles **(Waypoint 2)** walk along its spine in hallways of mountain laurel. Climbing higher, you have views of the valley to the east, and then reach the crest, where the forest is primarily shortleaf pine.

The trail then descends the western slope of Hickorynut Ridge, where pines give way to hardwoods and mountain laurel. Walk down a set of dirt and wood steps and cross a stream flowing through a flourish of ferns and rhododendron.

At 3.2 miles **(Waypoint 3)** you drop through a tunnel of foliage so thick that nearly all light is blocked out, and soon cross a tributary of Smith Creek. When you cross, the trail changes from a north-facing slope to south-facing, and the environment changes abruptly. The rhododendron and other cove plants disappear, and hardwoods thrive.

Walking among large oaks, circle around Smith Mountain and turn north to parallel Smith Creek. At 4 miles **(Waypoint 4)** you reach the first observation platform for Anna Ruby Falls. This 50-foot column of water is the final plunge of York Creek, which flows in from the east. Continue across the ravine to reach the platform near the bottom of the second set of falls. Formed by Curtis Creek, this 150-foot deluge crashes and kicks up a cloud of mist, which offers some cool relief on a warm day.

From the platforms, you can walk south on the Anna Ruby Falls National Recreation Trail. This 0.4-mile paved path follows Smith Creek and winds among large hardwoods. The swift stream shoots through rock piles, wells up in churning pools, and races off again down the ravine.

At 4.3 miles, the paved path ends at the Anna Ruby Falls parking area **(Waypoint 5)**, which has a restroom. To return to the trailhead at Unicoi State Park, retrace your steps on the paved path. At platforms for the smaller waterfall, turn right and retrace your steps on the Smith Creek Trail.

UTM WAYPOINTS

1. 17S 251308E 3846092N
2. 17S 252424E 3848453N
3. 17S 252505E 3849889N
4. 17S 251750E 3850166N
5. 17S 251929E 3849551N

Christmas ferns line the low trails in Unicoi State Park.

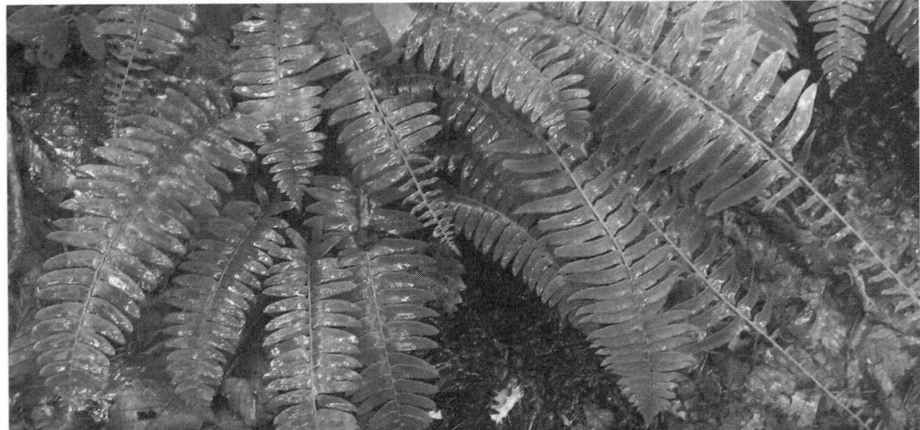

TRIP 21 Unicoi State Park: Bottoms Loop & Lake Trail

Distance	4.2 miles, loop
Hiking Time	2 hours
Difficulty	Easy
Elevation Gain/Loss	+/-420 feet
Trail Uses	Leashed dogs and good for kids
Best Times	Year-round
Agency	Unicoi State Park
Recommended Map	A *Unicoi State Lodge Park Trail Map* is available at the visitors center and online at www.gastateparks.org.

HIGHLIGHTS The Bottoms Loop Trail takes a quiet turn through rhododendron thickets, large hardwoods, and pines to visit rippling Smith Creek and an idyllic frog pond. Along the trail interpretive signs highlight its microhabitats and identify various tree species. From Bottoms Loop, you can cross GA Highway 356 to stroll around Unicoi Lake. Six fishing piers dot the lakeshore, though only two were occupied with folks casting their lines to reel in catfish and bream when I scouted this area. On the northwest shore, the lakeside beach was deserted, but I could imagine that it must be lively on a summer afternoon with swimmers splashing about and laughter carrying across the lake.

DIRECTIONS From Atlanta take Interstate 85 north to Interstate 985. Take I-985 to Exit 24 for GA Highway 369. Turn left onto GA 369 west, go 0.6 mile, and turn right onto U.S. Highway 129 north. Take U.S. 129 to Cleveland. From the town square in Cleveland, go 0.4 mile and turn right onto GA Highway 75. Travel east on GA 75 9.7 miles, passing through Helen, and turn right onto GA Highway 356. Go 1.8 miles on GA 356, and turn right at the sign for the UNICOI LODGE AND CONFERENCE CENTER.

FACILITIES/TRAILHEAD There are no facilities at the trailhead, but there is a restroom at the lodge and conference center as well as at the parking area at the lake's southwest end. There is a $3 parking fee for the park. You can purchase an Annual ParkPass for $30 by calling (770) 389-7401.

The Bottoms Loop Trail begins on the east side of the road that leads to the lodge, near the junction with GA 356 **(Waypoint 1)**. Enter the trail marked for the UNICOI TO HELEN TRAIL, BOTTOMS LOOP TRAIL, and TENNIS COURTS. You soon reach a junction with the Frog Pond Nature Trail. Continue straight and travel south on the trail marked with yellow and green blazes. Pass the tennis courts, and at 0.2 mile **(Waypoint 2)** the Frog Pond Nature Trail again intersects on the left. Rather than turning onto it, continue straight to travel south and cross Unicoi Bottoms Road. Enter the trail marked UNICOI HELEN TRAIL and ascend through mountain laurel and large hardwoods blanketed with moss.

A gradual descent takes you to a trail junction at 0.5 mile **(Waypoint 3)**. Take a sharp left turn and cross a stream to walk through ferns and poplars. Rising out of the bottomland, you enter a pine forest with a significant number of damaged trees. After crossing a low hill, the trail turns north and joins Smith Creek.

At 1.2 miles **(Waypoint 4)** there is a T junction where a long wood footbridge crosses Smith Creek. Turn right to take the trail marked LODGE and travel northeast following green and yellow blazes.

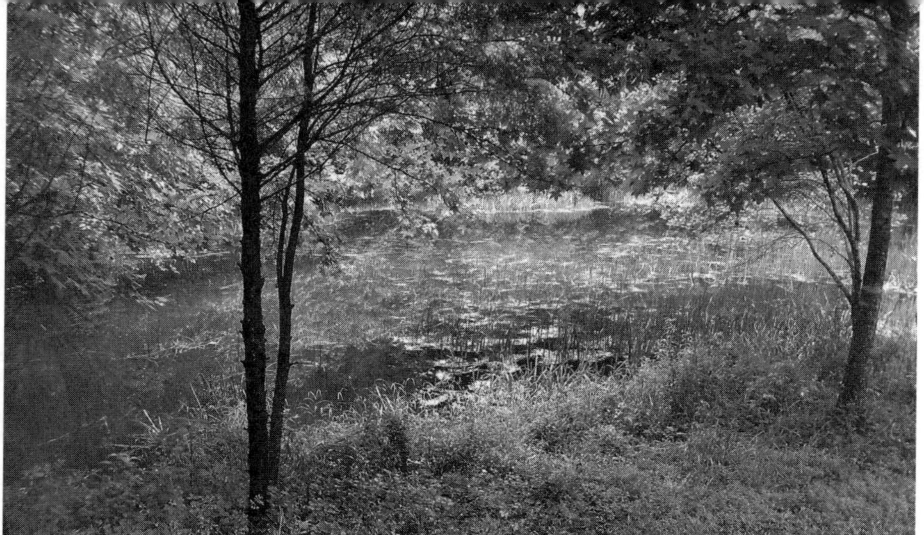

Frog Pond Trail

The trail cuts across a field and then enters dense pines and hardwoods.

Cross Unicoi Bottom Road again, and at 1.9 miles turn right at **Waypoint 2** to take the Frog Pond Trail. The marshy pool lies to the left at the edge of a sunlit clearing. From the pond, continue northeast across the grassy opening and enter the trees near an interpretive sign for microhabitats.

Ahead, look for markers that identify several types of trees. There is one especially attractive spot where a large pitch pine, sourwood tree, and eastern hemlock form a tight trio.

Back at **Waypoint 1**, cross GA 356 to enter the Lake Loop Trail at the sign marked COTTAGES/CAMPGROUND/LAKE TRAIL **(Waypoint 5)**. The yellow-blazed path takes the high ground, with Unicoi Lake visible below on your left. Shaded by hemlocks, pines, and hardwoods, the trail passes an odd collection of cylindrical cabins and rolls easily along a finger of the lake. As I walked the lakeside path when I scouted this hike, a couple in a canoe were out for a leisurely paddle, while the shadows of hemlocks and pines crept across the water.

At **Waypoint 6**, turn left and then take another left to walk the path on the eastern side of the Trading Post, a store with T-shirts and other gifts. The trail returns to the lake and follows the shoreline. At **Waypoint 7**, bear left at a Y junction and travel northwest, following yellow blazes. At the northern end of the lake, descend wood and gravel steps and take the wood bridge across the water.

Cross the sandy swimming beach and pick up the path at the LAKE TRAIL sign. At **Waypoint 8** bear left at the Y junction to wind along the western shore of the lake with clear views of the water. The path ends at a paved parking area with a restroom **(Waypoint 9)**. To return to the lodge parking lot, walk to GA 356 and turn left. Cross the lake dam, continue east along GA 356 and turn right at the sign for UNICOI LODGE AND CONFERENCE CENTER.

UTM WAYPOINTS

1. 17S 250814E 3845744N
2. 17S 250797E 3845453N
3. 17S 250821E 3845229N
4. 17S 250498E 3844829N
5. 17S 250807E 3845793N
6. 17S 250976E 3846279N
7. 17S 250593E 3846508N
8. 17S 250402E 3846459N
9. 17S 250300E 3845931N

TRIP 22 Unicoi State Park: Unicoi to Helen Trail

Distance	5.3 miles, out-and-back
Hiking Time	2–3 hours
Difficulty	Easy
Elevation Gain/Loss	+/-895 feet
Trail Use	Leashed dogs
Best Times	Year-round
Agency	Unicoi State Park
Recommended Map	A *Unicoi State Lodge Park Trail Map* is available at the visitors center and online at www.gastateparks.org.

see map on p. 149

HIGHLIGHTS A prime tourist destination, Helen draws thousands of visitors each fall when the mountain foliage beams red and gold, and the town hosts its annual Oktoberfest. Helen's Bavarian-style architecture sets it apart from other Georgia towns, and you will see the characteristic sloped brown roofs and timbering on everything from restaurants to souvenir shops.

From Unicoi State Park, you can walk to town on Unicoi to Helen Trail, which begins on the road to Unicoi State Park Lodge and Conference Center. The route first follows the Bottoms Loop Trail and departs it to cross Smith Creek. You'll walk through hardwoods and hemlocks, climb a ridge, and then drop into a creek drainage. Near town, the trail skirts White Strasse Road, which leads to GA Highway 17, the main street through Helen. After touching White Strasse, the trail bends to the southeast and ends at Unicoi Hill Park. From the park, you can walk south to meet GA 17.

DIRECTIONS From Atlanta take Interstate 85 north to Interstate 985. Take I-985 to Exit 24 for GA Highway 369. Turn left onto GA 369 west, go 0.6 mile, and turn right onto U.S. Highway 129 north. Take U.S. 129 to Cleveland. From the town square in Cleveland go 0.4 mile and turn right onto GA Highway 75. Travel east on GA 75 9.7 miles, passing through Helen and turn right onto GA Highway 356. Go 1.8 miles on GA 356 and turn right at the sign for the Unicoi Lodge and Conference Center.

FACILITIES/TRAILHEAD There are no facilities at the trailhead, but there is a restroom at the Unicoi Park Lodge and Conference Center. There is a $3 parking fee for the park. You can purchase an Annual ParkPass for $30 by calling (770) 389-7401.

The hike begins on the east side of the road that leads to the Unicoi Park Lodge and Conference Center, near the junction with GA 356 **(Waypoint 1)**. Enter the trail marked for the UNICOI TO HELEN TRAIL, BOTTOMS LOOP TRAIL and TENNIS COURTS. You soon reach a junction with the Frog Pond Nature Trail. Continue straight and travel south on the trail marked with yellow and green blazes. Pass the tennis courts and continue straight at the next junction with the Frog Pond Nature Trail. Travel south and cross Unicoi Bottoms Road. Enter the trail marked UNICOI HELEN TRAIL and ascend through mountain laurel and hardwoods.

A gradual descent takes you to a trail junction at 0.5 mile **(Waypoint 2)**. Continue straight on the Unicoi to Helen Trail, traveling southwest. At a broad clearing, turn left and walk along the edge of the field, passing wood posts with yellow and green markings.

At 0.9 mile **(Waypoint 3)** bear right and take the long wood footbridge across

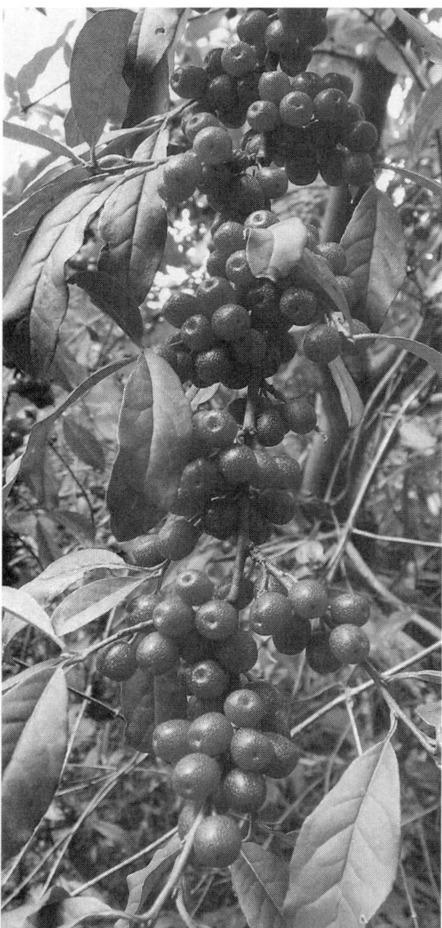

Autumn olives

the slow-flowing Smith Creek, traveling southwest. The dense trees and underbrush suddenly give way to a pleasing forest of hemlocks and high rhododendron. Smith Creek keeps you company, rolling through a stretch of boulders.

At 1.1 miles **(Waypoint 4)** bear left at a Y junction and cross a wood footbridge. The trail then swings past a wetland and rises into hardwoods and mountain laurel, moving up a ridge.

At 1.7 miles **(Waypoint 5)** you reach a high point at a four-way junction with a bike trail. Continue straight and descend through pines and oaks. A creek bed to the left lies beneath a shroud of rhododendron, while open hardwoods sprawl out to the right.

Just beyond the 2-mile mark, you drop into one of the prettiest spots along the trail where a mountain laurel grove shades a four-way trail junction **(Waypoint 6)**. Continue straight, and at the next Y junction bear left and follow the green-blazed path toward Helen. A small creek flows on your left, while the slope to the right is a wild mix of mossy rocks, laurel, pines, and hardwoods. The creek takes a quick, steep drop, forming a small waterfall.

At 2.5 miles **(Waypoint 7)** the trail reaches White Strasse Road and runs beside it briefly. Turn left to dive back into the forest and descend to the trail's end at Unicoi Hill Park **(Waypoint 8)**. From the park you can walk south on White Strasse to intersect GA 17, which runs through Helen. In the 1970s, Helen locals were searching for ways to increase tourist traffic, and they lit on an idea proposed by John Collack, an artist from Clarkesville. While in the U.S. Army, Collack has been stationed in southern Germany, and inspired by his time there, he suggested that Helen be redesigned to resemble a Bavarian village. This new style, which began to be implemented in 1969, turned the town into a prime tourist destination. From **Waypoint 7**, retrace your steps to return to the trailhead.

UTM WAYPOINTS

1. 17S 250823E 3845754N
2. 17S 250822E 3845226N
3. 17S 250500E 3844809N
4. 17S 250155E 3844726N
5. 17S 250009E 3844364N
6. 17S 249686E 3843936N
7. 17S 249902E 3843650N
8. 17S 249812E 3843512N

TRIP 23 Moccasin Creek State Park: Non-Game Interpretive Trail

Distance	1.0 mile, loop
Hiking Time	30 minutes
Difficulty	Easy
Elevation Gain/Loss	+70/-65 feet
Trail Uses	Leashed dogs and good for kids
Best Times	Spring, summer, and fall
Agency	Moccasin Creek State Park
Recommended Maps	An overview map of the park is available at www.gastateparks.org/info/moccasin; USGS 7.5-min. *Lake Burton*

HIGHLIGHTS Within just a mile, the Non-Game Interpretive Trail passes through several wildlife habitats, including streams that house the spotted salamander and open fields that draw raptors in their search for prey. Managed by the Georgia Department of Natural Resources, the trail is designed to not only display wildlife management techniques but also teach people about Georgia's natural resources. There are many signs along the trail that call out notable plants and animals, and this easy loop has plenty of features to keep kids engaged.

DIRECTIONS From Atlanta travel north on Interstate 85 to Interstate 985. Take I-985 north, and then U.S. Highway 23 to U.S. Highway 23/441. Take U.S. Highway 23/441 north to Clayton. From Clayton, take U.S. Highway 76 west 11.2 miles to the intersection with GA Highway 197. Turn left on GA 197 to travel south 3.6 miles and turn right into the fenced-in parking area (across GA 197 from the entrance to Moccasin Creek State Park).

FACILITIES/TRAILHEAD There are no facilities at the trailhead. Moccasin Creek State Park has restrooms, plus sites for tents, trailers, and RVs ($25).

From the parking area, walk 137 feet to the sign marked Wildlife Trail **(Waypoint 1)**. The narrow path follows Moccasin Creek, and you soon see an interpretive sign for river cane, which grows along the banks of many Georgia rivers and creeks. As you proceed, look to the left for a bat box as well as a box to attract bluebirds.

At 0.1 mile **(Waypoint 2)**, bear right at a Y intersection, and then cross the stream (keeping your eyes peeled for the spotted salamander). The trail is especially attractive as it once again skirts the creek, and then turns left at a large rosebay rhododendron. At 0.2 mile **(Waypoint 3)**, a small path on the right leads to an observation tower where you can scan the open field for wildlife.

Continue southwest across the field and you'll find an interpretive sign explaining that this open plot of land creates forest "edges." You're more likely to see a high volume of animals around edges because of the habitat diversity they create. To better understand the extent to which animals use this open ground, check out the "browse enclosure" (a square patch of ground enclosed in a wire fence) at the edge of the field. The grass inside the cage indicates just how high the vegetation in the field would be if it hadn't been grazed by local wildlife. The difference between the height of the grass in the cage and outside the cage can be eye-popping.

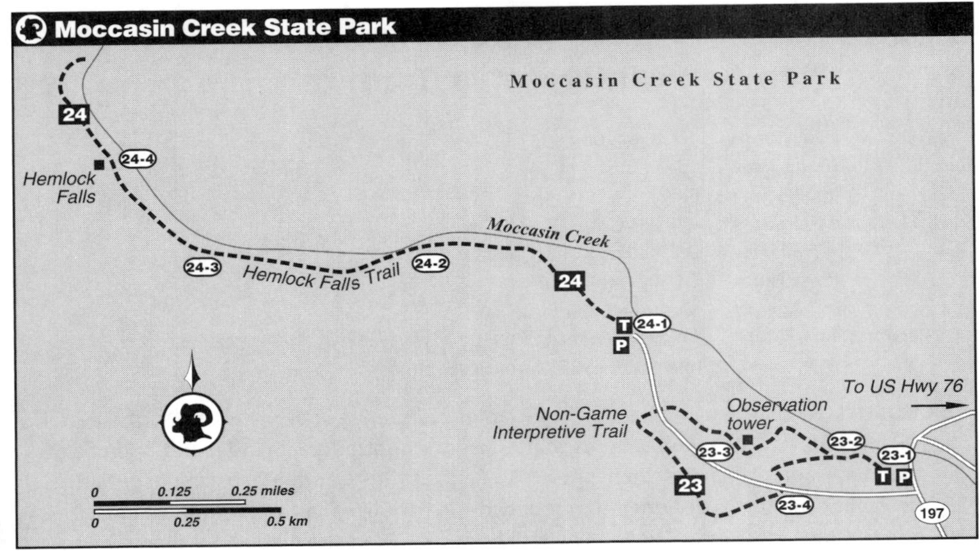

The trail then enters dense forest of pines and hardwoods, and you can scan the woods for trees riddled with holes created by pileated woodpeckers. At 0.4 mile, cross a gravel road and continue southwest. At 0.5 mile the path winds around a pond where you can see wood duck nesting boxes. The birds are attracted to these boxes because they typically nest in tree cavities.

The forest soon changes dramatically as you move from pines and hardwoods into a grove of eastern hemlock trees. Farther on, at the edge of a field, turn right to move along the edge of the opening. You reenter the forest, which now includes poplars and rhododendron. The land in this area serves as a watershed for a stream that you'll cross. Ferns, hemlocks, and laurel also thrive in this wet environment.

At 0.7 mile **(Waypoint 4)** turn left (west) onto the gravel road, walk 30 feet, and turn right to enter the forest going northwest. At the edge of the field turn right and go northeast. At the next intersection **(Waypoint 2)** bear right to return to the trailhead.

UTM WAYPOINTS

1. 17S 263169E 3858881N
2. 17S 263014E 3858927N
3. 17S 262914E 3858977N
4. 17S 262917E 3858863N

Non-Game Interpretive Trail

BAT
HOUSE
These flying mammals can consume more than half their weight in insects each night. Bats are protected in Georgia under State Wildlife Statutes and the Georgia Cave Protection Act. These valuable pest controllers may be attracted to your yard by the addition of a "bat box".

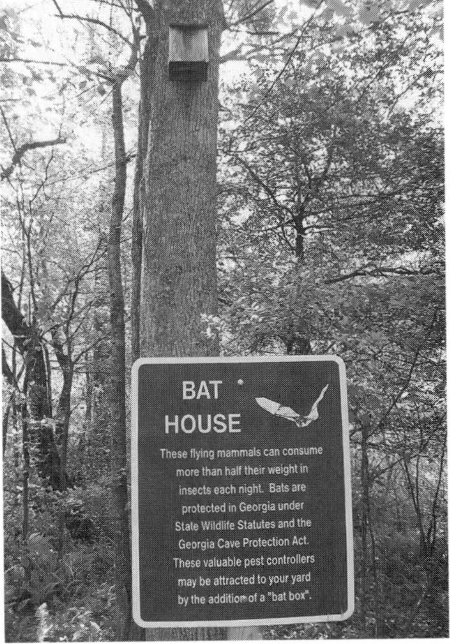

TRIP 24 Moccasin Creek State Park: Hemlock Falls Trail

Distance	1.8–2.3 miles, out-and-back
Hiking Time	1½ hours
Difficulty	Easy
Elevation Gain/Loss	+/-330 feet
Trail Uses	Leashed dogs and good for kids
Best Times	Spring, summer, and fall
Agency	Moccasin Creek State Park
Recommended Map	USGS 7.5-min. *Lake Burton*

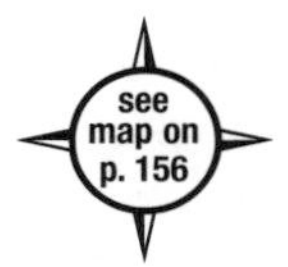
see map on p. 156

HIGHLIGHTS What makes the Hemlock Falls Trail so glorious is that Moccasin Creek is your constant companion—and a rowdy one at that. The wide stream doesn't just "flow" through this lush ravine, it slips, slides, tumbles, and falls in white heaps of churning water. Its roar fills the surrounding forest, which is sometimes bright green, and other times shaded and moody. The trail is not especially difficult, which makes it popular, but its greatest appeal is the set of falls a little less than a mile in. After a 15-foot drop, Hemlock Falls comes down like a hammer, pounding a broad, black and tan rock slab before fanning out into a pool.

DIRECTIONS From Atlanta travel north on Interstate 85 to Interstate 985. Take I-985 north, and then U.S. Highway 23 to U.S. 23/441. Take U.S. 23/441 north to Clayton. From Clayton, take U.S. Highway 76 west 11.2 miles to the intersection with GA Highway 197. Turn left on GA 197 to travel south 3.6 miles, and turn right into the entrance for Lake Burton Wildlife Management Area (across GA 197 from the entrance to Moccasin Creek State Park). At a Y junction in the road, bear left (to the right is the fenced parking area for the Non-Game Interpretive Trail). Travel 0.5 mile to the parking area for Hemlock Falls on the left.

FACILITIES/TRAILHEAD There are no facilities at the trailhead. Moccasin Creek State Park has restrooms, plus sites for tents, trailers, and RVs ($25).

At the northwest side of the parking area **(Waypoint 1)**, enter the Hemlock Falls Trail, which runs along a narrow berm a stone's throw from the creek. About 600 feet down the trail, a small side trail on the right leads to a wide clearing right beside the creek that can be used for camping. It has a fire ring and enough room for four to five tents. About 800 feet down the trail, there is another, less hidden campsite on the right.

The rush of the creek grows louder as you rise above the stream, and a gorgeous scene unfolds at 0.4 mile **(Waypoint 2)**. In the creek below, a band of whitewater squeezes through a small opening between boulders, while above on the far hillside a thin stream of water falls like a natural shower.

The trail rises gradually while Moccasin Creek continues in a string of cascades and grows louder. The drama continues at 0.6 mile **(Waypoint 3)** where the creek slides under a wood footbridge and immediately flows over a series of rock ledges. While walking over the narrow wood planks (when I scouted the area) I was struck by a sudden aroma—the rich smell of earth and creek water, which lingered only in this small pocket and disappeared as I climbed the far bank.

At 0.9 mile **(Waypoint 4)** Hemlock Falls lies to the left and below. Turn left and descend into a low, flat area of thinned forest to access the wide pool below the falls.

When you return to the main trail, you can turn left and continue northwest. About 700 feet farther you can turn left off the trail and descend to the base of the drainage where a small clearing has served as a campsite. About 0.2 mile beyond Hemlock Falls, the trail is practically impassable and disappears into dense brush.

From **Waypoint 4**, retrace your steps going southeast to return to the trailhead.

UTM WAYPOINTS

1. 17S 262557E 3859280N
2. 17S 261982E 3859554N
3. 17S 261621E 3859538N
4. 17S 261312E 3859779N

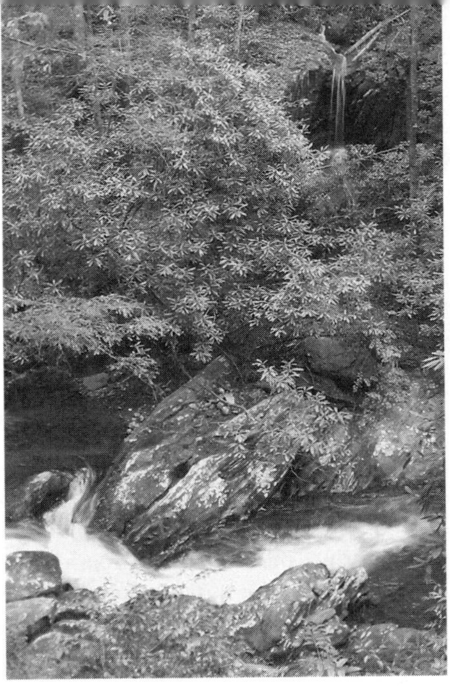

The ever lively Moccasin Creek

TRIP 25 High Shoals Falls Scenic Area & Falls Trail

Distance	2.4 miles, out-and-back
Hiking Time	1½–2 hours
Difficulty	Easy to moderate
Elevation Gain/Loss	+/-500 feet
Trail Uses	Swimming and good for kids
Best Times	Year-round
Agency	U.S. Forest Service, Blue Ridge District
Recommended Map	USGS 7.5-min. *Tray Mountain*

HIGHLIGHTS This is one of those places that you really should try to hit on a warm, sunny day—midweek if possible to avoid crowds—and be sure to bring your swimsuit. The High Shoals Trail snakes down through an inviting hemlock forest to two waterfalls. The first, Blue Hole Falls, gushes into a sunlit pool that makes a great swimming hole. The second waterfall, High Shoals Falls, drops at least 100 feet with water careening down a rough jumble of rock. The trail to the falls is not especially steep, but the sustained climb back to the trailhead makes it moderately difficult.

DIRECTIONS From Atlanta take Interstate 85 north to Interstate 985. Take I-985 to Exit 24 for GA Highway 369. Turn left onto GA 369 west, go 0.6 mile, and turn right onto U.S. Highway 129 North. Take U.S. 129 north to Cleveland, and turn right onto GA Highway 75 toward Helen. From the middle of Helen, continue traveling about 11.3 miles on GA 75 and turn right onto Indian Grave Gap Road (Forest Service Road 283). Travel 1.5 miles, fording the Hiawasee River (actually driving through it) and climbing steeply to the parking area at the sign marked HIGH SHOALS FALLS SCENIC AREA AND BLUE HOLE FALLS.

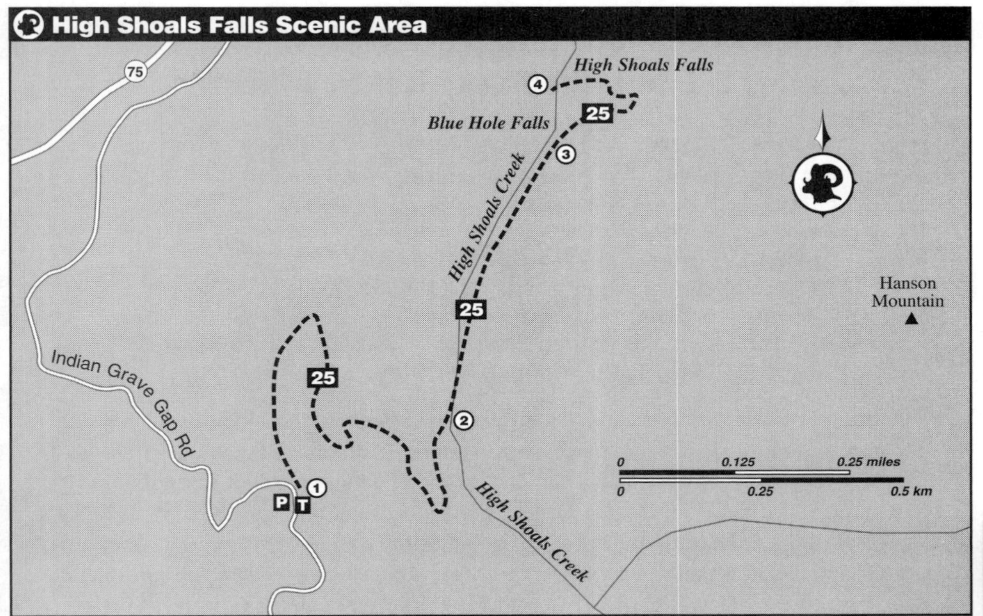

FACILITIES/TRAILHEAD There are no facilities at the trailhead, and there is no fee to use the area.

At the north corner of the gravel parking area **(Waypoint 1)**, descend the dirt path that immediately runs beneath bright orange flame azalea. The trail twists down a slope through mixed hardwoods with mountain laurel providing some shade. Widely spaced trees make for a clear forest, and Hanson Mountain is visible to the immediate northeast.

At 0.5 mile you cross the cove floor where huge hemlocks surround the trail. At 0.6 mile **(Waypoint 2)** cross High Shoals Creek on a wood footbridge. After walking another 0.2 mile, rhododendron forms a tunnel on the trail, and you descend with the creek visible to the left making a series of short but powerful drops.

Blue Hole Falls

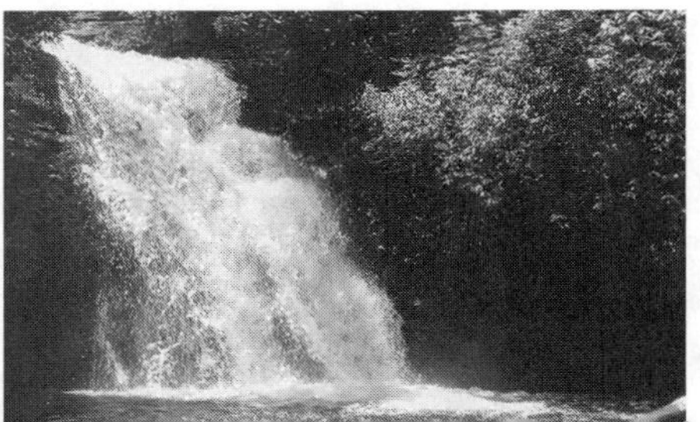

At 0.9 mile **(Waypoint 3)** the trail on the left descends to the observation platform for Blue Hole Falls. You can walk down and around the platform to take a dip in the pool. Back at **Waypoint 3**, turn left and continue descending to a trail junction at the 1-mile mark. Turn left and descend southwest for a little less than 0.2 mile to reach the observation platform for the High Shoals Falls **(Waypoint 4)**.

From the High Shoals Falls, retrace your steps to the trail junction, and turn right to hike back to the trailhead.

UTM WAYPOINTS

1. 17S 250573E 3856056N
2. 17S 250827E 3856154N
3. 17S 251048E 3856644N
4. 17S 251040E 3856720N

TRIP 26 Black Rock Mountain State Park: James E. Edmonds Backcountry Trail

Distance	7.2 miles, loop
Hiking Time	4 hours
Difficulty	Moderate to strenuous
Elevation Gain/Loss	+2095/-2065 feet
Trail Uses	Leashed dogs and backpacking
Best Times	Year-round (spring is best for wildflowers)
Agency	Black Rock Mountain State Park
Recommended Map	A park and trail map is available in the visitors center and online at www.gastateparks.org/info/blackrock.

HIGHLIGHTS Sitting at an altitude of 3640 feet, Black Rock Mountain State Park is the highest state park in Georgia. And its premier path, the James E. Edmonds Backcountry Trail, provides awesome views of the Appalachian Mountains. The must-see spot along the trail is the summit of Lookoff Mountain (3162 feet) where you can gaze across the pastoral Wolffork Valley to ridges that run for dozens of miles. Suitable for a dayhike or an overnight backpacking trip, the trail not only has lofty views but also explores a rich forest that blossoms into a wildflower garden in spring, from bright orange flame azaleas to dwarf irises that form purple bouquets beside the path.

DIRECTIONS From Atlanta take Interstate 85 north to Interstate 985 toward Gainesville. Take I-985 to GA Highway 365, north and travel north to where GA 365 connects with U.S. Highway 32/U.S. Highway 441. Take U.S. 441 north to Mountain City, follow signs to Black Rock Mountain Parkway, and turn left onto Black Rock Mountain Parkway. Go approximately 2.5 miles to reach the trailhead parking on the right at a horseshoe bend in the road. Continue on the road to reach the park office.

FACILITIES/TRAILHEAD There are facilities at the park office but not at the trailhead. There is a $3 parking fee for the park. You can purchase an Annual ParkPass for $30 by calling (770) 389-7401. Camping along the James Edmonds Backcountry Trail is permitted in four designated camping sites only ($5 per person), and reservations are required. Before you hike, obtain a camping permit in the park office. There are water sources along the trail.

At the northeast side of the parking lot, enter the woodchip path **(Waypoint 1)**. At a Y intersection, bear right onto the James Edmonds Backcountry Trail and follow orange blazes, descending on a narrow path lined with ferns. Soon the path becomes heavily shaded by rhododendron and mountain laurel, and in spring you can begin looking for the bright orange blossoms of flame azaleas. The forest transitions to pines and hardwoods, and at 0.7 mile **(Waypoint 2)** bear right at the Y intersection to begin the James Edmonds loop.

At 0.8 mile **(Waypoint 3)** you reach the path to the first designated campsite, Fern Grove. With room for a couple of three-person tents, the site has three wooden benches and a fire ring, plus it lies close to a creek. Continuing on the James Edmonds trail you take a brief walk across a ridge, and then descend steeply and cross Black Rock Road. As the rocky path crosses a northern slope, you're engulfed in heavy mix of hardwoods, laurel, and more rhododendron. At 2.4 miles a wood footbridge crosses a beautiful section of Taylor Creek whose

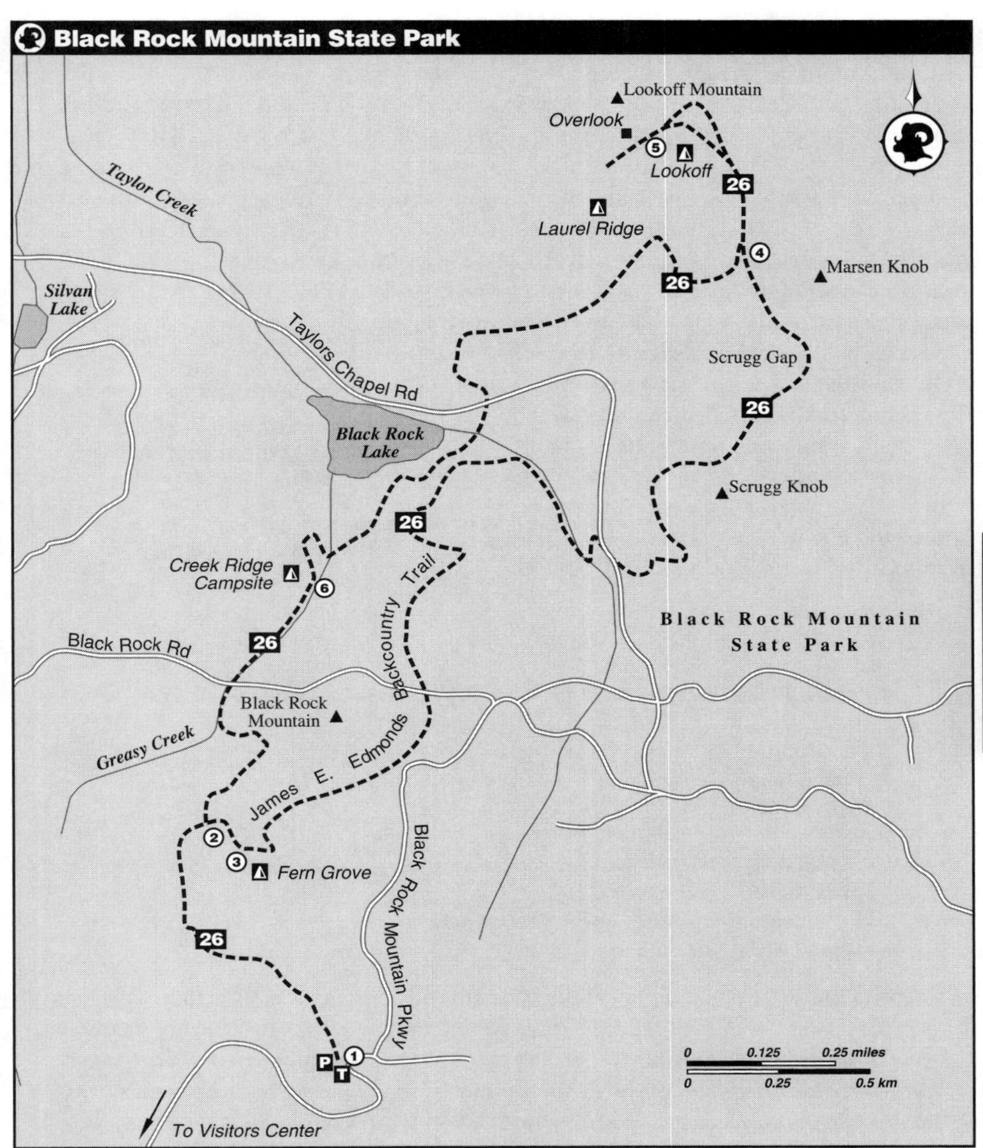

clear waters rush through mossy boulders.

The trail crosses a gravel road and becomes steeps as it climbs Scrugg Knob. It levels and circles Marsen Knob to a junction at 3.4 miles **(Waypoint 4)**. Continue straight here to travel north toward Lookoff Mountain. At the next Y intersection bear right to reach the Lookoff Mountain Overlook at **Waypoint 5**. From this wide slab of rock there is a clear view over the Little Tennessee River Valley, and beyond it, to the northwest, clusters of knobs and ridges roll like waves. On the southwest side of the overlook, a path leads to the Laurel Ridge designated campsite, which is sheltered among the trees. From the overlook, the trail loops back, going northeast and soon passes the Lookoff Mountain designated campsite. It's a little roomier than the Laurel Ridge camp, with bigger benches and space for about three tents.

Descend back to **Waypoint 4** and turn right to travel west. The trail crosses over the spine of a ridge and then drops moderately through younger hardwoods and pines. Cross the road that leads to Black Rock Lake and jog slightly to the right to enter the forest and continue. You climb to a waterfall that slides over rock slabs, and then cross the stream on a wood footbridge. Faint at first, the sounds of Greasy Creek grow louder as you round a bend. Take the wood bridge across Greasy Creek, and at 6.1 miles you reach a Y intersection **(Waypoint 6)**. To the right is the designated Creek Ridge campsite, which is long, narrow, and not very spacious. Bear left at the Y junction and travel southwest to continue. A high wood footbridge carries you across Greasy Creek. When you reach the end of the loop, back at **Waypoint 2**, go right and travel west to take a steep ascent back to the trailhead.

UTM WAYPOINTS

1. 17S 279628E 3865434N
2. 17S 279343E 3866085N
3. 17S 279420E 3866007N
4. 17S 280826E 3867604N
5. 17S 280584E 3867903N
6. 17S 279654E 3866785N

TRIP 27 Warwoman Dell & Becky Branch Falls Trail

Distance	1.1 miles, loop
Hiking Time	30 minutes
Difficulty	Easy
Elevation Gain/Loss	+/-90 feet
Trail Uses	Leashed dogs and good for kids
Best Times	Year-round
Agency	U.S. Forest Service, Chattooga River District
Recommended Map	USGS 7.5-min. *Rabun Bald*

HIGHLIGHTS The Warwoman Dell and Becky Branch trails take you on a quick tour of an area that has seen plenty of interesting history. Part of the Warwoman Dell Trail runs along a wide treadway built for the Blue Ridge Railroad, which was supposed to connect Charleston, South Carolina, with Cincinnati, Ohio, but was never finished because the Civil War interrupted construction. In the 1930s this site was a Civilian Conservation Corps camp from which men worked on reforestation projects, raised trout, and fought fires.

The Warwoman Dell Trail leads you through mountain laurel and rhododendron as well as hemlocks, beeches, and sycamores. Interpretive signs point out various natural features along the way. The Becky Branch Trail leads to a waterfall set back in a cove.

DIRECTIONS From Atlanta take Interstate 85 north to Interstate 985. Take I-985 to GA Highway 365/U.S. Highway 23 to U.S. 23/441. Go north on U.S. 23/441 to Clayton. Continue past the junction of U.S. Highway 76 and U.S. 23/441 and turn right onto Warwoman Dell Road. Go about 2.7 miles. Right after this road bends sharply to the right, look for the Warwoman Dell entrance on the right.

FACILITIES/TRAILHEAD There are picnic tables near the trailhead, and a privy sits near the pavilion above the parking area.

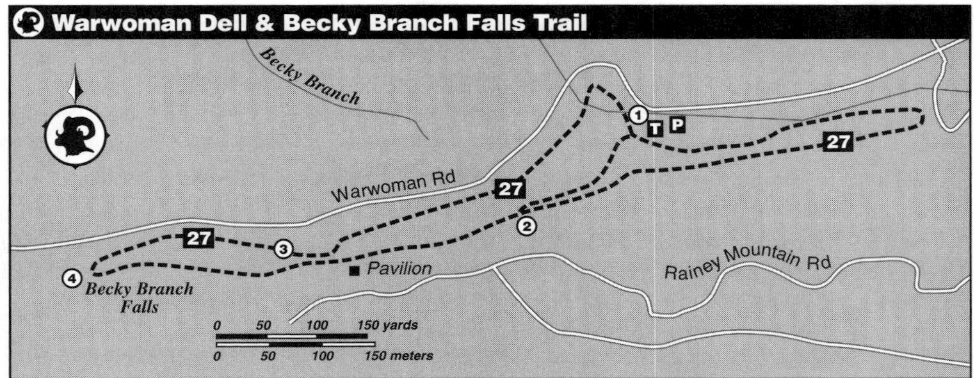

From the parking area (**Waypoint 1**) cross the creek and walk past the pavilion with a picnic table. Walk up 66 stone steps to what is reportedly part of the Blue Ridge Railroad bed. You soon reach a T intersection at a stone wall (**Waypoint 2**). Turn right and walk southwest on a wide trail shaded by hemlocks. At 0.1 mile you reach a trail junction where the Bartram Trail crosses and a sign displays information about the railroad. Bear right to pass through a large timber pavilion. To the right a sign tells the story of Warwoman Dell. Some people believe Warwoman Creek and this area are named for Nancy Ward, a Cherokee woman who fought alongside her husband in a battle with the Creeks in 1775. Typically, a female within a Cherokee tribe would make the decision to go to war, and she was referred to as the "warwoman." All that is known for sure is that this place refers to such a person.

Continue straight, and at 0.2 mile there is an interpretive sign that highlights how the fault zone here was created during the formation of the Appalachian Mountains. Cross the creek to reach a Y junction (**Waypoint 3**). Bear right to reach an interpretive sign that points out the plant life here. In addition to the mountain laurel, beech trees, and other species mentioned here, the ravine also gives life to a wide variety of plants such as resurrection ferns and bloodroot. Continue west up the creek ravine, and at 0.3 mile continue straight at a trail junction. At 0.4 mile you reach Becky Branch Falls (**Waypoint 4**). You can walk down into the small pocket to the base of the waterfall, which drops about 20 feet, sliding down a series of shelves.

Back on the trail, return east and bear right at the junction to descend on a leaf-covered path to the creek. Take the rolling trail back to **Waypoint 2** and turn right, passing through the pavilion once again.

Becky Branch Falls

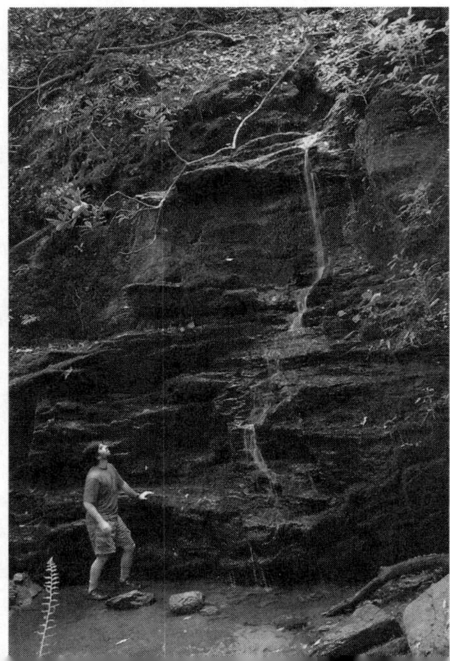

From here you could walk down to the gravel road below and take it back to the parking area, but it's probably more interesting to retrace your steps. Walk down the gravel path to the intersection with the Bartram Trail and bear right to walk east on the wide, flat path you came down before and return to **Waypoint 2**. Continue straight (northeast) to walk along the hillside where rhododendron droops low amid a mix of beeches and hemlocks.

The trail takes a sharp turn back to the west and descends toward the creek. Look left for the CULVERTS OF STONE sign. Lean down to peer through a small tunnel, which served a drainage culvert to preserve the railroad bed. Farther down you reach a picnic table beside the creek, as well as an interpretive sign for the area's many bird species, such as the brown thrasher and female hooded warbler. The path then returns you to the parking area.

There is one other feature you might want to check out. From the parking area, walk west down the gravel road about 170 feet. On the right a path leads to the old "trout rearing station" just inside the edge of the forest. The old stone tanks that held the fish remain, though they are now filled with leaves and covered in moss.

UTM WAYPOINTS

1. 17S 285199E 3862515N
2. 17S 285159E 3862461N
3. 17S 284856E 3862421N
4. 17S 284656E 3862399N

TRIP 28 Rabun Beach Recreation Area: Angel Falls Trail

Distance	1.8 miles, out-and-back
Hiking Time	2–3 hours
Difficulty	Moderate
Elevation Gain/Loss	+/-465 feet
Trail Uses	Leashed dogs and good for kids
Best Times	Spring, summer, and fall
Agency	U.S. Forest Service, Chattooga River District
Recommended Map	USGS 7.5-min. *Tiger*

HIGHLIGHTS Climbing the Joe Creek ravine through an exotic forest of magnolia, mountain laurel, and rhododendron, this brief walk leads to two waterfalls. The first, Panther Falls, stands about 50 feet high with water flowing down what resembles a stone staircase. At the end of the trail you reach Angel Falls, some 60 feet high, with streams slipping down countless thin layers of stone. The trail includes a bit of steep climbing, but for the most part the terrain is moderate, making this an enjoyable walk through exceptionally beautiful forest.

DIRECTIONS From Atlanta take Interstate 85 north to Interstate 985. Continue on I-985 to the junctions with U.S. Highway 23/441. Take U.S. 23/441 north, and 1.6 miles north of the Tallulah Gorge State Park entrance turn left onto Old U.S. Highway 441. Go 2.5 miles and turn left onto Lake Rabun Road. Go 4.5 miles on Lake Rabun Road and turn right into Rabun Beach Campground 2. Turn right, and travel 0.1 mile to the trail parking area.

FACILITIES/TRAILHEAD The parking area has a restroom. There is no fee for trailhead parking. The campground has 80 tent and trailer sites ($10–$20).

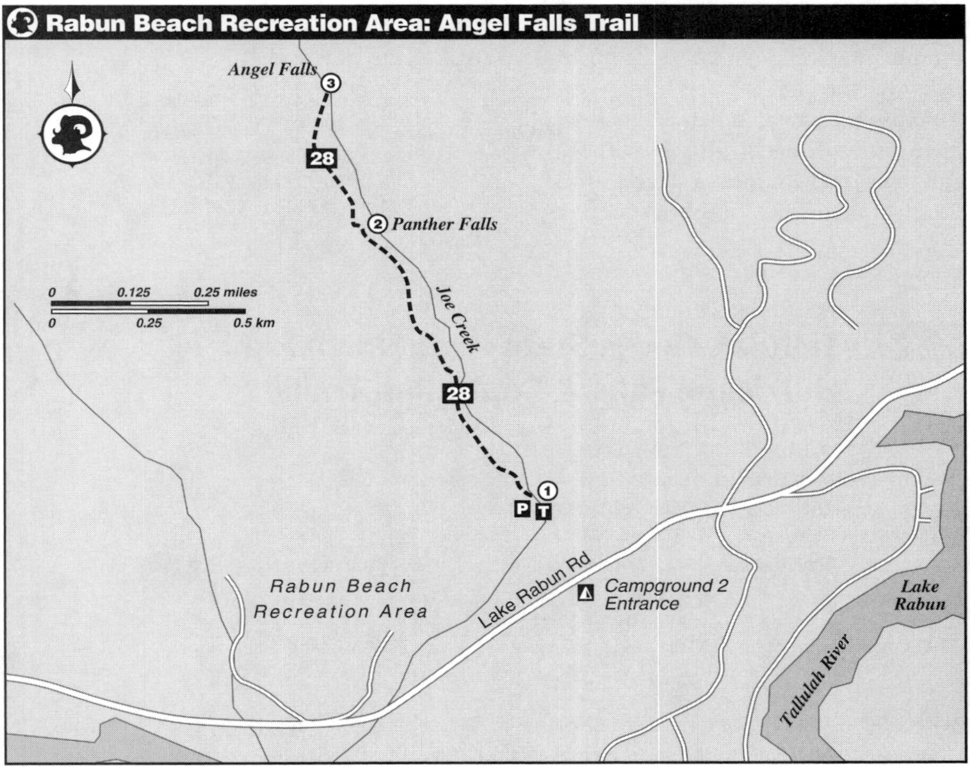

Rabun Beach Recreation Area: Angel Falls Trail

Angel Falls
Panther Falls
Joe Creek
0 0.125 0.25 miles
0 0.25 0.5 km
Rabun Beach Recreation Area
Lake Rabun Rd
Campground 2 Entrance
Lake Rabun
Tallulah River

From the parking area walk northwest to cross the road and enter at the Angel Falls Trail sign **(Waypoint 1)**. You soon cross a wood footbridge where the shallow creek rolls down rocky steps. The path climbs up the moss-covered creek bank shaded by hemlocks and magnolias. Look down and to your right to watch Joe Creek rushing beneath a canopy of rhododendron.

A steady climb through a mix of pines and hardwoods brings you to a wood footbridge where the trail crosses the creek and continues its gradual ascent. At 0.5 mile **(Waypoint 2)** Panther Falls lies to the right, and you can walk down to a shallow pool at its base.

The trail then takes a hairpin turn to the west and ascends steeply. On the slope, a cable is strung between wood posts to prevent falls. With the stream cascading

Angel Falls

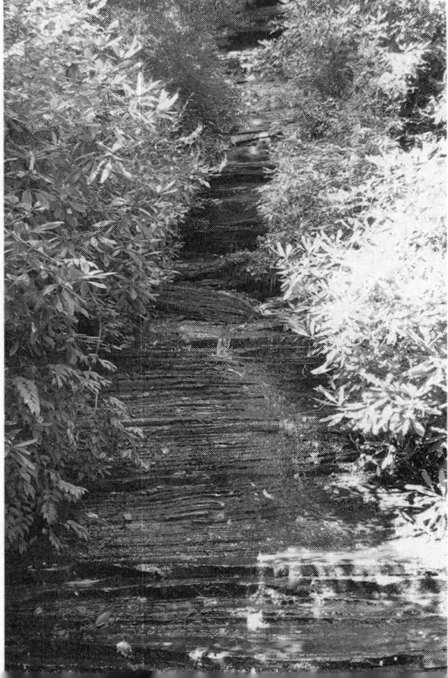

to your side, keep moving upward where mountain laurel boughs stretch horizontally over the path.

Cross the creek and walk to a wood platform **(Waypoint 3)**. To the right, Angel Falls sits tucked into a laurel thicket. From the falls, take the brief loop back to the trail you came up and retrace your steps to the trailhead.

UTM WAYPOINTS

1. 17S 273668E 3849366N
2. 17S 273298E 3850093N
3. 17S 273205E 3850459N

TRIP 29 Tallulah Gorge State Park: North Rim, Hurricane Falls, & South Rim Trails

Distance	2.1 miles, semiloop
Hiking Time	1½ hours
Difficulty	Moderate to strenuous
Elevation Gain/Loss	+/-850 feet
Trail Uses	Leashed dogs and good for kids (North Rim and South Rim trails)
Best Times	Year-round
Agency	Tallulah Gorge State Park
Recommended Map	A trail map is available at the visitors center and online at www.gastateparks.org.

HIGHLIGHTS The hike begins on the North Rim Trail where you have views of Oceana Falls and Bridal Veil Falls to the southeast as well as L'Eau d'Or (French for "water of gold") Falls to the northwest. Depending on your physical fitness, you have some options to reach the South Rim Trail. For an easy walk, go west and cross the dam to access the South Rim Trail. Or, if you're in good shape, descend the Hurricane Falls staircase and cross the suspension bridge. The Hurricane Falls Trail then climbs steeply to the South Rim. Walking along the edge of this side of the canyon you can see the beautiful Hawthorne Pool, Hurricane Falls, Tempesta Falls, Oceana Falls, and the Caledonia Cascade. Signs along the way point out exactly what you're viewing, and the many overlook points are marked and numbered on the park trail map.

DIRECTIONS From Atlanta take Interstate 85 north to Interstate 985. Continue on I-985 to the junction with U.S. Highway 23/441. Take U.S. 23/441 north to Tallulah Falls. Pass over the dam, and when the road bends to the right, look for the park entrance on the right. Take Jane Hurt Yarn Drive to the Interpretive Center.

FACILITIES/TRAILHEAD The Interpretive Center near the trailhead has restrooms. There is a $4 parking fee, and you can purchase an Annual ParkPass for $30 by calling (770) 389-7401. The park has 50 camping sites for tents, trailers, and RVs.

From the parking area, facing the Interpretive Center, go to the right side of the parking lot to enter the marked trail and travel northwest **(Waypoint 1)**. Loop around the west side of the center to a junction **(Waypoint 2)**. Turn left and walk east a quarter mile to Overlook 1 were you have the park's best view of the southern part of the gorge. Below you is Oceana Falls, while Bridal Veil Falls lies

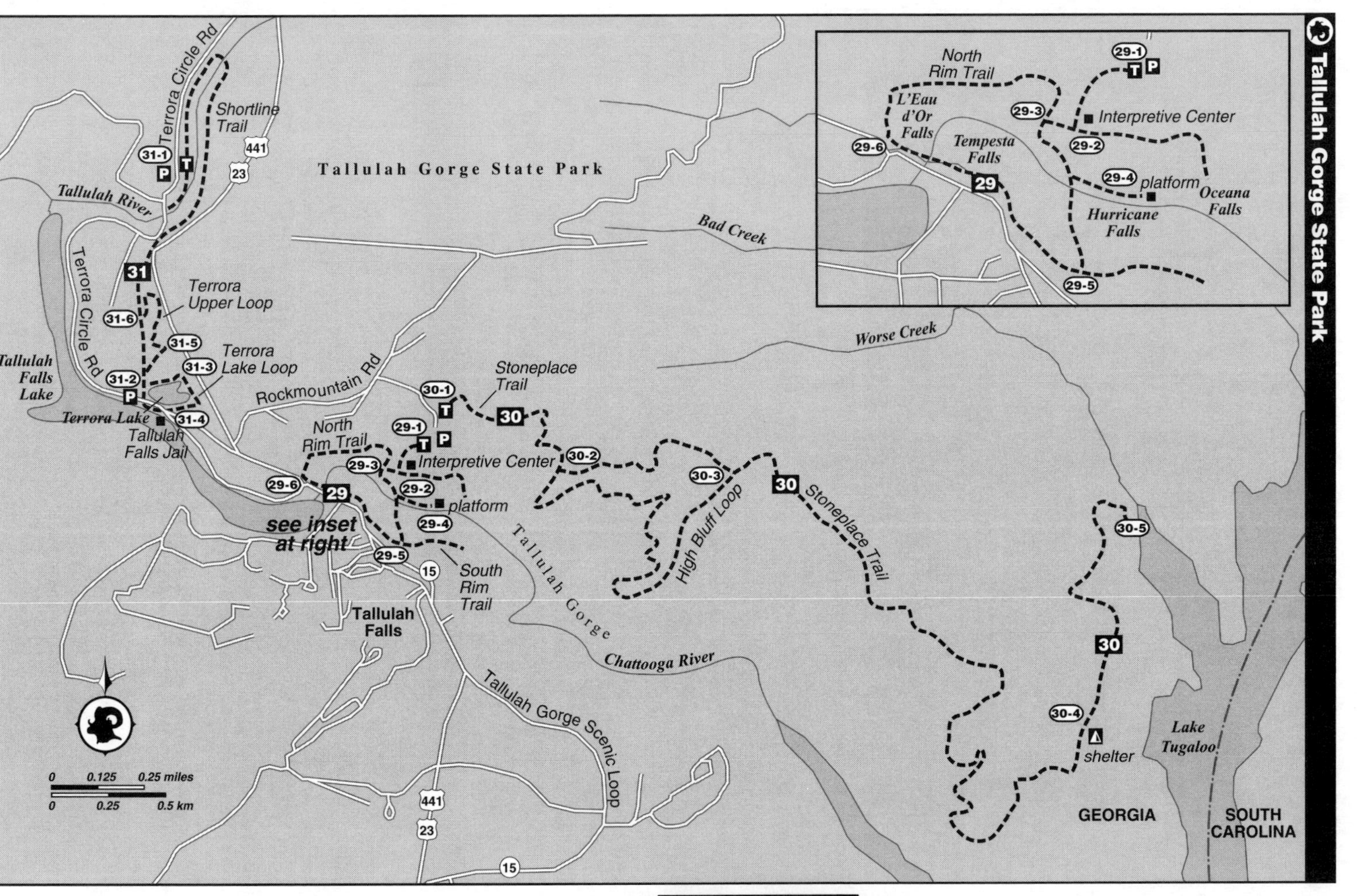
Tallulah Gorge State Park
North Rim Trail
L'Eau d'Or Falls
Tempesta Falls
Interpretive Center
platform
Oceana Falls
Hurricane Falls
29-1
29-2
29-3
29-4
29-5
29-6
29
Terrora Circle Rd
Shortline Trail
441
23
31-1
Tallulah Gorge State Park
Tallulah River
Bad Creek
31
Terrora Upper Loop
31-6
31-5
Terrora Lake Loop
31-3
Tallulah Falls Lake
31-2
Terrora Lake
31-4
Tallulah Falls Jail
Worse Creek
Rockmountain Rd
Stoneplace Trail
30-1
30
North Rim Trail
Interpretive Center
30-2
30-3
High Bluff Loop
Stoneplace Trail
platform
see inset at right
15
South Rim Trail
Tallulah Gorge
Tallulah Falls
Chattooga River
Tallulah Gorge Scenic Loop
30-5
30-4
shelter
Lake Tugaloo
GEORGIA
SOUTH CAROLINA
0 0.125 0.25 miles
0 0.25 0.5 km

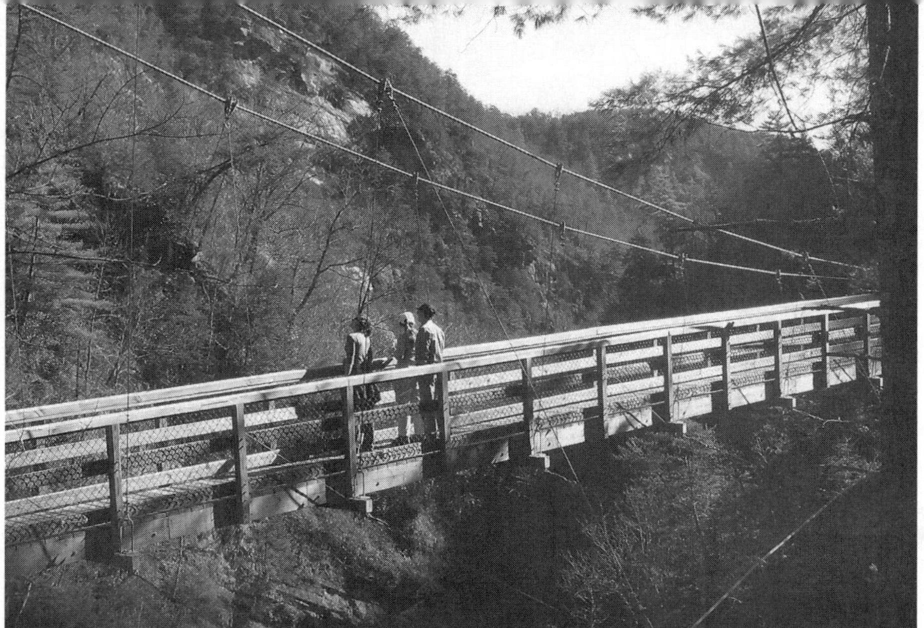
Suspension bridge spanning Tallulah Gorge

farther down the canyon. Backtrack to **Waypoint 2** and go straight (west) to reach Overlook 3 **(Waypoint 3)**. At this observation point you can see L'Eau d'Or Falls and Hawthorne Pool ahead.

Turn left to descend to Overlook 2 and look out at L'Eau d'Or Falls as well as Tempesta Falls and the Hawthorne Cascade. Continue descending on the Hurricane Falls staircase to cross the suspension bridge. You reach a set of stairs that descend through hemlocks to a wood platform **(Waypoint 4)** above a large pool in the gorge from which you can see the falls to the east. Backtrack up the stairs and turn left to continue on the Hurricane Falls Trail. The trail gets very steep as it climbs to the South Rim, and you'll likely be breathing heavily when you reach the lip of the canyon.

At **Waypoint 5** turn left and then bear left at a Y junction to proceed to Overlook 8, which offers a good look at Hurricane Falls and a rock outcrop called "Devil's Pulpit." From the next overlook you can see Oceana Falls and a sign indicates that the section of gorge you're viewing is 650 feet deep. At the final overlook a little farther ahead, the bluff visible to the right stands a whopping 1000 feet high.

From Overlook 10 retrace your steps to **Waypoint 4** and continue straight to Overlooks 7 and 6 for more views of the Hawthorne Pool as well as Tempesta Falls. Continue to where the trail meets U.S. 441 and turn right to take the walkway across the dam. Once across, turn right **(Waypoint 6)** and descend metal and wood stairs. Then turn left to take the North Rim Trail. Overlook 5 looks back south at Hawthorne Pool, while Overlook 4 gives you a chance to see the Tallulah Falls Dam.

Continue on the North Rim Trail to **Waypoint 3**. Bear left to return to **Waypoint 2**, from which you can turn left to return to the Interpretive Center, or go straight to access the back patio of the center.

UTM WAYPOINTS

1. 17S 281155E 3846843N
2. 17S 281046E 3846783N
3. 17S 280980E 3846800N
4. 17S 281166E 3846605N
5. 17S 281052E 3846481N
6. 17S 280616E 3846772N

TRIP 30 Tallulah Gorge State Park: Stoneplace Trail & High Bluff Loop

see map on p. 167

Distance	10.3 miles, semiloop
Hiking Time	5–6 hours
Difficulty	Moderate
Elevation Gain/Loss	+1200/-1205 feet
Trail Uses	Leashed dogs and mountain biking
Best Times	Year-round
Agency	Tallulah Gorge State Park
Recommended Map	A trail map is available at the Interpretive Center and online at www.gastateparks.org.
Note	A free permit is necessary to hike this trail and may be obtained at the Interpretive Center. Be aware that hunting is allowed in the surrounding area, so you should wear orange or brightly colored clothing while hiking in fall and winter.

HIGHLIGHTS The Stoneplace Trail is a wide, attractive path on former logging roads that descends to an inlet on Lake Tugaloo, winding through hardwood coves and slopes covered in mountain laurel and stands of hemlock. If you want to backpack it, a shelter sits just off the trail a little less than 4 miles in. Nestled in low rolling hills, the lake cove is a real reward after the long trek down; it's wonderfully sunny and an inspiring place to swim, fish, or just relax on the pier. From the Stoneplace Trail you can also access the brief High Bluff Loop, which wanders the hills on the north side of the Tallulah Gorge, and occasionally gives you a glimpse of the canyon.

DIRECTIONS From Atlanta take Interstate 85 north to Interstate 985. Continue on I-985 to the junction with U.S. Highway 23/441. Take U.S. 23/441 north to Tallulah Falls. Pass over the dam, and when the road bends to the right, look for the park entrance on the right. Take Jane Hurt Yarn Drive to the Interpretive Center.

FACILITIES/TRAILHEAD The Interpretive Center near the trailhead has restrooms. There is a $4 parking fee, or you can purchase an Annual ParkPass for $30 by calling (770) 389-7401. At 3.8 miles there is a backcountry shelter. Obtain a permit before hiking the trail.

After you enter the park, the Stoneplace Trailhead lies on the left, just beyond the payment kiosk **(Waypoint 1)** (north of the Interpretive Center parking area). The chipped bark trail descends into pines, poplars, and oaks and then climbs onto a ridge. At 0.8 mile the trail intersects with the High Bluff Loop **(Waypoint 2)**. Turn left and go east to continue on the Stoneplace Trail, rolling easily among sourwood trees and more oaks and pines.

Not far beyond the 1-mile mark, turn right onto an old roadbed and travel east. At a trail marker indicating 1.2 miles, go around a metal gate and enter the Tallulah Gorge Wildlife Management Area. At 1.3 miles **(Waypoint 3)** bear left at the Y intersection and travel northeast, following yellow blazes, to continue on the Stoneplace Trail. You cross a dry ridge where the path is sandier and moves into stands of young pines.

The trail then gradually descends through hardwood coves with poplars, rhododendron, dogwoods, and galax, which announces its presence with a strong, musky odor. A bit beyond the

3-mile mark the trail turns to the east, and you have views of the far side of Tallulah Gorge. Lake Tugaloo soon appears to your right, and the land you see on the far side of the water is South Carolina.

At 3.8 miles (**Waypoint 4**) a path on the right leads to the backcountry shelter, which sits within sight of Stoneplace Trail. Continuing on, the Stoneplace path grows noticeably cooler and shaded by hardwoods. At a T intersection with a gravel road, turn right onto the road and walk down it to cross a stream and reach the lake pier at **Waypoint 5**. The lake would be a great place to canoe or kayak. If you wanted to haul in a boat, the lake is accessible via Stoneplace Road, though this requires four-wheel drive.

From the lake, retrace your steps and at the 8-mile mark you reach **Waypoint 3**. Turn left onto the High Bluff Loop and travel southwest. The rutted trail drops to cross a power line break, and then continues downward through young pines where you have slight winter views of the gorge. The character of the forest changes dramatically at about 9 miles when you pass through a wet cove full of thick rhododendron, laurel, and poplars. In a little less than a half mile, the path makes a horseshoe bend to the northeast and returns you to the junction with the Stoneplace Trail at **Waypoint 2**. Bear left onto the Stoneplace Trail to return to the trailhead.

UTM WAYPOINTS

1. 17S 281266E 3847016N
2. 17S 281744E 3846725N
3. 17S 282483E 3846686N
4. 17S 284005E 3845571N
5. 17S 284236E 3846363N

TRIP 31 Tallulah Gorge State Park: Shortline & Terrora Trails

Distance	3.4 miles, out-and-back
Hiking Time	1½ hours
Difficulty	Easy
Elevation Gain/Loss	+155/-145 feet
Trail Uses	Leashed dogs and good for kids
Best Times	Year-round
Agency	Tallulah Gorge State Park
Recommended Map	A trail map is available at the visitors center and online at www.gastateparks.org.

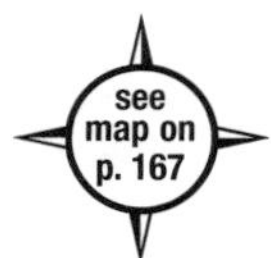

HIGHLIGHTS In the northwest section of Tallulah Gorge State Park, the Shortline Trail and two Terrora trails explore Tallulah Falls Lake and neighboring hills above the dam. The paved Shortline Trail (1.4 miles one-way) follows an old railroad bed through a peaceful stretch of forest, a good route for people with limited mobility or those who want to run or walk for exercise. The Terrora Lake Loop (0.5 mile) circles a small lake and runs through an array of habitats, including wetlands, rocky cliffs, hemlock stands, and pine-hardwood forest. The Terrora Upper Loop crosses a tributary stream and low hills east of the lake. The route I describe combines the three paths into an easy yet interesting dayhike.

DIRECTIONS From Atlanta take Interstate 85 north to Interstate 985. Continue on I-985 to the junction with U.S. Highway 23/441. Take U.S. 23/441 north to Tallulah Falls. Pass the main

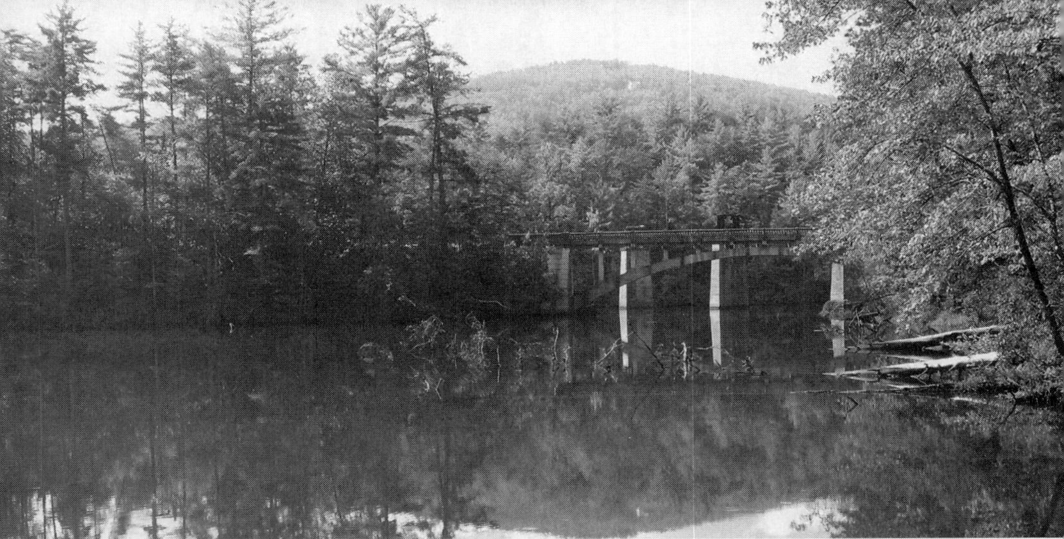

Skirting the shore of placid Terrora Lake

entrance for Tallulah Gorge State, go another 1.2 miles, and turn left onto Terrora Circle Rd. There are two parking areas for the trail on this road. Go 0.6 mile to the first parking area on the left. If you'd prefer to start at the other parking area, go an additional mile and turn left just before the bridge into the parking area.

FACILITIES/TRAILHEAD There are no facilities at the trailhead. There is a $4 fee for the park, or you can purchase an Annual ParkPass for $30 by calling (770) 389-7401.

Shortline Trail

From the parking area **(Waypoint 1)**, enter the paved path and turn left at the T junction. (To the right the path goes 780 feet and ends at the road.) The path skirts the river and at 0.3 mile turns right and crosses a sturdy footbridge.

Across the bridge the trail passes through a splendid corridor of hemlocks and hardwoods with a rocky slope at your left shoulder. After a power line clearing, the trail moves close to the road and then turns away to pass through a hallway of rocks where moss-covered boulders jut onto the trail.

At 1.3 miles the Shortline Trail ends at the second parking area **(Waypoint 2)**, the location of the trailhead for the Terrora Lake and Terrora Upper loops.

Terrora Lake Loop

To begin the Terrora Lake Loop from the Shortline Trail, go to the north end of the parking area and enter the trail to the right of the bulletin board. Descend the wood steps and follow green blazes through a mixture of pines, hardwoods, hemlocks, and mountain laurel.

The trail drops down to the shore of the lake where two benches provide a spot to enjoy the still water ringed by forest **(Waypoint 3)**. The trail turns left and rolls through dense laurel that brushes your shoulders and rhododendron boughs that you must duck beneath. As you circle the lake, you can see the shoreline trees and a distant hill reflected on its glassy surface.

From this wetland area, the trail rises into a pine-hardwood forest, and boulders on the slope provide habitat for snakes, foxes, and birds like the eastern phoebe. You then reach a bench with a nice view of the lake through the pines. Not far ahead, the trail ends at the Tallulah Falls Jail **(Waypoint 4)**. Constructed in 1913, this building originally overlooked

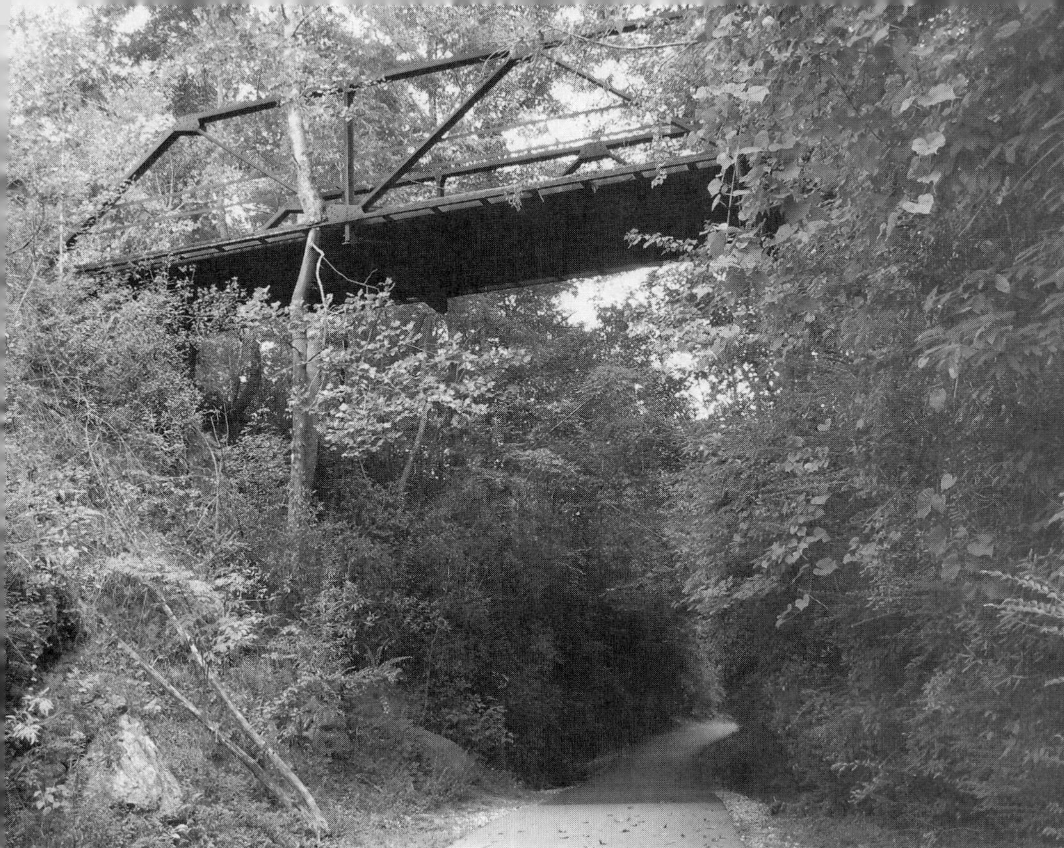

Shortline Trail

Tallulah Falls Lake and served as Tallulah Falls City Hall.

From the jail, go to the road and turn right to return the trailhead at the parking area where you started (**Waypoint 2**).

Terrora Upper Loop

From the north end of the parking area at **Waypoint 2**, take the orange-blazed Terrora Upper Loop, which goes north and parallels the Shortline Trail. Walk nearly 550 feet, turn right when you reach a sign marked HEMLOCK HAMMOCK, and walk 200 feet to reach a set of benches in a stand of tall hemlocks (**Waypoint 5**). The shade of the trees and a nearby gurgling stream make this a peaceful place to linger a while.

When you're ready to continue, return to the main trail and turn right. The path crosses a tributary stream of Tallulah Falls Lake, crosses a power line break and then drops to cross the stream again. Near the water the forest is wild with mountain laurel and rhododendron.

You then climb to meet an old roadbed where the dry slopes are thick with hickory trees and oaks. Turn left to travel west on the roadbed for 190 feet, and then turn left to go south and cross the power line break again. A final descent takes you to an intersection with the Shortline Trail (**Waypoint 6**). Turn right to return to the trailhead.

UTM WAYPOINTS

1. 17S 280190E 3848174N
2. 17S 279964E 3847204N
3. 17S 280039E 3847215N
4. 17S 280101E 3847107N
5. 17S 280042E 3847373N
6. 17S 279961E 3847509N

TRIP 32 Panther Creek Trail

Distance	11.0 miles, out-and-back
Hiking Time	5 hours
Difficulty	Moderate
Elevation Gain/Loss	+735 feet / -720 feet
Trail Uses	Leashed dogs and backpacking
Best Times	Year-round
Agency	Chattahoochee-Oconee national forests, Chattooga River District
Recommended Maps	USGS 7.5-min. *Tallulah Falls* and *Tugaloo Lake*.

HIGHLIGHTS With steep cliffs, waterfalls, rushing streams, and exotic forest, Panther Creek ranks as one of Georgia's most beautiful hiking paths. Since it's also easily accessible, it can be crowded during weekends and holidays. Just 3.4 miles in is the trail's main attraction, Panther Creek Falls, where multiple streams of water rush over a hulking bluff and collect in an immense pool. The flat patch of land at the pool's edge is one of the most scenic campsites in Georgia. Granted, there are usually plenty of people vying to get this spot, and the trail nearby can see heavy traffic, but if you can visit midweek or in the off-season, you might nab it for a great overnight trip.

DIRECTIONS From Atlanta take Interstate 85 to Interstate 985. Take I-985 to U.S. Highway 23/GA Highway 365. From the junction of U.S. 23 and U.S. Highway 441, take U.S. 23/441 north for 15 miles, and turn left on Glen Hardman Rd. Then turn right onto Old Highway 44, travel 1 mile to the parking area on the left.

FACILITIES/TRAILHEAD The trailhead has a restroom and picnic tables.

From the parking area cross Old Highway 44 and enter the Panther Creek Trail at a wooden sign **(Waypoint 1)**. The trail soon passes beneath two overpasses for U.S. 23/441 and descends slightly through pines, oaks, and hickories.

The forest grows more intense as ferns and rhododendron appear, and you walk along a rocky bluff with hemlocks lining the path. Thick foliage partially obscures your view of Panther Creek, but you can hear it rushing by below. Occasionally you can look down to see it flowing fast and swirling into pools. At 0.8 mile turn left just before the second rock overhang to climb up and around the rocks. Not far ahead **(Waypoint 2)** look to the right to see a small but powerful waterfall. Walk down to the bank to see the narrow, swift stream bend around rock, forming a natural flume.

After rolling along the slope, the trail drops to the creek, which you cross on a footbridge. The path stays within a few feet of the boulder-filled creek that courses through lush stands of hemlock and mountain laurel. The trail climbs away from the water, but you can peer down and see the creek running through interesting boulder formations. At 2.2 miles you round a big bend. Just below the next set of falls, the creek forms shallow pools where you'll likely see people fishing for trout.

In an especially tranquil area, the water slows in a wide channel, and a string of hemlocks line the bank. You then cross a rock outcrop that looks over at a series of small falls and a narrow creek channel that forms a water chute. At 3.4 miles **(Waypoint 3)** Panther Creek Falls lies to the left. Also on the left, at the edge of the

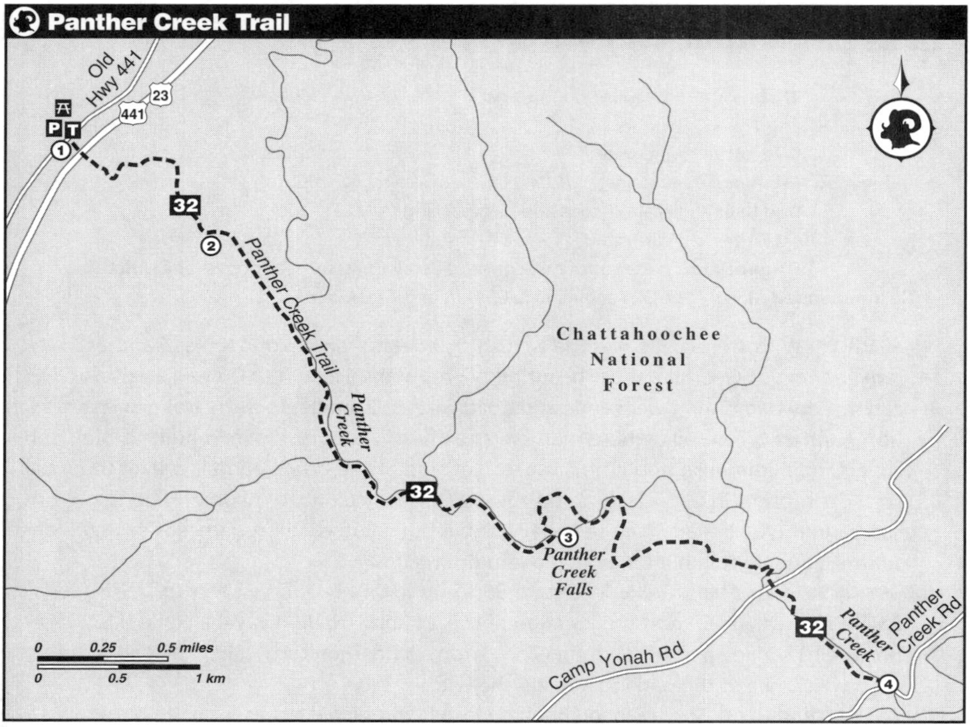

Panther Creek Trail

Old Hwy 441
23
441
P T
1
32
2
Panther Creek Trail
Panther Creek
Chattahoochee National Forest
32
3
Panther Creek Falls
32
Panther Creek
Panther Creek Rd
Camp Yonah Rd
4
0 0.25 0.5 miles
0 0.5 1 km

large pool is a flat area where you could set up camp with the falls as a magnificent backdrop.

From **Waypoint 3** continue northwest on a rugged path that cuts across a slope. The forest below the falls and farther

Panther Creek Falls

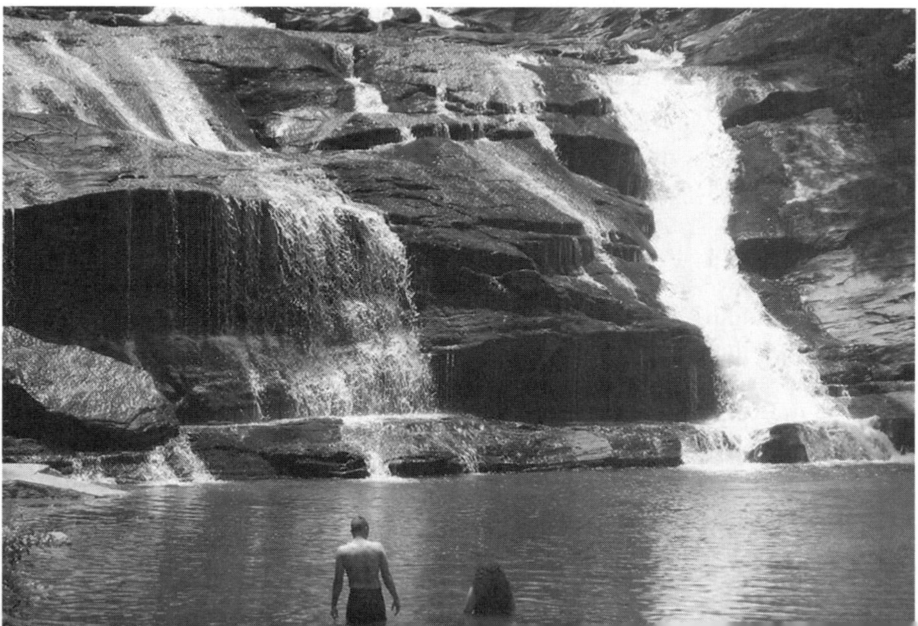

downstream is within the Panther Creek Botanical Area, which lies in a fault zone that supports an unusual number of rare plants. Many species in this heavily forested area, such as the yellowwood tree and the gaywings flower, which blooms a beautiful shade of lavender, appear rarely in Georgia.

At 4 miles the trail turns south and climbs steeply through dense forest following a creek tributary. This marks the end of the dramatic creek views, though the forest is pleasant with stretches of beech, oaks, and poplars, as well as hemlocks and mountain laurel. Be aware that the path traverses eroded slopes where the footing can be dicey, so watch your step to keep from twisting an ankle.

You drop to the creek bank again at 5 miles and descend on a wider treadway. After walking a little less than a half mile, you cross a metal and wood bridge to reach the end of the trail at Panther Creek Road **(Waypoint 4)**. Retrace your steps to return to the parking area

UTM WAYPOINTS

1. 17S 278391E 3842300N
2. 17S 279249E 3841679N
3. 17S 281244E 3839754N
4. 17S 283309E 3838739N

TRIP 33 Lake Russell Recreation Area: Sourwood Trail

Distance	3.8 miles, semiloop
Hiking Time	1½ hours
Difficulty	Easy to moderate
Elevation Gain/Loss	+/-330 feet
Trail Uses	Leashed dogs and good for kids
Best Times	Year-round
Agency	U.S. Forest Service, Chattooga River District
Recommended Map	USGS 7.5-min. *Ayersville*

HIGHLIGHTS This mellow loop trail leads to a beaver pond along Nancy Town Creek, as well as Nancy Town Falls, a secluded, 20-foot cascade. The trail takes you through diverse habitat, from your typical pine-hardwood mix to clearer areas of oaks and hickory trees to creekside corridors of mountain laurel and rhododendron.

DIRECTIONS From Atlanta take Interstate 85 north to Interstate 985. Continue on I-985 to GA Highway 365 toward Cornelia. Continue on GA 365 to the Clarkesville exit/GA Highway 197. Turn right onto GA 197 and travel south 2.5 miles. Turn right onto Dicks Hill Parkway (GA Highway 13), go 0.8 mile and turn left onto Lake Russell Road. Take Lake Russell Road for 2 miles and turn left onto Forest Service Road 591 at a sign for Nancy Town Lake. Go 0.1 mile to the parking area on the right at a road junction.

FACILITIES/TRAILHEAD There are no facilities at the trailhead. The Lake Russell Campground has 42 sites for RVs and tents, plus restrooms and showers.

From the parking area **(Waypoint 1)**, walk northeast on the paved road with the Nancy Town Lake below on your right. At 0.5 mile **(Waypoint 2)** turn left to enter the Sourwood Trail and travel northwest following blue blazes. Walk beside a stream branch of Nancy Town Lake for 0.2 mile and then turn east, away from the water.

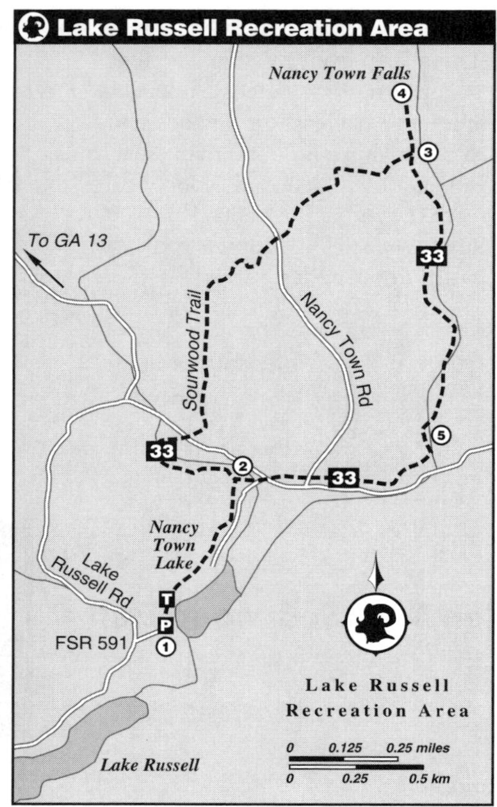

Nancy Town Falls

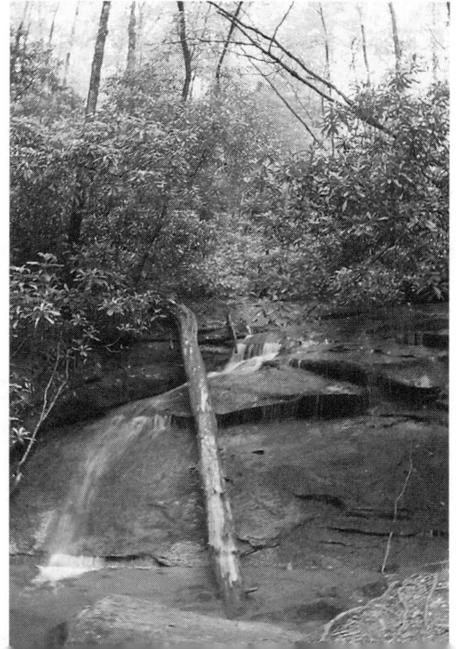

A steady climb through loblolly pines brings you to a large burn area where you can see charring at the base of pines. Rangers have conducted controlled burns here to reduce the fuel load, and when I walked through this area on a windy day it was rather spooky as thin trunks of trees left standing creaked and knocked together. At 1.3 miles into your walk you cross Nancy Town Road at the high point of the hike, 1324 feet. The forest is much more attractive as the trail drops through oaks and hickory trees, and a wood footbridge carries you across a feeder stream for Nancy Town Creek. Ahead on the left is a grassy opening, a patch of low ground that is actually part of the beaver pond along Nancy Town Creek.

At 1.8 miles you reach a trail junction at the bank of Nancy Town Creek **(Waypoint 3)**. Turn left to walk about a tenth of a mile to Nancy Town Falls **(Waypoint 4)**. This low cascade is modest but still appealing and offers solitude beneath a great crown of thick laurel.

From the falls, return to **Waypoint 3** and continue straight, walking south. As you move along the beaver pond look for wood duck nesting boxes standing in the water. The trail continues along the creek, which tumbles through a pleasant stretch of rhododendron and mountain laurel.

At 2.8 miles **(Waypoint 5)** the trail intersects with Red Root Road. Turn right onto the road and travel southwest. At a Y intersection in the road keep left to return to **Waypoint 2.** Take a left and retrace your steps to the parking area.

UTM WAYPOINTS

1. 17S 271881E 3820391N
2. 17S 272184E 3820863N
3. 17S 272872E 3822047N
4. 17S 272840E 3822200N
5. 17S 272876E 3820918N

TRIP 34 Victoria Bryant State Park: Perimeter Trail

Distance	3.6–4.0 miles, loop
Hiking Time	2 hours
Difficulty	Easy
Elevation Gain/Loss	+305/-295 feet
Trail Use	Leashed dogs
Best Times	Year-round
Agency	Victoria Bryant State Park
Recommended Map	A park map is available in the park office and online at www.gastateparks.org/info/vicbryant.

see map on p. 179

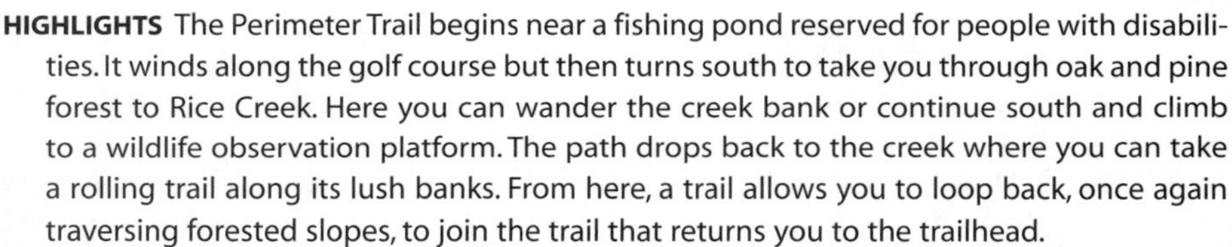

HIGHLIGHTS The Perimeter Trail begins near a fishing pond reserved for people with disabilities. It winds along the golf course but then turns south to take you through oak and pine forest to Rice Creek. Here you can wander the creek bank or continue south and climb to a wildlife observation platform. The path drops back to the creek where you can take a rolling trail along its lush banks. From here, a trail allows you to loop back, once again traversing forested slopes, to join the trail that returns you to the trailhead.

DIRECTIONS From Atlanta take Interstate 85 north and take Exit 160 toward Royston/Elberton. Turn right onto GA Highway 51 and travel southeast to GA Highway 145. Turn right onto GA 145, go 1.2 miles, and turn left onto U.S. Highway 29/GA Highway 8. Go 0.1 mile and turn left onto GA Highway 327/Park Rd. Go north about 1 mile, and turn left into Victoria Bryant Park. The parking area is on the left near the entrance. The trailhead is on the right about 400 feet from the entrance. Continue on the road to reach the park office.

FACILITIES/TRAILHEAD There are restrooms at the park office but not at the trailhead. The park charges a $3 parking fee. You can purchase an Annual ParkPass for $30 by calling (770) 389-7401.

Just past the attendant booth near the park entrance, turn right onto the paved path that skirts the fishing pond (**Waypoint 1**). Walk about 500 feet, turn right onto a dirt path, and ascend to the west, following red blazes. An uphill walk beside the golf course leads you to a Y junction (**Waypoint 2**). Bear right and follow orange blazes, climbing a hill of pines and hardwoods.

A little beyond the 1-mile point you reach a Y junction (**Waypoint 3**). Bear left to continue on the orange-blazed Perimeter Trail. (If you were to bear right you would enter the Broad River Loop.) A long descent takes you to Rice Creek at 1.3 miles. The path to the left goes southeast to the Pioneer Camping Area. But to continue, travel west along the lower flanks of a hill. The trail turns east and makes a gradual ascent to a hilltop and he observation platform (**Waypoint 4**), which overlooks a long, narrow grazing field where you can watch for deer, turkeys, and other animals. The path continues across a hill and eventually takes you past a fishing pond to a parking area. Though the trail ends at the parking area you can easily walk west down the road to continue and access the creek.

At **Waypoint 5** there is a creek ford. From here, Victoria's Path forms a small loop that rolls along the banks of Rice Creek. This undulating path is surrounded by oaks, poplars, and sourwood trees, as well as dense mountain laurel, giving it an exotic feel. From an overlook platform, you can see the creek rushing through a corridor of heavy laurel. From Victoria's Path you join the Perimeter Connector at **Waypoint 6**. The connector carries you through more forest to the trail junction at **Waypoint 2**. Bear right and travel northeast to return to the trailhead.

UTM WAYPOINTS

1. 17S 301239E 3797401N
2. 17S 300687E 3797443N
3. 17S 300619E 3797655N
4. 17S 300495E 3796938N
5. 17S 300851E 3797851N
6. 17S 300595E 3797029N

TRIP 35 Victoria Bryant State Park: Broad River Loop

Distance	5.0 miles, loop
Hiking Time	2 hours
Difficulty	Easy
Elevation Gain/Loss	+290/-285 feet
Trail Use	Leashed dogs
Best Times	Year-round
Agency	Victoria Bryant State Park
Recommended Map	A park map is available in the park office and online at www.gastateparks.org/info/vicbryant.

HIGHLIGHTS The Broad River Loop wanders to the more remote northwestern section of the park, winding through bottomland forest. The trail intersects a path that visits a beaver pond where there is an observation platform. Returning to the Broad River Loop you'll swing northwest to touch the bank of the Broad River. After enjoying a view of this wide channel, climb to a hilltop where quiet woods make it easy to forget that a golf course and busy campground lie close by. On your way back, you'll return to the low forest and cross a small river tributary before retracing your steps to the trailhead.

DIRECTIONS From Atlanta take Interstate 85 north, and take Exit 160 toward Royston/Elberton. Turn right onto GA Highway 51, and travel southeast to GA Highway 145. Turn right onto GA Highway 145, go 1.2 miles, and turn left onto U.S. Highway 29/GA Highway 8. Go 0.1 mile and turn left onto GA Highway 327/Park Rd. Go north about 1 mile and turn left into Victoria Bryant Park. The parking area is on the left near the entrance. The trailhead is on the right about 400 feet from the entrance. Continue on the road to reach the park office.

FACILITIES/TRAILHEAD The park office has restrooms, but the trailhead does not. There is a $3 parking fee for the park. You can purchase an Annual ParkPass for $30 by calling (770) 389-7401.

Just past the attendant booth near the park entrance, turn right onto the paved path that skirts the fishing pond (**Waypoint 34-1**). Walk about 500 feet and turn right onto a dirt path and ascend to the west, following red blazes. An uphill walk beside the golf course leads you to a Y trail junction (**Waypoint 34-2**). Bear right and follow orange blazes, climbing a hill of pines and hardwoods. A little beyond the 1-mile point bear right at a Y junction (**Waypoint 34-3**) to take the Broad River Loop and travel northwest, ascending slightly among small oaks and pines. You soon cross a paved road and travel southwest.

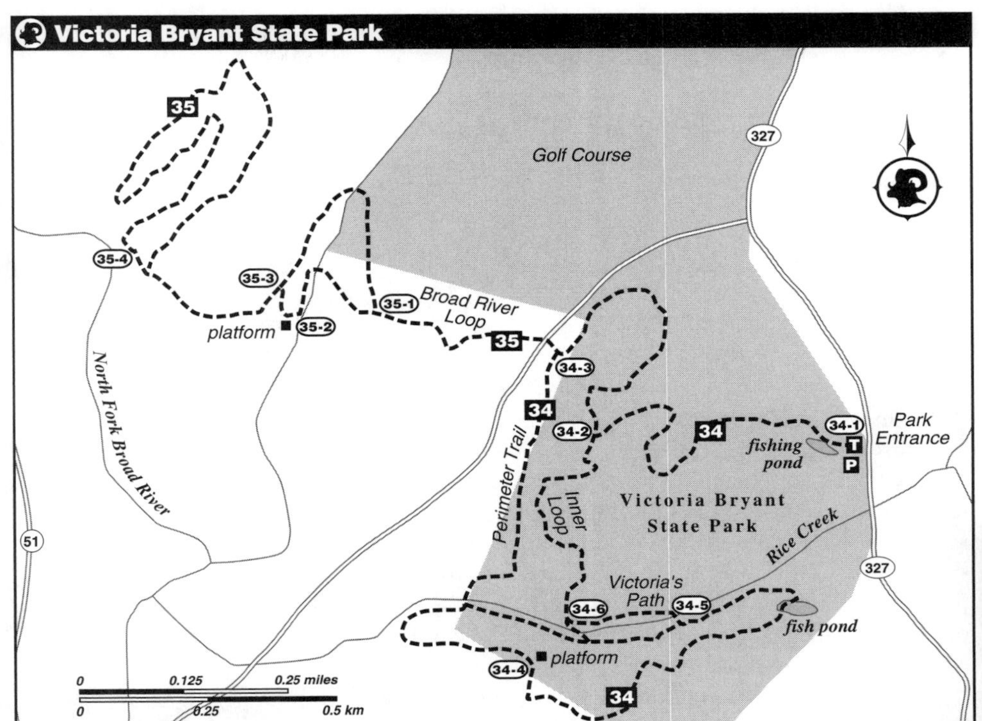

A winding descent leads to a creek surrounded by dense brush. Now out of sight of the golf course, the trail begins to feel more secluded, and a bench makes a good place to sit and look out over the bottomland forest. At 1.3 miles **(Waypoint 35-1)**, bear left at a trail junction and take the Pond Overlook Loop to the platform at 1.6 miles **(Waypoint 35-2)**.

Continue to a T intersection (**Waypoint 35-3**) and turn left to ascend southwest on the Broad River Loop. At a Y junction, bear left and walk down to the bank of Broad River **(Waypoint 35-4)**. Beside the trail there is a bench with a view to the south of the tranquil, slow-flowing water. The trail immediately turns away from the river and climbs moderately through open hardwood forest to a hilltop. Enjoy an easy walk on the level path as it crosses the hill covered in pines.

Descending the ridge, the path runs near the edge of the golf course. Turn left at the next trail junction to continue to **Waypoint 35-3**. Continue straight, traveling northeast, with the creek drainage to your right. Cross the drainage, and at 3.7 miles turn right to travel south. At **Waypoint 35-1**, turn left, go southeast, and return to **Waypoint 34-3**. Then turn left to go northeast and return to the trailhead.

UTM WAYPOINTS

1. 17S 300206E 3797776N
2. 17S 299997E 3797770N
3. 17S 299993E 3797857N
4. 17S 299661E 3797968N

Chapter 4

West of Atlanta

Resting in the shade of an oak high atop Kennesaw, you can hardly imagine the chaos that engulfed the mountain in the summer of 1864. It is a sublime place. But, if you care to look, the shadows of history are all around. The parks, battlefields, and greenways west of Atlanta offer hikers serene escapes, as well as the opportunity to examine important events in Georgia's history. While the cannons and interpretive signs at Kennesaw sketch out a Civil War battle, Sweetwater Creek State Park recalls early pioneer efforts to harness Georgia's rivers to generate power. And, not far from Atlanta's western edge, a long ribbon of asphalt that now hums with bicycle tires traces the path of the once mighty Silver Comet railway line. Whether you want to feed your mind or get your outdoor fix, just head west.

Pickett's Mill Battlefield

On the evening of May 27, 1864, a wooded ravine turned into a killing field as 10,000 Confederate troops repelled 14,000 attacking Union soldiers, forcing a weeklong delay in the Union march on Atlanta. Unlike some battlefields that are dotted with monuments, Pickett's Mill Battlefield remains a wild plot of forestland, largely unchanged since the days of the Civil War. Well-marked trails travel old roads used by the troops and carry you past an old mill site, earthworks used for fighting positions, and an old cornfield, which was the scene of a bloody clash during the battle. Most notable is the ravine, which is part of the Blue Loop Trail. Hundreds of federal troops charged up the steep slope of the deep cut, only to be cut down by Confederate musket fire.

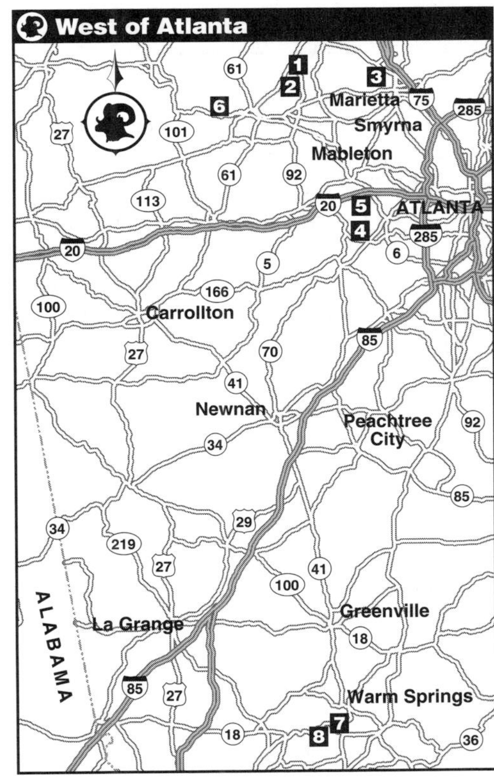

This rare night battle in the Civil War resulted in the loss of 1600 federal troops and 500 Confederates. When you hike, be sure to carry the brochure available at the visitors center. It has interpretive information that corresponds to trail markers located throughout the battlefield.

F. D. Roosevelt State Park

In 1921, President Franklin D. Roosevelt was stricken with polio, and eleven years later he established a home, known as the Little White House, in Warm Springs, Georgia, where he sought treatment in the area's natural mineral springs. While in the area, he would frequent nearby Pine Mountain, an extensive ridge set in the otherwise gently rolling Piedmont region of central Georgia. Roosevelt took a personal interest in preserving this natural area, which led to the creation of F. D. Roosevelt State Park on Pine Mountain. Covering some 9000 acres, it is Georgia's largest state park and includes diverse forest, from high ridges of pines and hardwoods to rocky coves with waterfalls.

The National Audubon Society considers Pine Mountain an important bird area, which would please Roosevelt; he was a birding enthusiast all his life. A *Birds of F. D. Roosevelt* brochure (available online) has a checklist of species in the area.

The 23-mile Pine Mountain Trail, which traverses the ridge, is considered one of the best backpacking treks in Georgia, with 13 backcountry campsites. Each year, about 60,000 people hike the trail, which is maintained by the hardworking Pine Mountain Trail Association. If you're not interested in a multiday backpacking trip, you can dayhike one of the many loops along the trail. The 6.7-mile Wolfden Loop at the east end of the park is one of the most attractive hikes, while a shorter option is the Dowdell Loop Trail that circles through the oak and hickory forest near the top of Dowdell's Knob.

Wolfden rock formation on Wolfden Loop Trail (Trip 7)

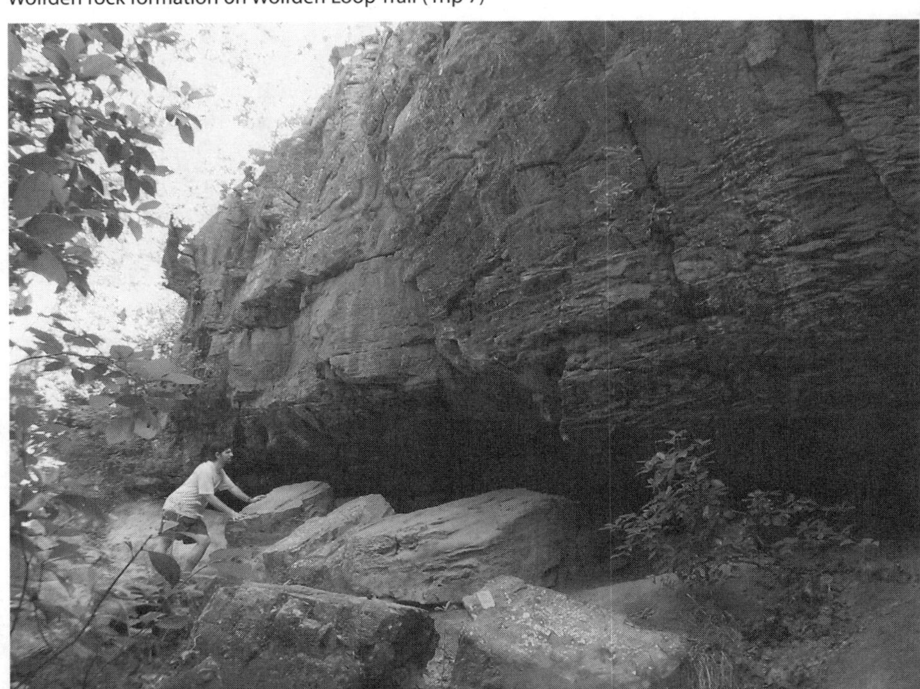

TRIP 1 Pickett's Mill Battlefield: Red, Blue, & Brand House Trails Loop

Distance	3.2 miles, loop
Hiking Time	2 hours
Difficulty	Easy to moderate
Elevation Gain/Loss	+/-610 feet
Trail Use	None
Best Times	Spring, fall, and winter
Agency	Pickett's Mill Battlefield Historic Site
Recommended Map	*The Battle of Pickett's Mill: A Complete Trail Guide* is available at the visitors center.

HIGHLIGHTS This long loop hike begins at the ravine overlook and passes the point where federal troops charged out of the ravine and met a hail of Confederate fire on May 27, 1864. You then follow the Red Trail, along a stream, past the site of Pickett's Mill and then the old cornfield. You ascend a hill where trenches dug by federal troops are still visible. After a brief walk on the White Trail, the orange-blazed Brand House Trail takes you to the more remote northern section of the battlefield site where a field hospital was located. A raised piece of ground indicates the site of the Brand family house.

DIRECTIONS From Atlanta, travel north on Interstate 75 and take Exit 267B for U.S. Highway 41 and GA Highway 5 south. Merge onto the Canton Road Connector, go 0.2 mile, and take U.S. Highway 41 north. Travel 11.6 miles, and turn left onto Old Acworth Dallas Highway/GA Highway 92. Go 4 miles, and stay straight to take the Dallas Acworth Highway/GA Highway 381. Go 2.2 miles and turn left onto Mt. Tabor Church Rd.

FACILITIES/TRAILHEAD The visitors center has restroom facilities, which is open Tuesday–Saturday, 9 AM–5 PM. Admission fees are $3 per adult, $2.50 per senior, and $1.75 per child. There are picnic tables and a group shelter.

Begin at the Ravine Overlook located at the rear of the visitors center **(Waypoint 1)**. To the left the ravine lies somewhat hidden in the dense forest to the left. Turn right and walk east on the trail marked red and blue. After walking some 530 feet, turn right at the Y intersection to go southeast on the Red Trail. You pass the site of an old cornfield bordered by a wood rail fence as well as trenches constructed after the battle. The path drops gradually until about the half-mile mark where it climbs a hill. On this high ground, Confederates formed a line and attacked the Union troops in the cornfield below.

Descend the hill, cross a wood footbridge and turn right at the next trail junction to continue on the Red Trail. At 0.7 mile you reach the place where the Pickett family had a home, which was likely destroyed during the war. Turn right at the trail junction to continue on the Red Trail. About 400 feet farther is the former location of Pickett's Mill **(Waypoint 2)** where only a few foundation ruins remain. At this gristmill, corn and wheat were ground to supply local people with meal and flour. You roll alongside the gently flowing creek and cross a wood footbridge at a bend in the stream. The edge of a former wheat field comes into view, and the trail climbs a steep slope. At the 1-mile mark **(Waypoint 3)**, as you ascend the hill, look right to see the trenches dug by Union troops.

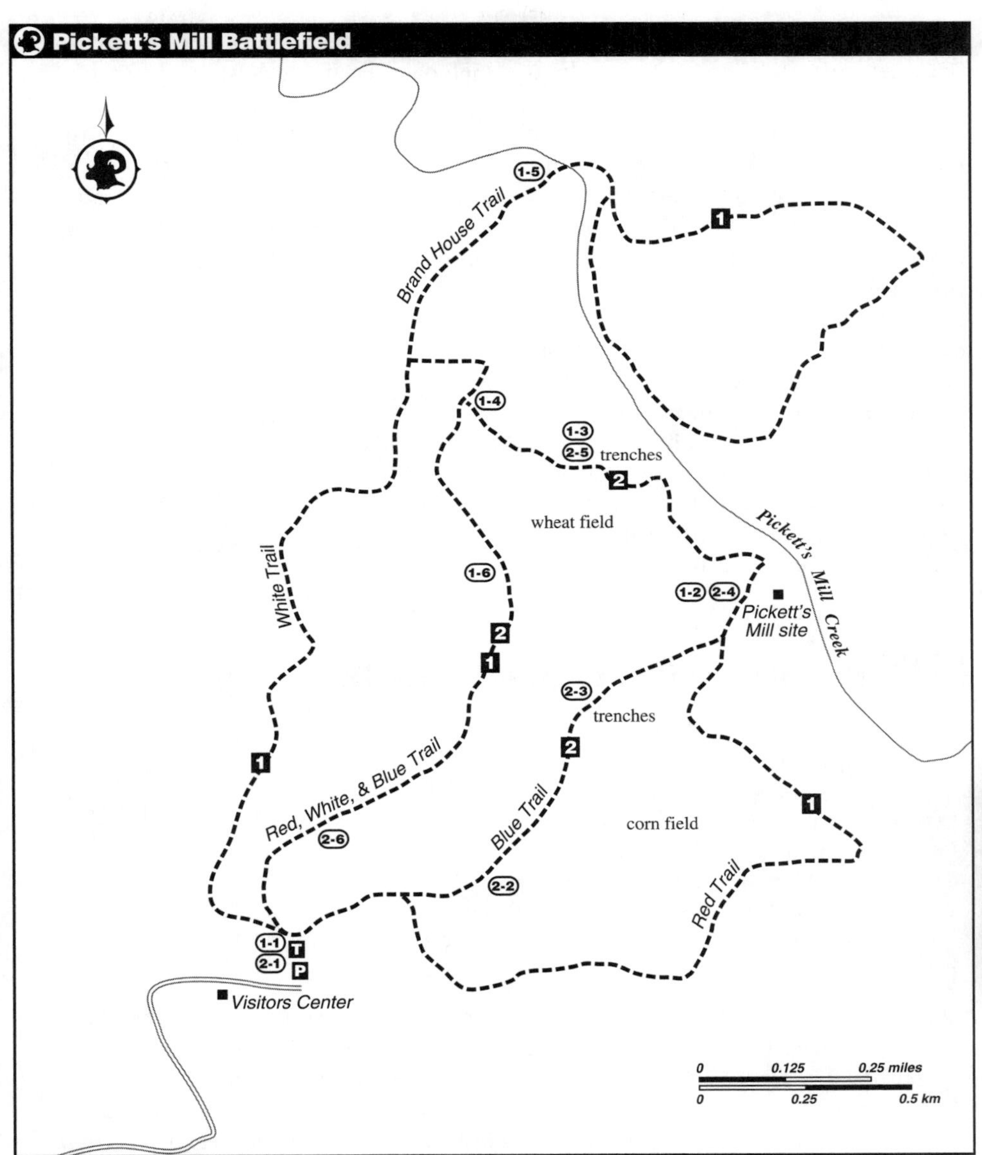

This rugged hill is another reminder that federal troops chose a formidable piece of ground for their attack, and to stumble across this ground at night must have been a severe challenge.

At 1.1 miles, turn right at a T intersection, and turn right at the next intersection **(Waypoint 4)** to walk northeast on the White Trail. After going another 0.1 mile, turn right near the top of Hazen's Hill and travel northeast on the orange-blazed Brand House Trail. This path descends moderately toward Pickett's Mill Creek, passing the former site of a Union field hospital **(Waypoint 5)** at 1.4 miles. Continue on the shaded Brand House Trail, dropping through thick pine forest. Cross the creek, and at 1.5 miles bear right at the Y intersection. After climbing, look carefully to see the mound of earth that marks where the Brand family had a home. Turn right, traveling southwest to cross the ridge. The trail soon moves down the side of the ridge, and during the descent (at 2 miles) you reach a side trail that leads to a secluded wood bench overlooking a thin burbling stream. From here, the trail drops to the creek and follows it north to complete a loop and return to **Waypoint 4** (2.6 miles).

From **Waypoint 4**, turn southeast onto the trail marked red, white, and blue and wind down through one of the more attractive sections of the battlefield, where sunlight shoots through the crowns of high oaks. Farther below, the forest dims to a dark green where ferns envelop a thin stream. You then move through the wide ravine (**Waypoint 6**), where it's easy to imagine the desperation of the troops who faced withering fire while charging out of this shooting barrel.

UTM WAYPOINTS

1. 16S 707022E 3761560N
2. 16S 707610E 3762055N
3. 16S 707410E 3762169N
4. 16S 707237E 3762272N
5. 16S 707294E 3762514N
6. 16S 707264E 3761924N

TRIP 2 Pickett's Mill Battlefield: Blue Trail Loop

Distance	1.5 miles, loop
Hiking Time	1 hour
Difficulty	Moderate
Elevation Gain/Loss	+280/-230 feet
Trail Use	Good for kids
Best Times	Spring, fall, and winter
Agency	Pickett's Mill Battlefield Historic Site
Recommended Map	*The Battle of Pickett's Mill: A Complete Trail Guide* is available at the visitors center.

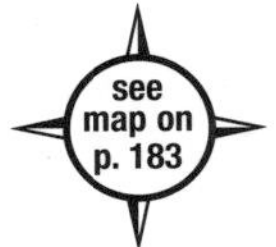
see map on p. 183

HIGHLIGHTS This short loop gradually descends through forest with thickets and considerable ground cover where Brig. Gen. William B. Hazen's Union soldiers traded attacks with Confederates under Col. G. F. Baucum and Brig. Gen. Mark P. Lowry. The action through here was pivotal in the battle. When the Union troops failed to secure the ground south of the cornfield (which you pass during the first part of the loop) they had to withdraw, which ruined their opportunity to succeed. At the site of the Pickett family house, you follow the trail blazed blue and red, climbing west past the former location of a wheat field as well as trenches dug by Union troops. The path then turns south to explore the ravine where waves of Union troops were cut down as they scrambled up the steep slopes to meet the Confederates.

DIRECTIONS From Atlanta, travel north on Interstate 75 and take Exit 267B for U.S. Highway 41 and GA Highway 5 south. Merge onto the Canton Road Connector, go 0.2 mile, and take U.S. Highway 41 north. Travel 11.6 miles and turn left onto Old Acworth Dallas Highway/GA Highway 92. Go 4 miles and stay straight to take the Dallas Acworth Highway/GA Highway 381. Go 2.2 miles and turn left onto Mt. Tabor Church Road.

FACILITIES/TRAILHEAD The visitors center has restroom facilities and is open Tuesday–Saturday, 9 AM–5 PM. Admission fees are $3 per adult, $2.50 per senior, and $1.75 per child. There are picnic tables and a group shelter.

Begin at the Ravine Overlook located at the rear of the visitors center **(Waypoint 1)**. Turn right and walk east on the trail marked red and blue. After walking 530 feet, bear left at the Y intersection and descend on the blue-blazed trail. On a blue-sky day, sun pours in here and heats the wide path covered in pine needles. At 0.2 mile **(Waypoint 2)** the cornfield lies to the right; it was on this land that Brig. Gen. Hazen's Union soldiers stopped one Confederate attack but finally withdrew when the rebels massed reinforcements and attacked a second time. At the Y intersection bear left to continue north.

At 0.3 mile **(Waypoint 3)**, look to the right of the trail for a long, narrow depression. Dismounted cavalry soldiers used these pits for protection when they held off a Union attack, which prevented Hazen from defeating the Confederates in his assault in the cornfield. At 0.4 mile you reach an intersection, which was the site of the Pickett family residence. Turn left and take the blue- and red-blazed trail northeast. About 400 feet farther is the former location of Pickett's Mill **(Waypoint 4)** which produced corn meal and flour for locals. You roll alongside the gently flowing creek and cross a wood footbridge at a bend in the stream. After passing an old wheat field, make a steep climb up a hill and look right to see the trenches dug by Union troops.

At 0.8 mile turn southeast onto the trail marked red, white, and blue. You begin beneath tall oaks and descend into a creek drainage with ferns lining a narrow stream. You then take a rolling trail through the wide ravine **(Waypoint 5)** with attractive, open forest. In such a serene setting it's hard to imagine the violence and chaos that unfolded here in May 1864, but the steep ravine wall visible on your left is a monument to the extreme nature of fighting in Georgia's rugged landscape.

UTM WAYPOINTS

1. 16S 707022E 3761560N
2. 16S 707315E 3761684N
3. 16S 707453E 3761907N
4. 16S 707610E 3762055N
5. 16S 707410E 3762169N

TRIP 3 Kennesaw Mountain National Battlefield Park Loop

Distance	7.2 miles, loop
Hiking Time	4–5 hours
Difficulty	Moderate to strenuous
Elevation Gain/Loss	+/-1385 feet
Trail Use	Leashed dogs
Best Times	Year-round
Agency	National Park Service, Kennesaw Mountain National Battlefield Park
Recommended Map	A trail map is available at the visitors center.

HIGHLIGHTS Toil and trouble. Those two words come to mind as you hike across Kennesaw Mountain and imagine the Confederates and Union soldiers battling to control the rocky slopes. In June 1864, General William T. Sherman maneuvered his army south of Kennesaw Mountain, hoping to flank the Confederate line and capture the Western and Atlanta Railroad, a critical supply line in Marietta. Confederate soldiers who were dug in on the mountain first clashed with Union troops on June 19, and fighting continued on this 2888-acre battlefield until July 2. There are more than 17 miles of trails on the battlefield, and this hike includes a good sampling of what's available. This hike crosses Kennesaw Mountain and Little Kennesaw Mountain, which offer dramatic views, interpretive signs concerning the battle, and remnants of battlefield earthworks. You'll descend to fields to get the perspective of the attacking Union soldiers, and wind through a hardwood forest with trails built for hiking, walking, or running.

DIRECTIONS From Atlanta take Interstate 75 to Exit 269 (Barrett Parkway), and at the light go west onto Barrett Parkway. Go 3 miles and turn left onto Old Highway 41. At the next light turn right onto Stilesboro Road. The visitors center is on the left.

FACILITIES/TRAILHEAD Restrooms are available at the visitors center, which is open from dawn until dusk everyday, except Thanksgiving, Christmas, and New Year's Day. There is no fee. Be sure to carry all the water and food you will need for a full day's hike.

From the south side of the visitors center, enter the wide dirt and gravel trail that winds upward through oak and hickory **(Waypoint 1)**. Very steep in some sections, the path reaches an overlook with an expansive view of the broad valley below. Continue to a second, higher overlook platform and take the asphalt path that climbs to the southwest. At the 1-mile mark you arrive near the crest of the mountain (elevation 1808 feet) where there are cannons, plus interpretive signs explaining the fall of Atlanta in the war **(Waypoint 2)**.

The hike continues southwest across Kennesaw Mountain and then drops steeply over a narrow, rocky, and eroded section (watch your step!). As you cross a road, Little Kennesaw Mountain stands prominently before you. Dense forest closes in on the wide gravel trail that climbs moderately to the summit of Little Kennesaw at an elevation of 1600 feet.

Descending the boulder-strewn path on the flank of the mountain, you have seasonal views of lowlands to the west, and then follow switchbacks down through pines to a trail junction at 2.4 miles. Continue straight, traveling east to

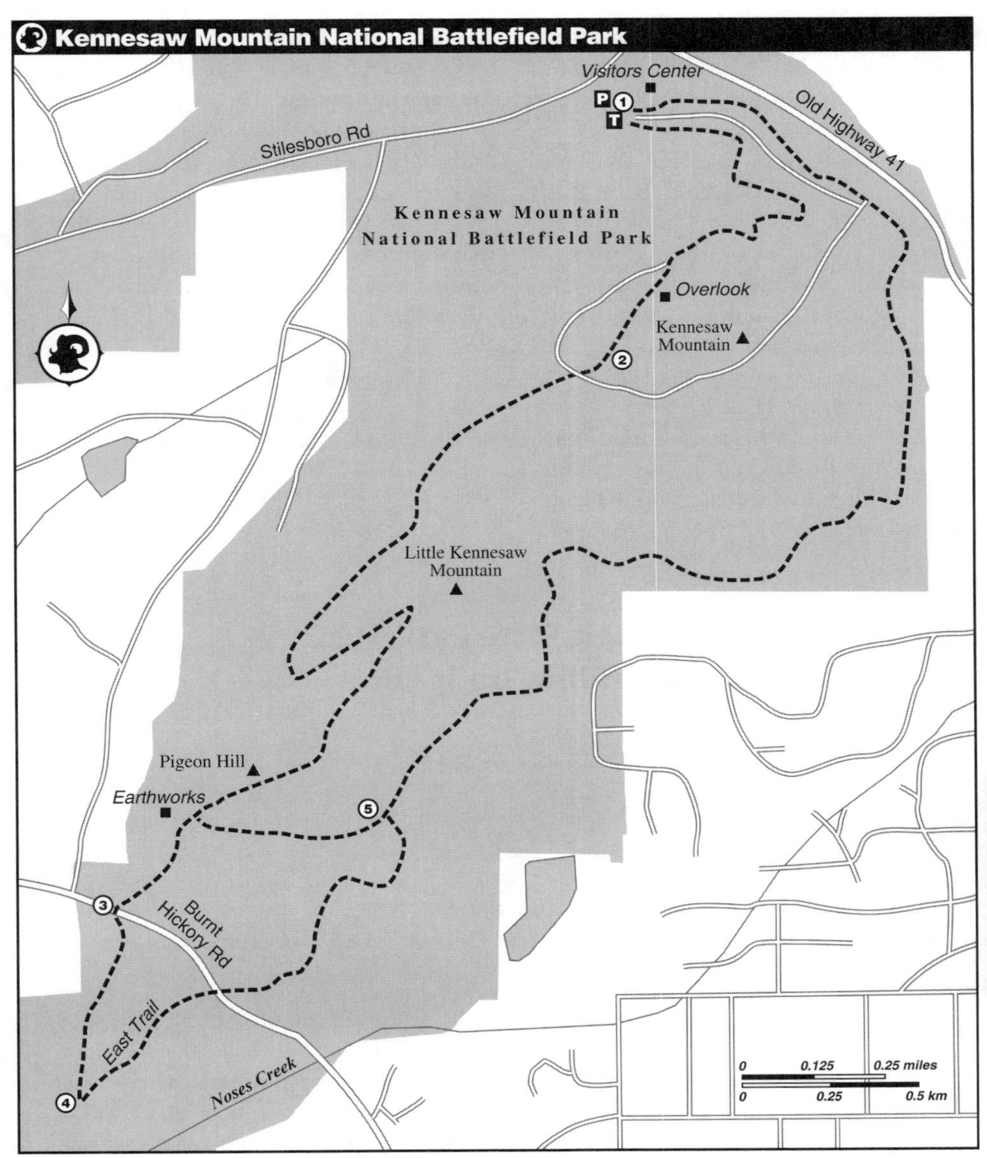

cross Pigeon Hill where 5500 Union soldiers launched a bloody but unsuccessful assault on the well-entrenched rebels.

Continue on an especially attractive section of trail where large oaks shade a field of boulders and then drop down to a wide rock outcrop where you can soak in the sun and enjoy long views to the west. Descending the outcrop, a trail intersects on the left. Rather than taking this trail, continue southwest and see if you can spy the battlement earthworks, or trenches, carved into the land beside the trail.

Cross Burnt Hickory Road to enter the field from which Union soldiers launched their assaults **(Waypoint 3)**. The field has been preserved to appear much like it did during the battle, and an interpretive sign at the edge of the field details troop movements.

Skirt the edge of the field and enter a wide, well-shaded gravel path that's popular with walkers and trail runners. This part of the hike gives a glimpse of the recreational trails in the area and serves as a nice cooldown. At 3.3 miles **(Waypoint 4)**, turn left onto the East Trail and take the low rise to the north. You then cross Burnt Hickory Road—watch carefully for cars whipping around sharp curves. At 4.1 miles you can turn left at a trail junction to further explore Pigeon Hill **(Waypoint 5)**. Backtrack to **Waypoint 5** and turn left to continue toward the visitors center on a mellow trail lined with oaks and sweetgums. The walking is easy as you take a wide path in a forest that transitions to mostly pine. At 6.5 miles, bear left at a Y intersection, following a sign that indicates it's 0.7 mile to the visitors center. At 6.6 miles bear left at another Y junction to walk the final half mile to the trailhead.

UTM WAYPOINTS

1. 16S 723737E 3762832N
2. 16S 723653E 3762178N
3. 16S 722349E 3760729N
4. 16S 722196E 3760054N
5. 16S 723031E 3760867N

TRIP 4 Sweetwater Creek State Park: History & Non-Game Wildlife Trails Loop

Distance	2.8–5.4 miles, semiloop
Hiking Time	2 hours
Difficulty	Easy to moderate
Elevation Gain/Loss	+315/-305 feet
Trail Uses	Leashed dogs and good for kids
Best Times	Year-round
Agency	Sweetwater Creek State Park
Recommended Map	A Sweetwater Creek State Park trail map is available at the Interpretive Center.

HIGHLIGHTS Sweetwater Creek State Park not only holds the remains of a historic manufacturing facility but its interpretive hiking trails lead to a set of falls as well as quiet, remote spots on Sweetwater Creek. In 1846, a mill was constructed along this stretch of the creek where the gradient changes abruptly. The mill produced thread, yarn, and fabric, including Osnaburg cloth (a rough cotton used to make uniforms for Confederate soldiers) until Union troops burned the mill in 1864. As you hike the red-blazed History Trail, you'll see where slaves piled stones to form the millrace, a long, narrow channel that directed water to a 16-foot-wide wheel, which, in turn, powered a series of gears to run machinery. Farther down, the History Trail overlooks Sweetwater Falls, and the Non-Game Wildlife Trail further explores the creek bank before winding through the pine and hardwood forest to the west.

DIRECTIONS From Atlanta take Interstate 20 west to Exit 44 at Thornton Road. Turn left onto Thornton Road, go 0.2 mile, and turn right on Blairs Bridge Road. Go 2 miles and then turn left on Mount Vernon Road. Go 1.4 miles and turn left at the sign for the visitors center. Continue on this road 0.6 mile to the parking area.

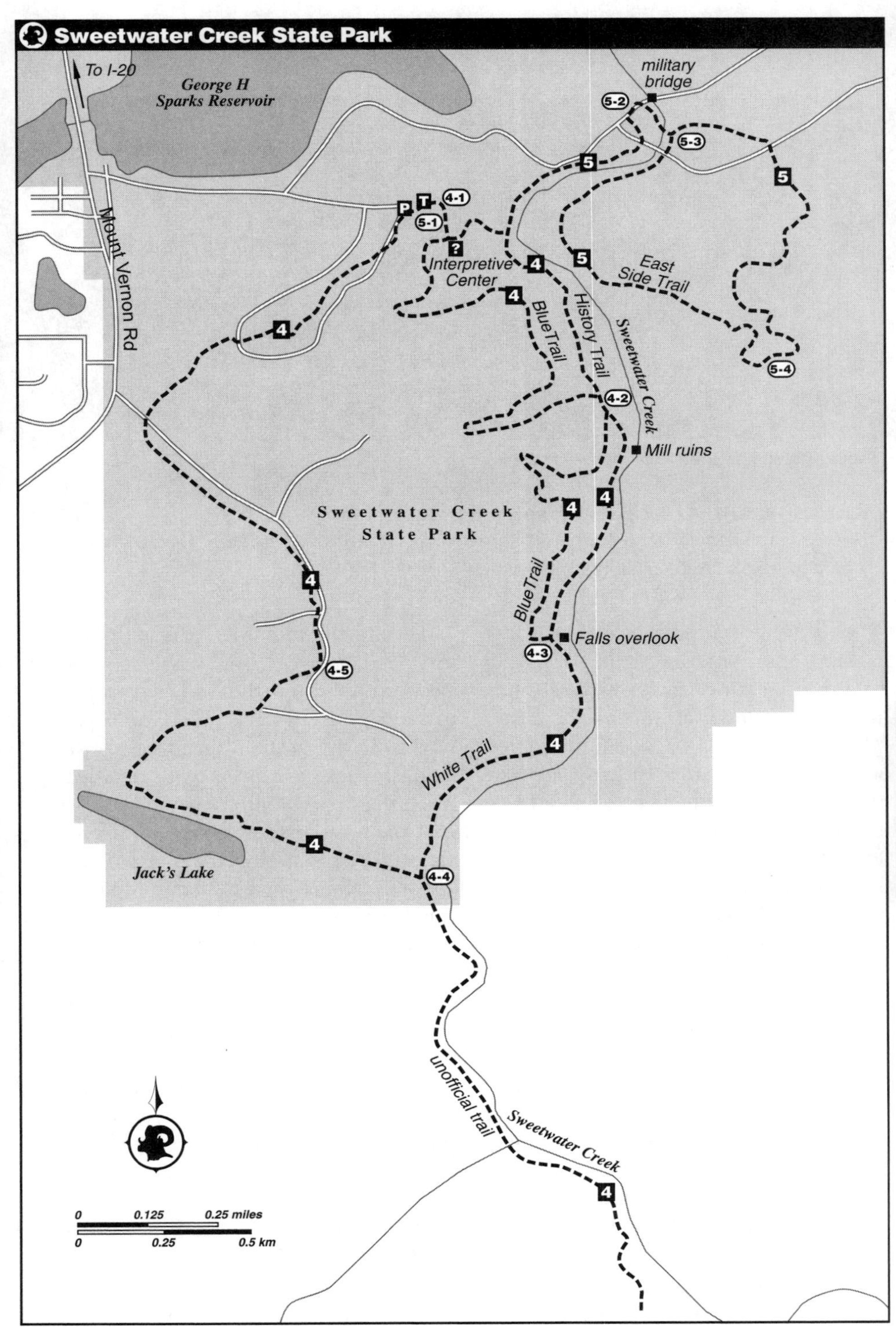
Sweetwater Creek State Park
To I-20
George H
Sparks Reservoir
military
bridge
Mount Vernon Rd
Interpretive
Center
East
Side Trail
History Trail
Blue Trail
Sweetwater Creek
Mill ruins
Sweetwater Creek
State Park
Blue Trail
Falls overlook
White Trail
Jack's Lake
unofficial trail
Sweetwater Creek
0
0.125
0.25 miles
0
0.25
0.5 km

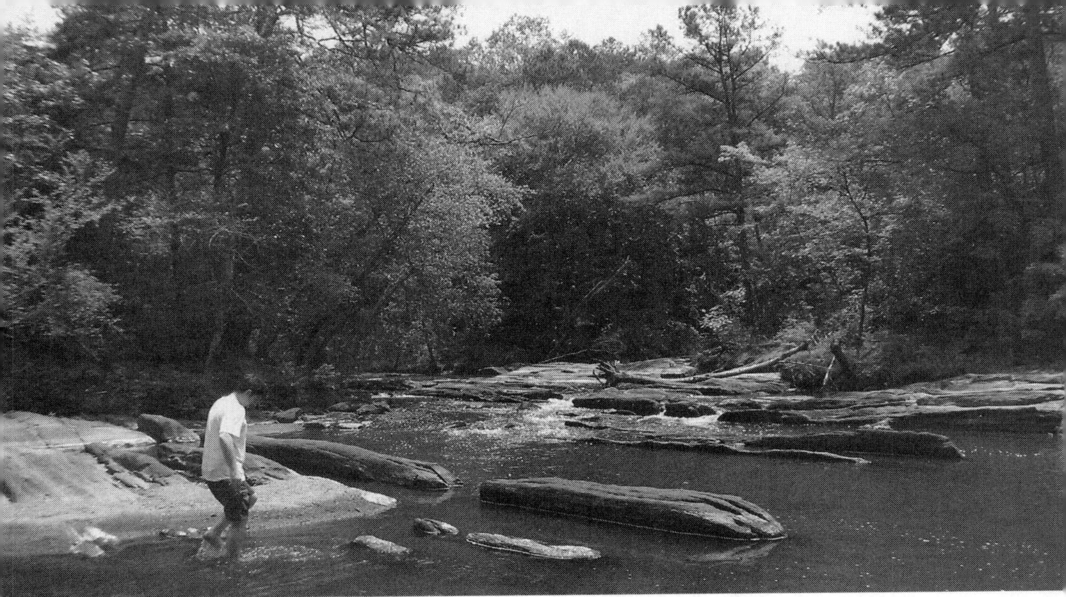

Wading in a remote stretch of Sweetwater Creek

FACILITIES/TRAILHEAD The Interpretive Center, restroom facilities, and picnic areas are all near the trailhead. The park is open 7 AM–10 PM and charges a $3 parking fee. You can also purchase a $30 Annual ParkPass by calling (770) 389-7401.

Begin at the southeast side of the parking area **(Waypoint 1)** and take the Sweetwater History Trail, which descends through oaks to a trail junction at 242 feet. The yellow-blazed East Side Trail is to the left, and the red-blazed History Trail is to the right. Turn right and go south following red blazes, passing interpretive signs for raccoons and blue jays. The path soon runs alongside Sweetwater Creek. As you walk among a forest of oaks, poplars, and beeches, look for the interpretive sign for New Manchester, which explains that a post office and company store were once located here. At 0.3 mile turn left to leave the red trail and take a connector trail, which crosses a wood footbridge. The bridge spans the millrace and leads to a small island that lies between the millrace and the main channel of Sweetwater Creek. After a brief walk across the island, at 0.5 mile return to the main trail, turn left, and go south. Ahead you soon see a set of wood steps to the left that give you a close view of the mill ruins **(Waypoint 2)**.

Beyond the mill, the red-blazed History Trail turns left, and a set of wood steps heads down to the creek. Follow this path 0.5 mile to Sweetwater Falls. If you can, avoid this section during peak visitation because it can be quite crowded. Also, the trail becomes what I call a goat path—an ankle-twisting jumble of rocks, roots, and sloped terrain. There are cables lining parts of the trail to keep you balanced. You reach wooden steps that ascend to platforms overlooking the broad swath of turbulent water **(Waypoint 3)**. Ascend the steps to the intersection with the blue and white Non-Game Wildlife trails.

From **Waypoint 3**, you can complete a short loop via the blue-blazed Non-Game Wildlife Trail, or walk a long loop via the white-blazed Non-Game Wildlife Trail.

Short Loop: Blue Non-Game Wildlife Trail

From **Waypoint 3**, to complete a 2.8-mile loop, go right to take the blue-blazed trail west. You climb steeply and then roller coaster through pines and hardwoods. The creek bellows far below and out of sight, and the trail drops down to intersect with the red-blazed History Trail at 1.8 miles into your trek. Stay on the blue trail, which turns west, and take the wide, rocky trail up into oaks. Having explored the rocky creek bank and high hardwoods, you now follow a stream through bottomland forest of beech and ferns. Look for an interpretive sign for the red-bellied woodpecker as well as trees riddled with holes. Beech trees appear as you follow a creek and then cross it to rise steeply into hardwoods and loblolly pines. An interpretive sign indicates that you might see a Carolina wren whose whistle sounds like "tea kettle, tea kettle, tea kettle." Benches along here offer good places to sit, rest, and listen for their song. The path continues to rise and fall as it turns west and then finally northwest to meet the sidewalk skirting the visitors center.

Long Loop: White Non-Game Wildlife Trail

This option allows you to complete a longer 5.4-mile loop. From the intersection of the white and blue trails, go left to follow the white-blazed trail south. Hug the creek for 0.6 mile and reach a wood footbridge at Jack's Branch, which flows into Sweetwater Creek **(Waypoint 4)**. A sign on the bridge cautions hikers that the path on the other side of the bridge is not a designated trail. Nevertheless, it passes an excellent spot on the creek, so cross the bridge and go south. After walking a little over 0.2 mile, look left for a wide section of the creek where it looks like two creeks are converging. (Actually, these are two branches of Sweetwater Creek that flow around an island.) Depending on water levels, you may have a wide gravel creek bank where you can rest and wade into the water to recline on exposed boulders. You can continue south along the creek for another half mile, but you soon move from attractive creekside views to less appealing forest. However, if you do visit here in summer, and you like blackberries, you might want to at least go as far south as the power line break, where you can feast among berry thickets lining the path.

A Fowler's toad

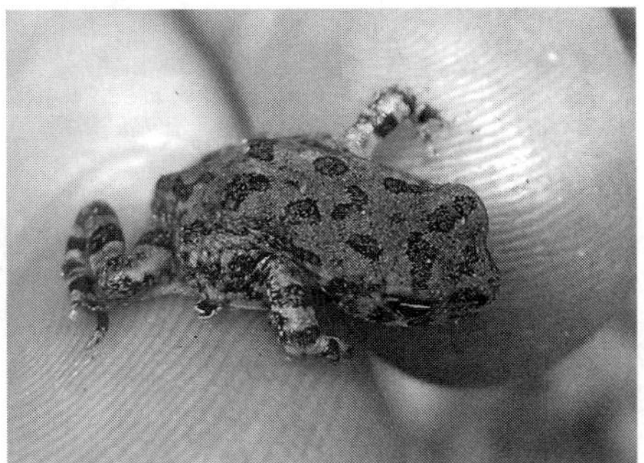

Return to the wood footbridge, turn left, and go west on the white-blazed trail. The trail stays close to Jack's Branch and soon reaches Jack's Lake, a small body of water to the left, which is home to mallard ducks. After climbing up through hardwoods, you reach the top of Jack's Hill where pockets of trees dot open grassland. At **Waypoint 5**, turn left and go north on the jeep road. At the next Y intersection with a jeep road, bear left. With small pines and dense brambles, the forest surrounding the path becomes less scenic. However, the path is easy and flat—welcome after your long walk—to the southwest end of the parking area.

UTM WAYPOINTS

1. 16S 719715E 3737194N
2. 16S 720130E 3736742N
3. 16S 720001E 3736005N
4. 16S 719547E 3735317N
5. 16S 719319E 3735941N

TRIP 5 Sweetwater Creek State Park: East Side Trail

Distance 2.6 miles, semiloop
Hiking Time 1–1½ hours
Difficulty Moderate
Elevation Gain/Loss +330/-325 feet
Trail Use Leashed dogs
Best Times Year-round
Agency Sweetwater Creek State Park
Recommended Map A Sweetwater Creek State Park trail map is available at the interpretive center.

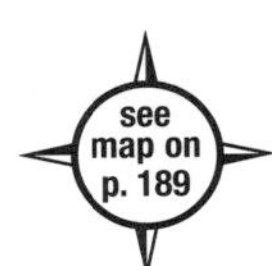

HIGHLIGHTS Compared to Sweetwater Creek State Park's other trails, the East Side Trail offers a bit more solitude and the opportunity to work your lungs. After taking an old military bridge across Sweetwater Creek, the trail takes a steep turn and rises to an elevation of more than 1000 feet. The hardwood forest is free of dense underbrush giving you clear views across the leafy ground. From the high, drier flank of the hill, the trail drops into a drainage where the moist soil supports lush ferns. The path levels out as it skirts the creek bank and completes the loop.

DIRECTIONS From Atlanta take Interstate 20 west to Exit 44 at Thornton Road. Turn left onto Thornton Road, go 0.2 mile, and turn right on Blairs Bridge Road. Go 2 miles and then turn left on Mount Vernon Road. Go 1.4 miles and turn left at the sign for the visitors center. Continue on this road 0.6 mile to the parking area.

FACILITIES/TRAILHEAD Near the trailhead parking area there is an interpretive center, restroom facilities, and a picnic area. The park is open 7 AM to 10 PM, and there is a $3 parking fee. You can also purchase a $30 Annual ParkPass by calling (770) 389-7401.

Begin at the southeast side of the parking area **(Waypoint 1)** and take the Sweetwater History Trail, which descends through oaks to a trail junction at 242 feet. The yellow-blazed East Side Trail is to the left and the red History Trail is to the right. Turn left and take the sandy path north alongside the slow-flowing river bordered by high brush. After walking 600 feet, bear right at a Y intersection.

At 0.3 mile, turn right to cross an old military bridge **(Waypoint 2)**. Just before you cross, look left for a yellow and red sign that offers a few details about the bridge's history.

After crossing, turn right and go southeast in bottomland forest of oaks, beeches, and poplars. The loop portion of the trail begins at 0.5 mile **(Waypoint 3)**. Turn left and climb to the east, leaving the shadier woods below and entering more open terrain dominated by chestnut oaks. As you ascend the hill, look for the leathery fins of shelf fungi sprouting from the bark at the base of trees.

At 1.4 miles, you reach the high point on the loop **(Waypoint 4)** and then drop steeply through a drainage, which is shaded by multiple canopy layers. Muscular vines stretch between trees, and smaller tendrils hang like curtains.

As you continue an easy descent, the creek comes into view and the trail levels out at 1.7 miles. In a low flow, the water is dead calm, and the rocks below the surface are green shadows. The trail breaks into sunlight, goes right, and then parallels the river. A few steps farther the level path turns away to the northeast, but you soon walk beside the water again and reach the beginning of the loop at 2.1 miles. Go northwest back to the bridge and retrace your steps to the trailhead.

UTM WAYPOINTS

1. 16S 719710E 3737192N
2. 16S 720208E 3737597N
3. 16S 720336E 3737514N
4. 16S 720604E 3736831N

TRIP 6 Silver Comet Trail: Rambo to McPherson Road

Distance	10.4 miles, out-and-back
Hiking Time	4–5 hours
Difficulty	Easy
Elevation Gain/Loss	+/-475 feet
Trail Uses	Road biking, horseback riding, and leashed dogs
Best Times	Year-round
Agency	Path Foundation
Recommended Map	A Silver Comet Trail map is available online at www.pathfoundation.org.

HIGHLIGHTS From 1947 to 1969, the Silver Comet Train carried passengers between New York City and Birmingham, Alabama, with service to Atlanta. Its early days marked the great age of rail travel, and the shining Silver Comet offered all the bells and whistles including luxury sleeping accommodations and observation cars. The portion of the rail line that ran through Cobb County to the Georgia/Alabama border closed in 1989. Then, in 1998, this corridor was transformed into a 60-mile paved, multiuse trail that draws cyclists and hikers, and includes 17 access points for people with disabilities. The section of the Silver Comet that begins at the Rambo Nursery in Dallas and runs west to McPherson Road is especially peaceful, as forest buffers much of the path from U.S. Highway 278. Also, small changes in elevation make the path comfortable for people of all abilities.

DIRECTIONS From Atlanta, take Interstate 20 west to Exit 44. Take GA Highway 6 west (which becomes GA Highway 6/U.S. Highway 278) 20.2 miles and then turn left onto Bonnie Lane. Go 0.2 mile and turn left onto Tucker Blvd. Go 0.2 mile to the parking area, which lies just before the entrance to Rambo Nursery.

FACILITIES/TRAILHEAD There is a privy in the parking area. There are no water sources along this section of the trail, so carry all that you will need.

For this hike, the only trailhead is near Rambo Nursery, so you can simply walk as far as you'd like, and then turn back. An interesting group of boulders just beyond McPherson Road makes a nice place to rest before returning.

From the southwest side of the parking area, enter the two-lane, paved Silver Comet Trail **(Waypoint 1)**, which runs though a mix of pines and hardwoods. Stay alert as you walk, as you'll likely encounter a large number of cyclists. In some areas, the shoulder of the trail is wide enough to walk on. At 0.7 mile, you reach a rest area with benches beside the path. Also, an interpretive sign points out the types of plants and animals you'll find along the old rail corridor.

At 0.8 mile **(Waypoint 2)**, cross the 700-foot-long bridge that was once a train trestle and sits 100 feet above the forested basin for Pumpkinvine Creek. To the

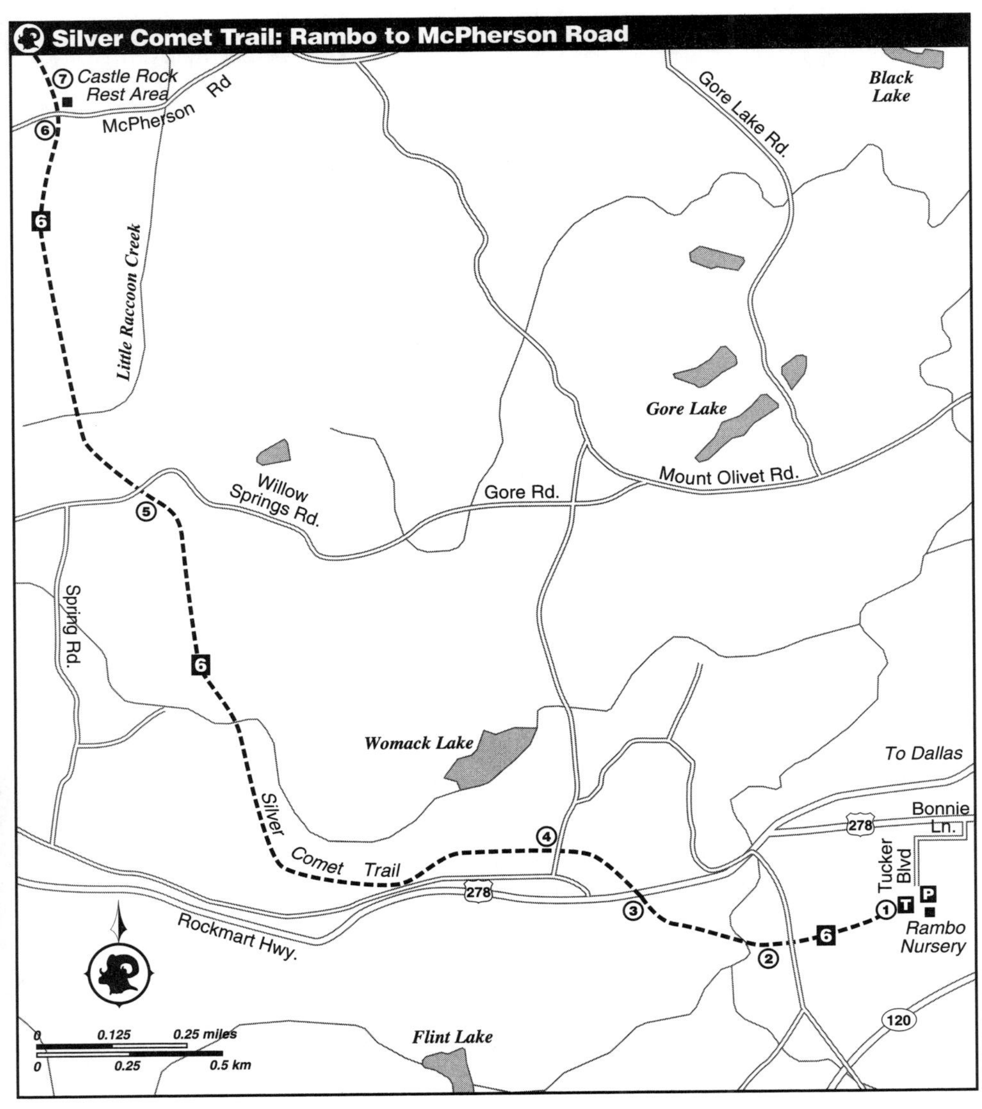

right the land is wild, though a housing subdivision fills your view to the left.

Walk another tenth of a mile and take a tunnel beneath U.S. 278 **(Waypoint 3)**. From here, the path is lined with dense poplars and pines, which buffer the highway noise. At 1.4 miles **(Waypoint 4)**, the path runs through a short tunnel that sits beneath Mount Olivet Rd. The trail takes its first noticeable rise, though it soon levels out, and you begin to walk through attractive forest.

Civilization intrudes again briefly as you pass through a power line break, but the thick woods soon close in. I scouted this trail on a blue-sky Saturday, and though there were plenty of people wheeling down the Silver Comet, traffic grew lighter as I continued west.

At 3.8 miles **(Waypoint 5)**, the trail runs beneath a wood trestle, which supports a

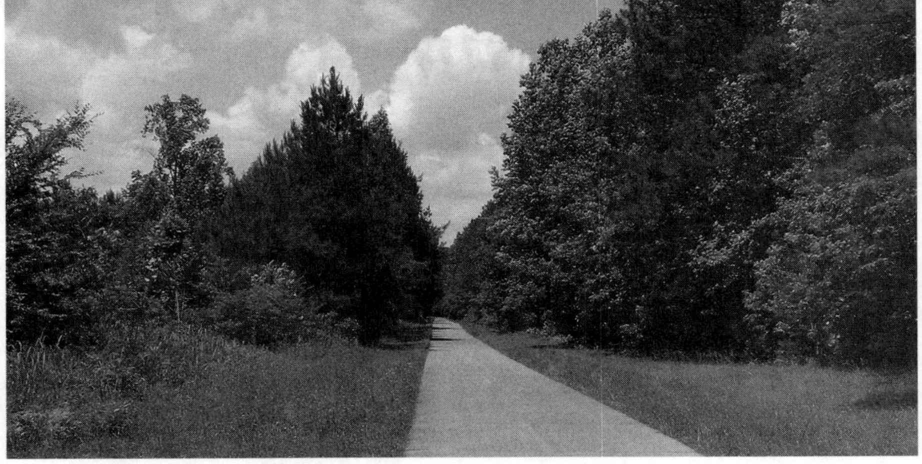

Silver Comet Trail between Rambo Nursery and McPherson Road

stretch of Willow Springs Road. As you pass beneath the trestle, the sweet and heavy aroma of aged wood hangs around its thick wood beams.

The Silver Comet Trail crosses McPherson Road at 4.9 miles **(Waypoint 6)**. If you continue, you reach the Castle Rock Rest Area at 5.2 miles **(Waypoint 7)**. The rest area is a wide shoulder to the right of the trail where benches sit beneath high boulders. If it's warm and the benches are covered in sun, you can scramble to the top of the boulders to rest in the shade. From the rest area, retrace your steps to return to the trailhead.

UTM WAYPOINTS

1. 16S 697012E 3754762N
2. 16S 696127E 3754534N
3. 16S 695599E 3754660N
4. 16S 694962E 3754909N
5. 16S 693153E 3756773N
6. 16S 692575E 3758018N
7. 16S 692594E 3758577N

TRIP 7 F. D. Roosevelt State Park: Wolfden Loop, White Candle, & Beaver Pond Trails

Distance	6.7–7.1 miles, loop
Hiking Time	4 hours
Difficulty	Moderate
Elevation Gain/Loss	+/-690 feet
Trail Uses	Leashed dogs and backpacking
Best Times	Year-round
Agency	F. D. Roosevelt State Park and Pine Mountain Trail Association
Recommended Map	A trail is available in the visitors center and online at www.gastateparks.org.

HIGHLIGHTS A little more than a mile into the Wolfden Loop Trail, you'll wind through groves of azalea, laurel, and rhododendron to visit several small falls and pools. The most impressive water feature is Cascade Falls, which is nestled beside the Wolfden rock crag. The Wolfden Loop meets the White Candle Trail on a western-facing slope with views of Pine Mountain Valley. Running between the White Candle and Woldfen trails, the Beaver Pond Trail crosses the wetland habitat along Wolfden Branch.

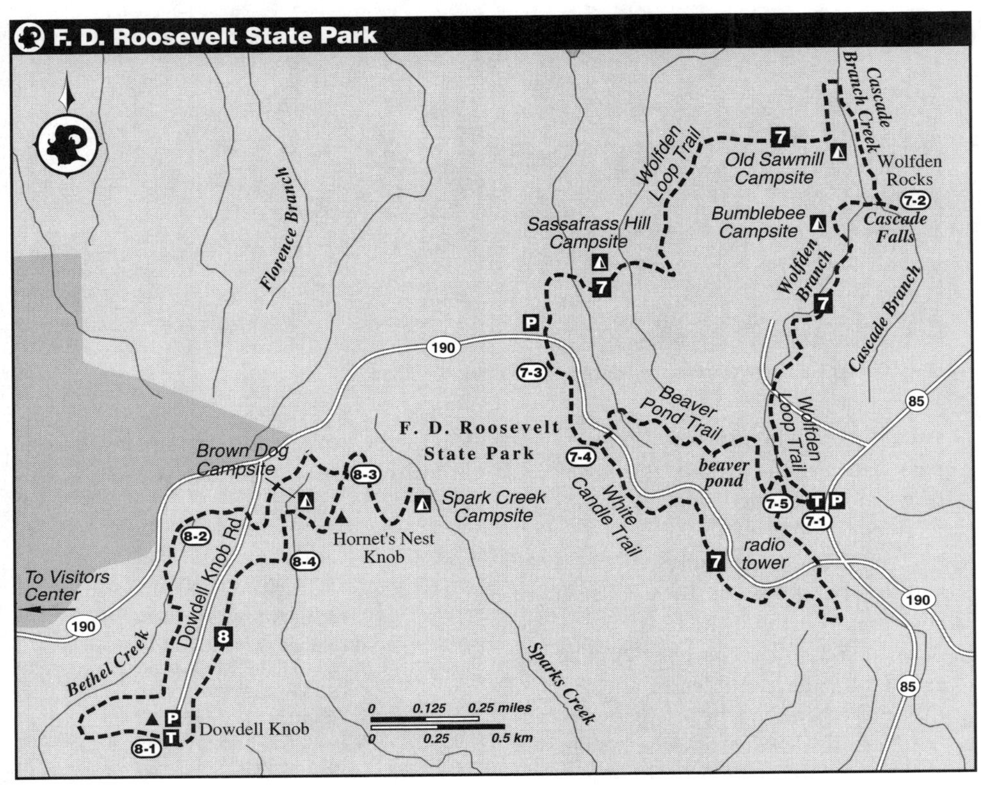

DIRECTIONS From Atlanta take Interstate 85 south to Interstate 185. On I-185 take Exit 42 for U.S. Highway 27 and turn left onto U.S. 27 east. Go 13.8 miles and turn left onto GA Highway 190. Travel on GA 190 about 3 miles to reach the visitors center on the right. To reach the trailhead from the visitors center, travel east on GA 190 to the intersection with U.S. Highway 85 ALT. Turn left and travel on U.S. Highway 85 ALT 0.2 mile and turn left into the parking lot near the WJSP-TV tower.

FACILITIES/TRAILHEAD There are no facilities at the trailhead. The park charges a $3 parking fee. You can purchase an Annual ParkPass for $30 by calling (770) 389-7401. Obtain a permit at the visitors center to camp in the backcountry ($5 per person per day). The park has 140 tent, trailer, and RV sites ($24) and 22 cottages ($95–$130).

At the northwest end of the parking area, enter the trail at the PINE MOUNTAIN TRAIL sign **(Waypoint 1)**. Walk 430 feet to the junction with the White Candle Trail, and continue straight to follow the Wolfden Loop Trail. In a forest of pines and poplars you skirt Wolfden Branch, and keep a lookout for deer and eastern box turtles on the trail. Ferns and mountain laurel grow thick as you wind through rolling terrain on a rocky and rooted path.

At the 1-mile mark, cross Wolfden Branch in a heavily forested pocket and climb up through an alcove of laurel. The trail quickly leaves the stream basin, rises to a rocky hilltop, and soon descends to the creek to wind among a series of small

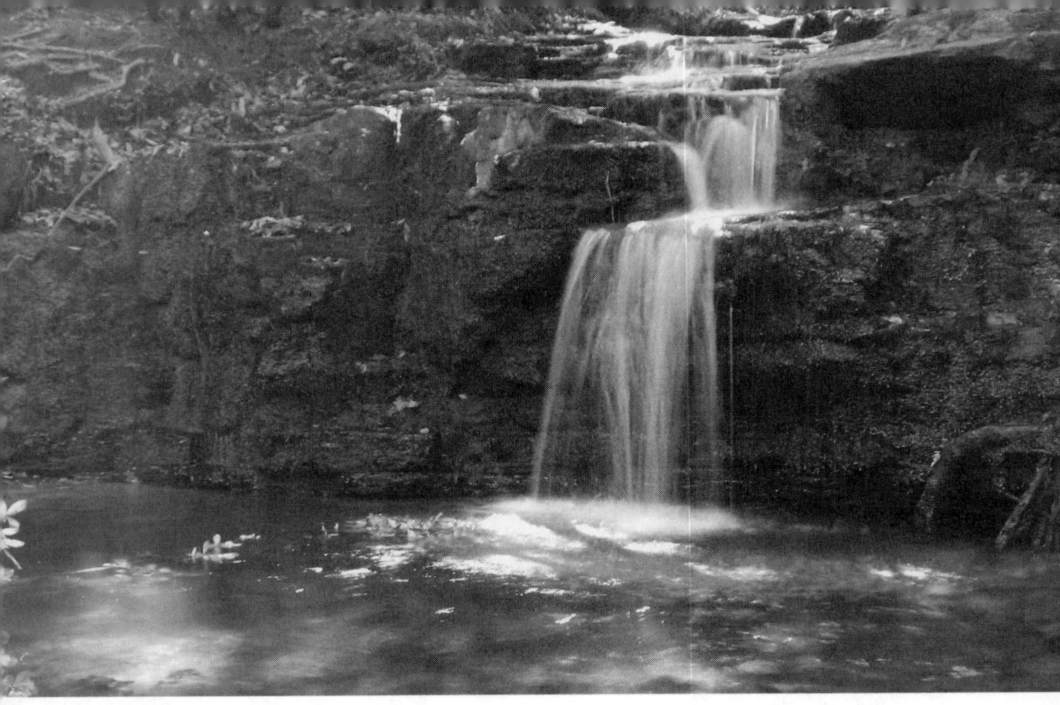

Cascade Falls on the Wolfden Loop Trail

waterfalls. The first is Csonka Falls, and 886 feet farther is Big Rock Falls where water pours over a low rock shelf into a large, tea-colored pool. At 1.5 miles Slippery Rock Falls rushes over a table of rock to cruise across a wide stone floor.

At 1.6 miles, the trail to the Bumblebee Campsite enters on the left. Turn right and travel north to continue on the Wolfden Loop. At mile 2 **(Waypoint 2)** you reach one of the best places to hang out for a while. At Cascade Falls a stream drops down a series of rock ledges, emptying into a sunlit pool of clear water. On a warm day it's difficult to resist the urge to wade in. From here, the trail turns left and passes the Wolfden rock outcrop, which has a long shallow opening at its base.

The trail proceeds over a pine-hardwood slope before dropping to cross Cascade Branch. At 2.3 miles the Old Sawmill Campsite lies to the left of the trail. After crossing a low area with some massive pines, the trail continues to alternate between hills with oaks and lower forest dominated by pines. At 4.4 miles you pass the spacious Sassafrass Hill Campsite.

At 4.9 miles cross the road to the Rocky Point Parking area. On the east side enter the blue-blazed trail. At 5 miles **(Waypoint 3)** bear left at the trail junction to continue on the Wolfden Loop Trail following white blazes. Here the path cuts across a southwest slope covered in oaks with intermittent views of forested terrain stretching to the horizon.

At 5.4 miles **(Waypoint 4)** bear left at the trail junction to take the Beaver Pond Trail 1.3 miles back to the parking area, or bear right to take the White Candle Trail 2.4 miles to the parking area. The White Candle Trail rolls easily along the slope, and at 7.1 miles the Odie Overlook provides a panoramic view of Pine Mountain Valley.

The trail then passes through an area where Roosevelt planted 5000 longleaf pines from 1929 to 1930, though half the stand was destroyed by a tornado in the 1950s. The trail crosses the road and winds northwest to a T junction **(Waypoint**

5). You can turn left onto the Beaver Pond Trail, or turn right onto the White Candle Trail for a quick trip back to the parking area.

From **Waypoint 5**, if you bear left onto the Beaver Pond Trail, you'll walk through bottomland forest and reach the pond at about 0.3 mile. You never know what you might see in here—I once spied an armadillo just before it dove into a hole at the base of a tree. From the pond, the trail continues for about a mile, climbing through hardwood forest and finally meeting the White Candle Trail at **Waypoint 4**. From **Waypoint 4**, you can take either the White Candle or Beaver Pond trails back to the trailhead.

UTM WAYPOINTS

1. 16S 715136E 3637248N
2. 16S 715650E 3639254N
3. 16S 713388E 3638297N
4. 16S 713700E 3637741N
5. 16S 714947E 3637396N

TRIP 8 F. D. Roosevelt State Park: Dowdell Loop Trail

Distance	4.4 miles, loop
Hiking Time	2–3 hours
Difficulty	Moderate
Elevation Gain/Loss	+665/-765 feet
Trail Use	Leashed dogs
Best Times	Year-round
Agency	F. D. Roosevelt State Park and Pine Mountain Trail Association
Recommended Map	A trail map is available in the visitors center and online at www.gastateparks.org.

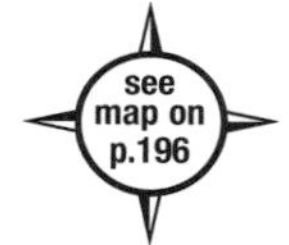

HIGHLIGHTS The highest point on Pine Mountain, Dowdell Knob sits at an elevation of 1395 feet and overlooks the low, rolling Piedmont hills. This was one of President Franklin Roosevelt's favorite places on the mountain to relax, and an interpretive sign explains that DOWDELL'S KNOB WAS ONE OF THE FEW PLACES WHERE HE FELT AT EASE AND COMFORTABLE ENOUGH TO WEAR HIS LEG BRACES OUTSIDE HIS PANTS. Having asked his Secret Service detail to wait down the road and leave him alone for a while, Roosevelt sat on this peaceful peak just two days before he died on April 12, 1945. Walking clockwise, you begin the Dowdell Loop Trail on the dry ridge of oaks and hickory trees. The path traverses rock slopes, dips into the Bethel Creek basin, and regains high ground before dropping to a shaded creek. On the final stretch, you climb the ridge again, with breaks in the trees providing views of distant hills.

DIRECTIONS From Atlanta take Interstate 85 south to Interstate 185. On I-185 take Exit 42 for U.S. Highway 27 and turn left onto U.S. Highway 27 east. Go 13.8 miles and turn left onto GA 190. Travel on GA Highway 190 about 3 miles to reach the visitors center on the right. To reach the trailhead from the visitors center, travel east on GA 190 5.7 miles and turn right onto Dowdell Knob Rd. Go 1.3 miles to the parking area.

FACILITIES/TRAILHEAD There are no facilities at the trailhead. The park charges a $3 parking fee. You can purchase an Annual ParkPass for $30 by calling (770) 389-7401. The park campground has 140 tent, trailer, and RV sites ($24) and 22 cottages ($95–$130). Obtain a permit at the visitors center to camp in the backcountry on the Pine Mountain Trail ($5 per person per day).

On the west side of the parking area, begin your hike at the PINE MOUNTAIN TRAIL sign **(Waypoint 1)**. Walk 360 feet to a T junction and turn right to travel northwest. As you walk along the crest of the ridge, the oak and hickory forest shrouds your views of the Piedmont lowlands to the south. Pine Mountain has some of the highest-elevation ridges in the state, and Georgia birders believe the mountain may be home to a couple of species usually found farther north, like the scarlet tanager and ovenbird, but the good hardwood forest has lots of other interesting breeders too, like the summer tanager, wood thrush, and great crested flycatcher.

At 0.4 mile you might see lizards, chipmunks, or even snakes in the rocky outcrops along the slope. As you move along a north-facing slope, moss adds a little flair to side of the path, and about a mile farther along, switchbacks take you down through a series of rock piles.

At 1.4 miles **(Waypoint 2)** turn right at the trail junction and travel northeast following white blazes. The path climbs to a hardwood forest where breaks in the tree canopy allow ample sunlight in. On the Pine Mountain slopes, the plentiful chestnut oak and hickory trees produce acorns and nuts that serve as rich food for deer, turkeys, squirrels, and birds.

At 1.9 miles, cross Dowdell Knob Road and follow moderate climbs and descents to a trail junction at 2.5 miles **(Waypoint 3)**. Turn right (the blue-blazed path to the left leads to the Spark Creek Campsite and travel south to continue on the Dowdell Loop. Cross the ominously named Hornet's Nest Knob and descend a rock-strewn path.

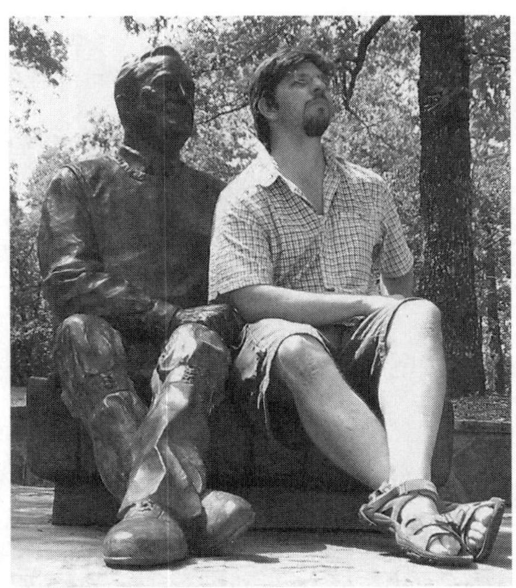

The author and FDR at Dowdell Knob

At 3.1 miles, the Brown Dog Campsite is to the right. Turn left to enter a creek basin where the forest is suddenly crawling with ferns and mossy rocks. Decidedly more lush and shaded than the majority of the trail, this is a good place to cool your heels **(Waypoint 4)**.

The trail climbs steeply from the creek and cuts across high ground. Oaks crowd the path as you ascend steadily across the east-facing slope of the mountain. Look left as you climb to catch glimpses of the lowlands to the east. At 4.4 miles, turn right at the trail junction to return to the trailhead.

UTM WAYPOINTS

1. 16S 710981E 3635868N
2. 16S 710933E 3636820N
3. 16S 712080E 3637553N
4. 16S 711708E 3637291N

Chapter 5
Central Atlanta

From the low banks of the Chattahoochee River to the towering granite peak of Stone Mountain, the central Atlanta area offers great contrasts in hiking trails. Certainly, a hot spot such as the Stone Mountain Walk-Up Trail can become a crowded human highway on a sunny Saturday. But the peak of exposed granite undoubtedly offers a view of Atlanta that you shouldn't miss. And even on a weekend, you can enjoy a peaceful walk along the Cherokee Trail that circles the mountain. Southeast of the city, Panola Mountain is a smaller but no less intriguing hulk of exposed granite where hikers can examine early forms of plant life growing in the harsh, rocky terrain. Also lying to the southeast, the William H. Reynolds Memorial Nature Preserve provides a decidedly different experience, where lowland woods are teeming with toads, turtles, beavers, and a variety of birds, including herons and geese.

Chattahoochee River National Recreation Area

From a remote spot high in the mountains of north Georgia, the Chattahoochee River begins its long journey to the Gulf of Mexico, skirting the western side of Atlanta along the way. In 1978, President Jimmy Carter authorized the formation of the Chattahoochee River National Recreation Area, which preserved 48 miles of river corridor from Buford Dam at Lake Sidney Lanier to Peachtree Creek northwest of Atlanta. Part of the National Park System, the Chattahoochee River NRA includes waterways and trails, split into 14 units, that not only offer Atlanta residents an escape from urban sprawl, but also trace the area's history. Some units, such as Island Ford, include paths along the riverbank that provide a picturesque backdrop for hiking, while also visiting rock outcrops formerly used by Native Americans. The forested trails in the Sope Creek unit explore the former sites of mills that established Atlanta as an industrial center in the South. And at Vickery Creek, where Gen. William Sherman left a path of destruction during the Civil War, a waterfall and rushing waters drown out troubles of the past and present.

Canada goose on "The Hooch"

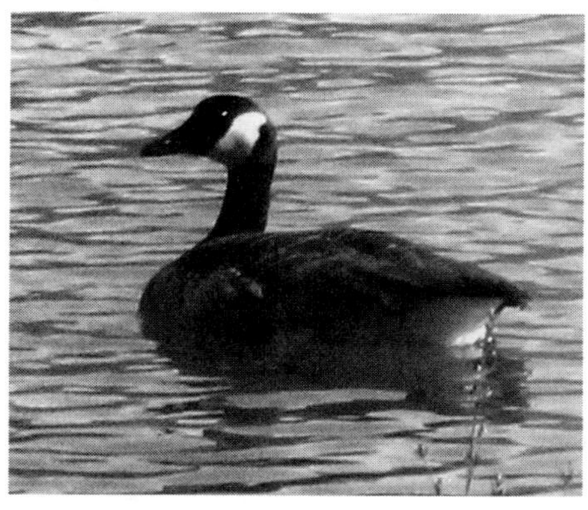

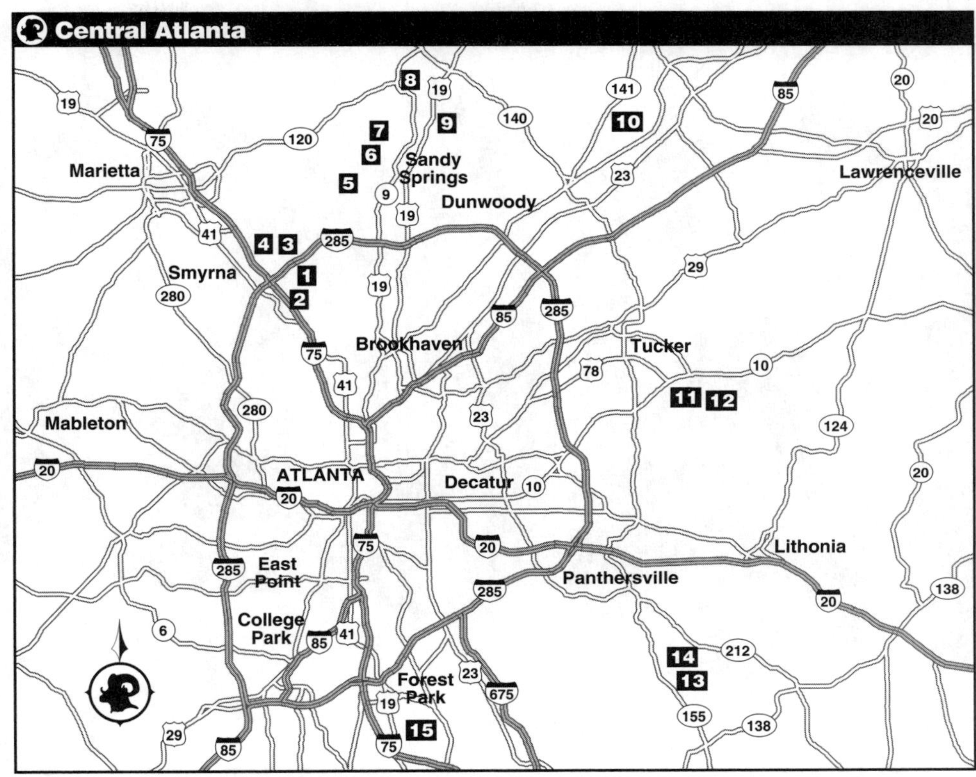

Stone Mountain Park

For at least 9000 years people have been drawn to the hulk of granite known as Stone Mountain. Archaeologists have unearthed artifacts from Ancient Woodland Indians who lived in the forest at the base of the mountain, and it's suspected that ancient people constructed a rock wall around the top of the mountain. The largest exposed piece of granite in the world, Stone Mountain became a tourist attraction in the 1850s and now draws 4 million visitors a year. It is most recognized for the carved mural depicting Robert E. Lee, Thomas "Stonewall" Jackson, and Jefferson Davis on horseback. The mural was begun in 1915, but disputes over the design and funding problems delayed its completion until 1972. Stone Mountain's other great attraction, its 1683-foot summit, offers an impressive 360-degree view of the surrounding landscape, including the Atlanta skyline and Appalachian Mountains.

Panola Mountain State Park

A miniature version of Stone Mountain, Panola Mountain is a 100-acre granite mountain where small communities of plants such as diamorpha remarkably survive in the harsh stone environment. Often, you must literally get down on your knees to see the hairlike stems of these minute plants that sprout in small patches of shallow soil on the rock slabs. A designated National Natural Landmark, Panola Mountain offers the opportunity to see the earliest stage of plant "succession." The plant life that takes hold on the

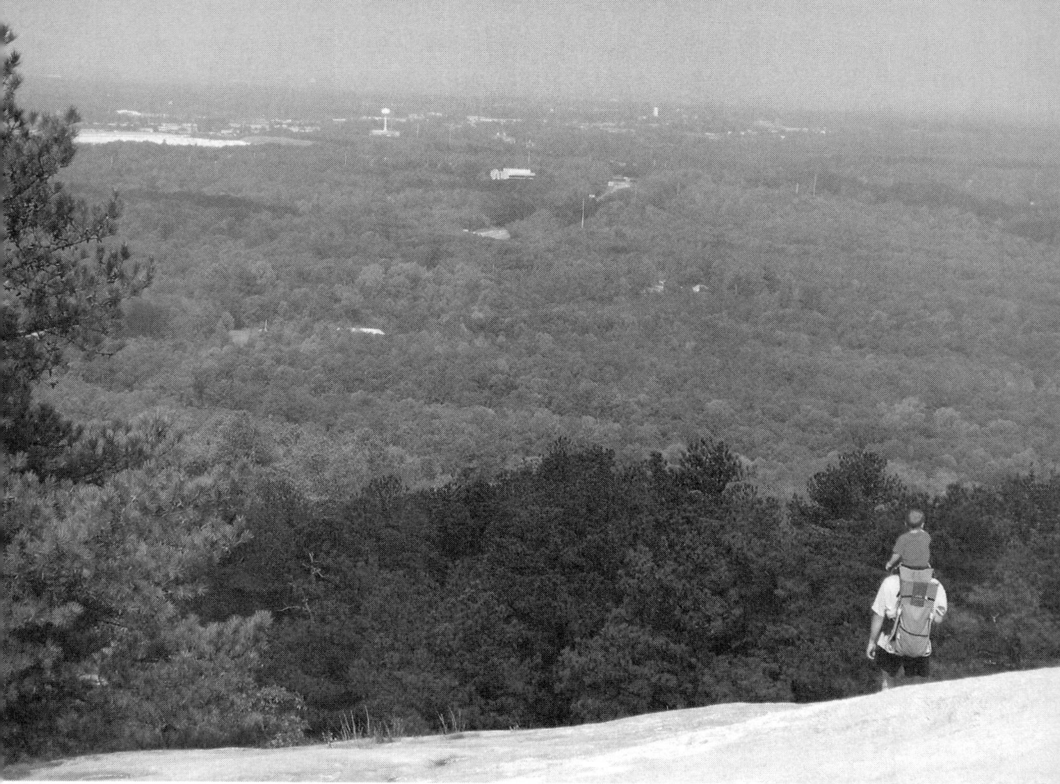

The view near the summit of Stone Mountain

bare granite ground over time leads to the growth of weeds, shrubs, and then trees. Portions of Panola Mountain are accessible to the public only through ranger-led hikes. These treks (hosted Wednesday–Saturday) offer the best opportunity to see Panola's fragile plant communities up close. On your own you can take the Rock Outcrop Trail to view one of the mountain's wide areas of exposed granite, while the Watershed Trail loops through maples, loblolly pines, sweetgum trees, and hardwoods to visit a creek.

Reynolds Nature Preserve

With 146 acres of forest and wetlands, including five ponds, the William H. Reynolds Memorial Nature Preserve supports a great variety of wildlife, including turtles, salamanders, toads, and beavers. Many bird species, such as Canada geese, green herons, and Kentucky warblers, live here, as well as numerous wildflowers, including American beauty berry, red trillium, and lizards' tail. The preserve has 4.5 miles of easy trails with several loops that you can link for long or short walks.

TRIP 1 Chattahoochee River National Recreation Area: East Palisades Trail

Distance	5–5.8 miles, semiloop
Hiking Time	2–3 hours
Difficulty	Easy to moderate
Elevation Gain/Loss	+895/-860 feet
Trail Use	Leashed dogs
Best Times	Year-round
Agency	National Park Service, Chattahoochee River National Recreation Area
Recommended Map	U.S. Forest Service *Cohutta and Big Frog Wilderness Georgia-Tennessee*

HIGHLIGHTS The East Palisades Trail gets its name from the high walls of granite rising above the Chattahoochee River. From atop these bluffs you can look down on rapids coursing through a broad section of the river strewn with boulders. Kayakers run these shoals, but as far back as the 1800s boaters found the rapids hair-raising enough to dub this gauntlet the Devil's Race Course. While the East Palisades Trail leads to bluff views, much of it runs flat beside the water, providing a comfortable path for throngs of walkers and joggers. The 393-acre forest also includes trails that loop through rolling hills of oak and poplar. Navigation here is not difficult as maps are posted at most trail junctions, making it easy to find your way. There are approximately 5 miles of trails in the area, so the round-trip hiking distance and time can vary.

DIRECTIONS From Interstate 285 east, take Exit 22 for Northside Drive, New Northside Drive, and Powers Ferry Road. Turn right onto Northside Drive, and continue to the intersection with Powers Ferry Road. Go through this intersection and travel 1.1 miles to Indian Trail. Turn right onto Indian Trail, and take this road to where it ends at the trail parking area.

From I-285 west, take Exit 22 for Northside Drive, New Northside Drive, and Powers Ferry Road. Continue straight to the second traffic light, and turn left onto Northside Drive. Take Northside Drive to the intersection with Powers Ferry Road. Go through the intersection and travel 1.1 miles to Indian Trail Road. Turn right onto Indian Trail Road, and take this road to where it ends at the trail parking area.

FACILITIES/TRAILHEAD There are no facilities at the trailhead. The park is open dawn to dusk year-round, except Christmas Day. The park charges a $3 parking fee, which you can pay at the kiosk at the trailhead. You can purchase a $25 annual pass for the recreation area by calling (678) 538-1200 or visiting www.nps.gov/chat/index.htm.

At the southwest corner of the parking area (**Waypoint 1**), enter the trail and follow the dirt path through thick stands of pines. The hike begins with an easy walk down a ridge, and then a trek through thick brush beside Long Island Creek, which empties into the Chattahoochee River. At 0.2 mile bear right at a Y intersection to go west, and at 0.5 mile

East Palisades overlooking the Chattahoochee

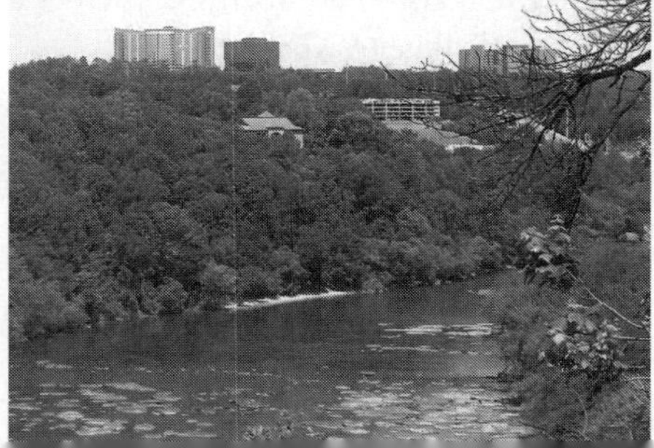

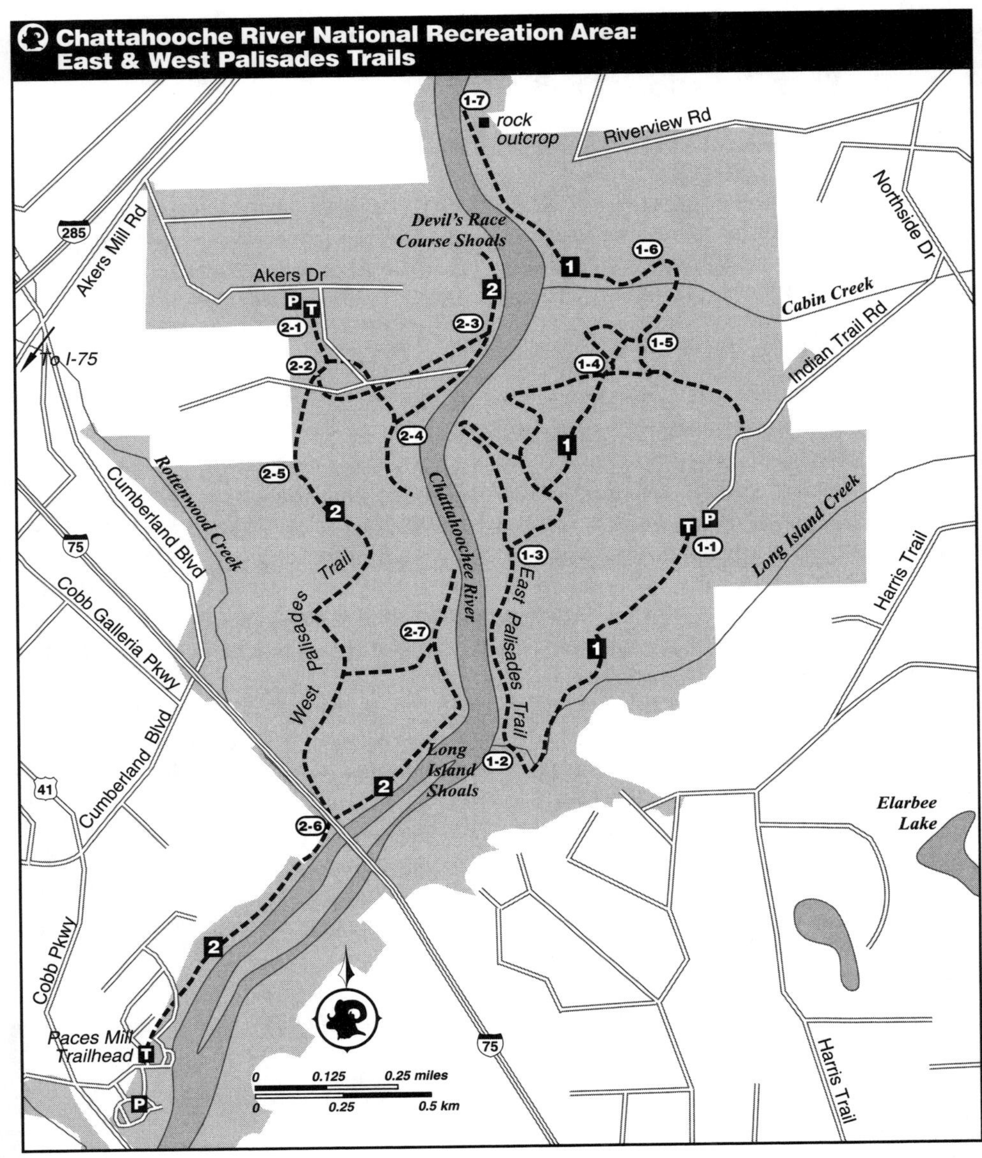

bear right again to go northwest across a wood footbridge **(Waypoint 2)**.

The Chattahoochee's Long Island Shoals come into full view to the left, and you'll likely see ducks paddling close to the bank and gathering on small islands of exposed rock. You cover flat ground and reach a trail junction just beyond the 1-mile mark **(Waypoint 3)**. From here you can continue straight along the river, or turn right to walk inland.

I recommend that you continue moving inland to explore the ridge covered in hardwoods. Make your way northeast to the trail junction marked **Waypoint 4** on the map above (marked E9 on the posted trail marker). From here you have several options. To the right (east) a series of paths proceeds a little less than a half mile, ending at Indian Trail Road. Or you can continue straight and explore smaller loops that wander the ridge top. Eventually, you should make your way to the junction marked **Waypoint 5** because it connects to the banks of the river north of here. From **Waypoint 5**, turn east and take the dramatic twisting descent past massive oaks into the Cabin Creek drainage.

After crossing the creek, bear left at the next trail intersection **(Waypoint 6)**. A little more than 800 feet in the distance, the trail meets a big bend in the Chattahoochee River. Turn north and walk upstream 0.2 mile to a remarkable stand of bamboo with stalks so thick you can't fully wrap a hand around one. The path crawls up the flank of the bluff, finally reaching a rocky point with a grand view of the Devil's Race Course Shoals **(Waypoint 7)**. Though rough trails continue along the bluff, they grow faint and you must bushwhack, making this a good point to turn back and retrace your steps to the trailhead.

UTM WAYPOINTS

1. 16S 737054E 3752305N
2. 16S 736590E 3751619N
3. 16S 736558E 3752245N
4. 16S 736835E 3752750N
5. 16S 736921E 3752845N
6. 16S 736959E 3753082N
7. 16S 736439E 3753531N

View from the East Palisades Trail along the shore of the Chattahoochee

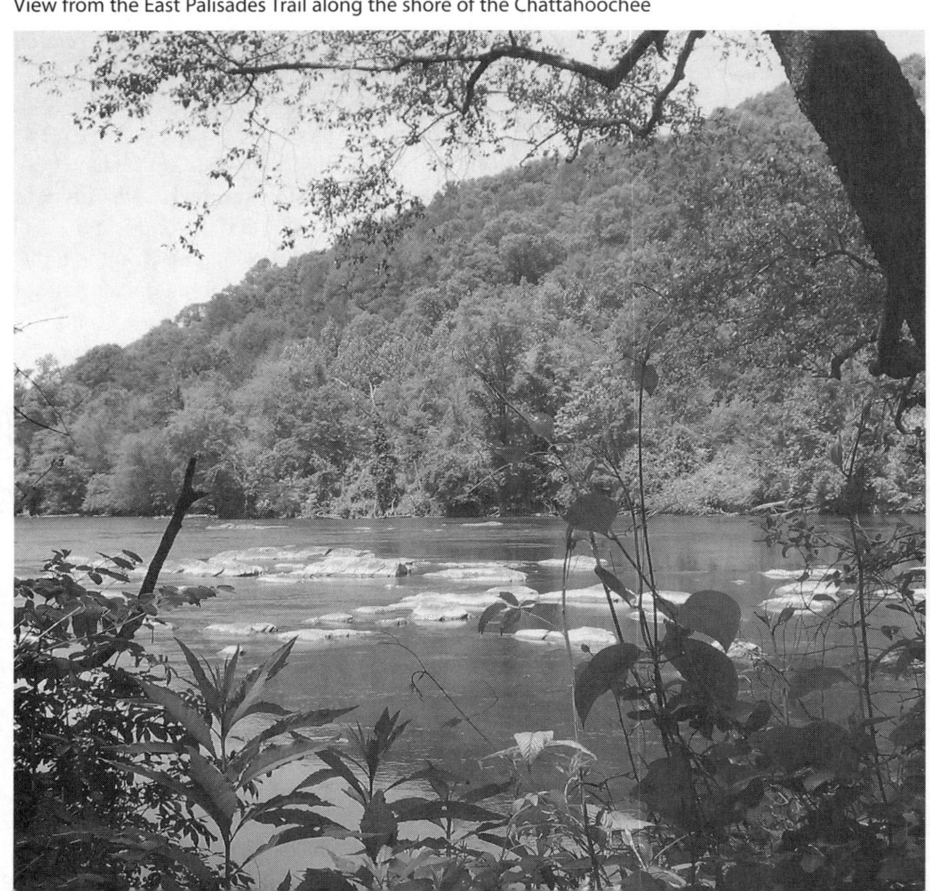

TRIP 2 Chattahoochee River National Recreation Area: West Palisades Trail

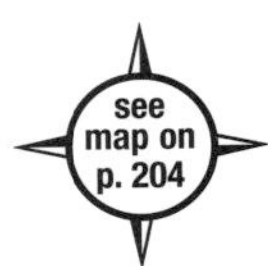

Distance	4.5–5.5 miles, out-and-back
Hiking Time	3 hours
Difficulty	Easy to moderate
Elevation Gain/Loss	+/-580 feet
Trail Use	Leashed dogs
Best Times	Year-round
Agency	National Park Service, Chattahoochee River National Recreation Area
Recommended Maps	A National Park Service map is available online at www.nps.gov/chat/planyourvisit/directions.htm.

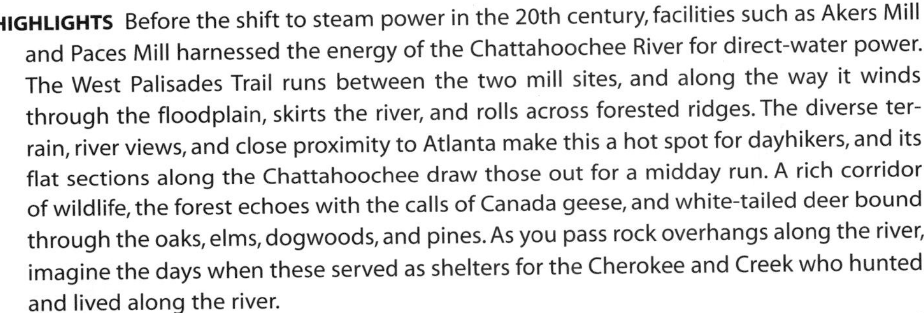
HIGHLIGHTS Before the shift to steam power in the 20th century, facilities such as Akers Mill and Paces Mill harnessed the energy of the Chattahoochee River for direct-water power. The West Palisades Trail runs between the two mill sites, and along the way it winds through the floodplain, skirts the river, and rolls across forested ridges. The diverse terrain, river views, and close proximity to Atlanta make this a hot spot for dayhikers, and its flat sections along the Chattahoochee draw those out for a midday run. A rich corridor of wildlife, the forest echoes with the calls of Canada geese, and white-tailed deer bound through the oaks, elms, dogwoods, and pines. As you pass rock overhangs along the river, imagine the days when these served as shelters for the Cherokee and Creek who hunted and lived along the river.

DIRECTIONS There are two access points for the West Palisades Trail, one at Akers Mill, and one at Paces Mill. The hike detailed below begins at the Akers Mill Trailhead.

To reach the Akers Mill Trailhead, take Interstate 75 north to Exit 258, Cumberland Boulevard. At the end of the exit ramp, turn right and go 0.5 mile to Akers Mill Road. Turn right onto Akers Mill Road and go 0.3 mile to Akers Drive. Turn right at the wood waterwheel and take the second left at the Palisades West entrance. The parking area is on the right.

To reach the Paces Mill Trailhead, take I-75 north to Exit 25, Mt. Paran Road. Turn right onto Mt. Paran Road and go to U.S. Highway 41 (Cobb Parkway). Turn right onto U.S. 41 and go 1 mile. Cross the Chattahoochee River and take an immediate left onto the entrance road.

FACILITIES/TRAILHEAD There are no facilities at the Akers Mill Trailhead. A restroom is available at the northern end of the trail (at Waypoint 3). The Paces Mill Trailhead has a restroom and picnic area. The recreation area charges a $3 parking fee, which you pay at a kiosk at each trailhead. You can purchase a $25 annual pass for the recreation area by calling (678) 538-1200 or by visiting www.nps.gov/chat/index.htm.

From the east side of the Akers Mill parking area, enter the path that begins beneath pines and drops through oaks and maples (**Waypoint 1**). After about 600 feet, bear right at the Y intersection and take the gravel path going southwest across the ridge. After another 250 feet you reach a trail junction with a trail marker labeled W8 (**Waypoint 2**) where you can bear right and go southwest to cross the ridge, or bear left to reach the river. If the river is calling you, bear left on the gravel path that dives to a trail junction in a flat clearing at 0.4 mile. Bear left, and a restroom facility lies on the left near a spot where the path nears the river (**Waypoint 3**). Move upstream, where mountain laurel drapes over the trail and the wide water comes into full view. Ahead, a small, sandy beach is a great spot to sit and watch the river rush on. At 0.8 mile, the path peters out, so return to **Waypoint 3**.

From **Waypoint 3**, I continued south to further explore the riverbank and saw a great blue heron gliding over the Chattahoochee with wings wider than a person's outstretched arms. At a T junction (**Waypoint 4**) at 1.3 miles, you can turn left to skirt the river for another tenth of a mile until the trail plays out. If you turn right at **Waypoint 4**, the trail crosses Trout Lily Creek in woods singing with birds, like a natural aviary. After traveling 380 feet, a path intersects on the left. Turn onto this trail and climb northwest about 390 feet to reach the road you originally descended. At the road, turn left and climb to the trail junction at 1.5 miles (**Waypoint 2**).

Rather than returning to the trailhead, you may want to turn south to hike the ridge and then descend to explore more of the riverbank. From **Waypoint 2**, go south, descend the gravel path, and then wind up a hill to a T intersection with a paved path (**Waypoint 5**). Turn left and go south to begin a long ridge walk on a shaded path beneath oaks and other hardwoods. If you're looking for solitude, this stretch feels more secluded than the paths along the river. At 2.2 miles, it's time to leave the high ground and drop to the river. (At 2.3 miles, continue straight, passing the trail that enters to the left).

At 2.6 miles (**Waypoint 6**) you can turn right to cross the bridge and proceed another 0.5 mile to the Paces Mill Trailhead. Or, turn left to once again follow the riverbank. Unlike the previous riverside trails, this path is rough, rooted, and eventually takes you scrambling over boulders. At 3 miles (**Waypoint 7**) a trail intersects on the left. You can continue north a little less than 1000 feet until the trail virtually disappears. Or, turn onto the trail on the left for a steep 900-foot ascent to a T junction. Turn right at the T junction, and travel north to traverse the ridge and return to the trailhead.

UTM WAYPOINTS

1. 16S 735984E 3752955N
2. 16S 736021E 3752746N
3. 16S 736497E 3752856N
4. 16S 736186E 3752529N
5. 16S 735957E 3752471N
6. 16S 736041E 3751452N
7. 16S 736327E 3751919N

TRIP 3 Chattahoochee River National Recreation Area: Powers Island

Distance	2.4 miles, semiloop
Hiking Time	1 hour
Difficulty	Easy
Elevation Gain/Loss	+150/-160 feet
Trail Uses	Leashed dogs and good for kids
Best Times	Year-round
Agency	National Park Service, Chattahoochee River National Recreation Area
Recommended Maps	A National Park Service map is available online at www.nps.gov/chat. Another map is available online at www.us-parks.com/chattahoochee/maps.html.

HIGHLIGHTS In the 1800s, the Power family owned a substantial amount of land along the Chattahoochee River. In 1832, James Power set up a ferry operation on the river (where Interstate 285 now crosses), and he likely farmed the surrounding land and harvested timber. As you walk the trails at Powers Island, you will see no trace of James Power's work—the trees and brush have reclaimed the land. There are really two areas to walk here. From the southwest corner of the parking lot, you can walk west to Powers Island, a narrow strip of land with a boat launch and good view of the river. From the north end of the parking lot, a trail leads to the lush hills and riverbank on the east side of the Chattahoochee.

DIRECTIONS From Interstate 285 east, take Exit 22 for Northside Drive, New Northside Drive, and Powers Ferry Road. Go to the second traffic light and turn left onto New Northside Drive. Cross over I-285 and go through the traffic light to take Interstate North Parkway. Go 0.6 mile, and the entrance is on the right before the river.

From I-285 west, take Exit 22 for Northside Drive, New Northside Drive, and Powers Ferry Road. Turn right onto New Northside Drive. Cross over I-285 and go through the traffic light to take Interstate North Parkway. Go 0.6 mile, and the entrance is on the right before the river.

FACILITIES/TRAILHEAD In the parking lot you will see the Chattahoochee Outdoor Center, but it has been closed since 2002. The recreation area charges a $3 parking fee, which you can pay at a kiosk at the trailhead. You can purchase a $25 annual pass for the recreation area by calling (678) 538-1200 or by visiting www.nps.gov/chat/index.htm.

Beginning at the north corner of the lot **(Waypoint 1)**, take the wide path that was once a road. No one is really sure if James Power built structures here, but in more recent years an odd mix of cabins and homes have occupied this bank of the river. These buildings were razed by the National Park Service, but you can still find the stone remains of old gravity-fed plumbing systems on the slopes. As you begin the trail, the river is not immediately visible, but you may hear the distant calls of geese mixed with the sounds of car traffic. At 0.2 mile turn right at the Y intersection **(Waypoint 2)** and climb a narrow path choked with underbrush.

At 0.3 mile, a path to the left drops 460 feet to the trail along the river. If you continue straight and pass this side trail, you move up a ridge where wildflowers add a touch of purple to the green forest palette. The path rises to about 1000

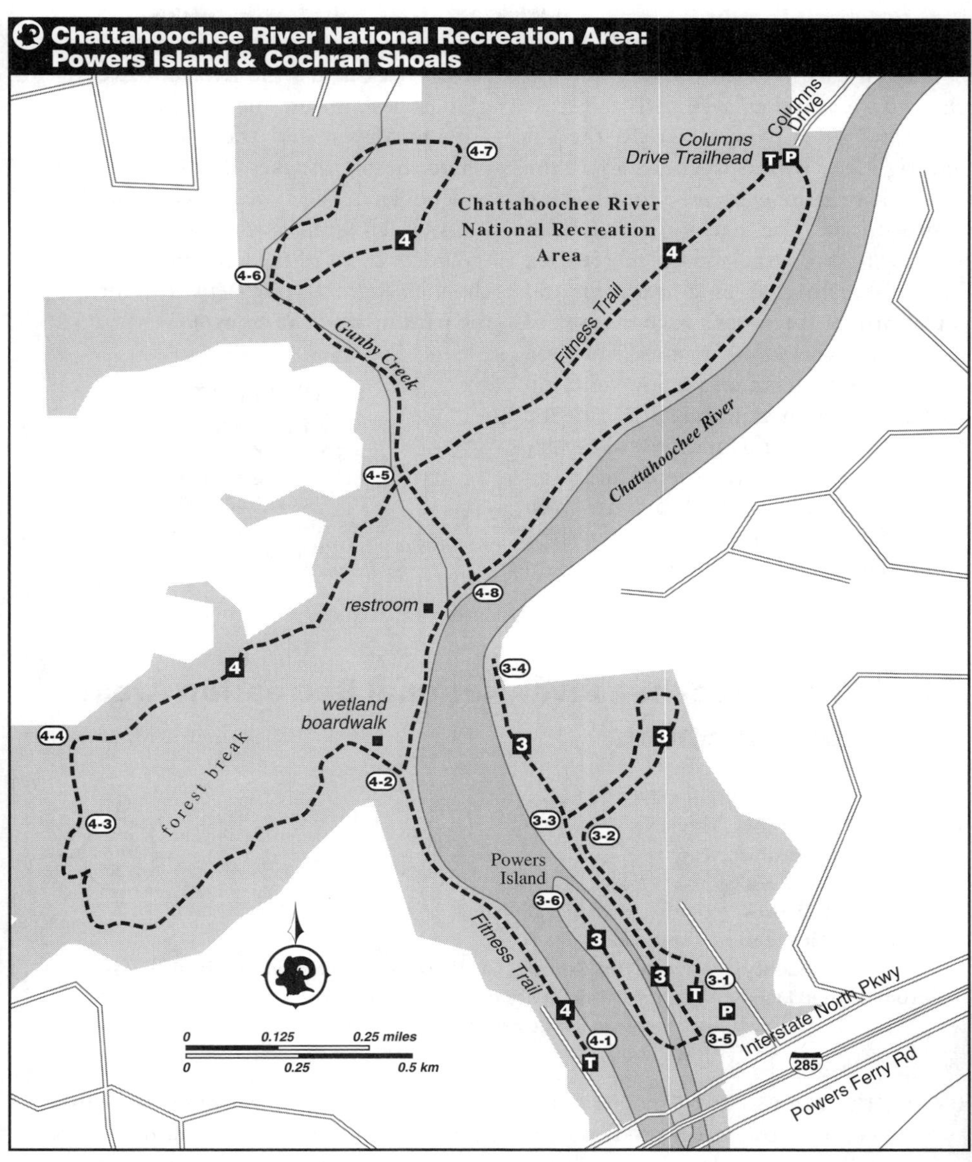

feet of elevation at 0.6 mile and then drops quickly down a drainage. As if you've stepped into a jungle, the forest drips with vines, and bright ferns blanket decaying logs.

At 0.8 mile, bear right, traveling west, and at the next trail junction **(Waypoint 3)** turn right to go northwest. Now visible on your left, the Chattahoochee River takes a big bend to the southeast. You can follow the river for another 0.2 mile until the path crawls over a rock outcrop and effectively ends **(Waypoint 4)**. You can walk a bit farther, but the trail plays out, so retrace your steps to **Waypoint 2**. Bear right to walk through brush and briars that border the river, and return to the parking lot.

To reach Powers Island, walk to the southwest corner of the parking lot, and then go west on the paved path and cross the iron bridge **(Waypoint 5)**. To the left and right, the wires suspended above the water channel are gates used for kayaking competitions. The narrow island takes no time to cross, and you quickly reach a bench beneath a tall pine near steps and a platform at the water's edge that serves as a canoe and kayak launch. This is a good place to relax and enjoy views up and down the Chattahoochee. During the Civil War, the federal infantry and cavalry forces crossed the river here during an assault, and came under heavy fire from a Confederate outpost atop a nearby ridge. The Union troops had to lie on the bank of the island until nightfall and retreat back across the river under cover of darkness. From the bench you can walk northwest and traverse the island where the path snakes through tall oaks and poplars. The trail stretches another 0.2 mile across the island and ends where the north point of the land meets a water channel. Retrace your steps to return to the parking area **(Waypoint 6)**.

UTM WAYPOINTS

1. 16S 736453E 3754485N
2. 16S 736257E 3754849N
3. 16S 736225E 3754879N
4. 16S 736077E 3755164N
5. 16S 736508E 3754399N
6. 16S 736222E 3754718N

TRIP 4 Chattahoochee River National Recreation Area: Cochran Shoals

see map on p. 209

Distance	5.7 miles, semiloop
Hiking Time	3 hours
Difficulty	Easy
Elevation Gain/Loss	+/-395 feet
Trail Uses	Leashed dogs and good for kids
Best Times	Year-round
Agency	National Park Service, Chattahoochee River National Recreation Area
Recommended Maps	A National Park Service map is available online at www.nps.gov/chat. Another map is available online at www.us-parks.com/chattahoochee/maps.html.

HIGHLIGHTS With a 3.1-mile Fitness Trail that skirts the Chattahoochee River, Cochran Shoals is one of the most heavily used outdoor areas near Atlanta and draws 3 million visitors a year. The gravel path is well maintained, and the river provides some great scenery for walkers, runners, or those in wheelchairs. Although Cochran Shoals receives heavy pressure from walkers and joggers, it also offers superb birding for migrant landbirds in spring and fall on the trails along the river. The hike detailed here begins on the Fitness Trail and then turns onto a short boardwalk where you can look for birds feeding in the marshy areas. The path then crosses woodland hills west of the river and returns to more bottomland forest before reconnecting with the Fitness Trail. You can then complete the long Fitness Trail loop, and even detour along the way to escape the crowds and explore a tucked-away creek.

DIRECTIONS Two trailheads serve the Cochran Shoals trails, one west of the river off Columns Drive and one east of the river off Interstate North Parkway, as described below. From Interstate 285 East, take Exit 22 for Northside Drive, New Northside Drive, and Powers Ferry Road. Go to the second traffic light, and turn left to go north on New Northside Drive. Cross over I-285 and go through the traffic light to take Interstate North Parkway. Take this road across the Chattahoochee River and go 0.8 mile. The entrance is on the right.

From I-285 west, take Exit 22 for Northside Drive, New Northside Drive, and Powers Ferry Road. Turn right at the first light to go north on New Northside Drive. Cross over I-285 and go through the traffic light to take Interstate North Parkway. Take this road across the Chattahoochee River and go 0.8 mile to the entrance on the right.

FACILITIES/TRAILHEAD At the time of publication, restrooms at the trailhead were under construction. There are restrooms at the Columns Drive parking area and near Waypoint 8 on the Fitness Trail. The recreation area charges a $3 parking fee, which you can pay at a kiosk at the trailhead. You can purchase a $25 annual pass for the recreation area by calling (678) 538-1200 or by visiting www.nps.gov/chat/index.htm.

At the end of the parking lot, take the wide gravel path and proceed northwest with Powers Island visible to your right **(Waypoint 1)**. At 0.4 mile **(Waypoint 2)** turn left off the gravel path and go west to cross a boardwalk. This marshy area is a prime destination for birding, and a bench along the walkway provides a good place to rest, look, and listen. "There are always a lot of woodpeckers, including red-headed around the dead trees, and wood ducks breed here," according to birding expert Giff Beaton. At 0.6 mile, continue straight at the trail junction to go southwest. Then, bear left at the next Y intersection to go southwest and climb the steep, rooted path onto a ridge. Here you leave the dense brush of the bottomland forest and rise into a crisp, leafy forest of hardwoods.

At 1 mile the trail reaches a wide, grassy break. From here, a series of trails crisscross the ridges west of the Chattahoochee River as well as the low forest surrounding Gunby Creek. Turn left (southwest), walk a few feet, and then turn right on a very narrow path to cross the wide forest break. At the opposite side of the break, a steep rocky path winds down to a trail junction (marked C56 on the map stand). Turn left and travel southwest.

At 1.2 miles (C55 on the map stand), turn right and turn sharply back to the northeast, climbing over the ridge. After the bustling Fitness Trail, this portion of Cochran Shoals seems much more quiet and calm, and the forest is ever more peaceful as you move west. At the next trail junction (C54 on the map stand) turn right to travel northeast on the top of the ridge. At **Waypoint 3** (C53 on the map stand), the trail to the right (northeast) leads to a shaded walk across a ridge of pines and hardwoods, but to continue your loop, turn left (southwest) to descend toward a creek basin.

At the bottom of the hill, cross a wood footbridge. Then, at 1.3 miles **(Waypoint 4)**, turn right (east) at the T intersection to begin a stroll on a flat and wide path that traverses bottomland forest and runs parallel with the creek.

At 1.7 miles the trail ends at an intersection with the gravel Fitness Trail. Turn left and go northeast passing an emergent wetland to the right. In 2006, nonnative plant species were removed to protect the habitat for a small population of the endangered Henslow's and Leconte's

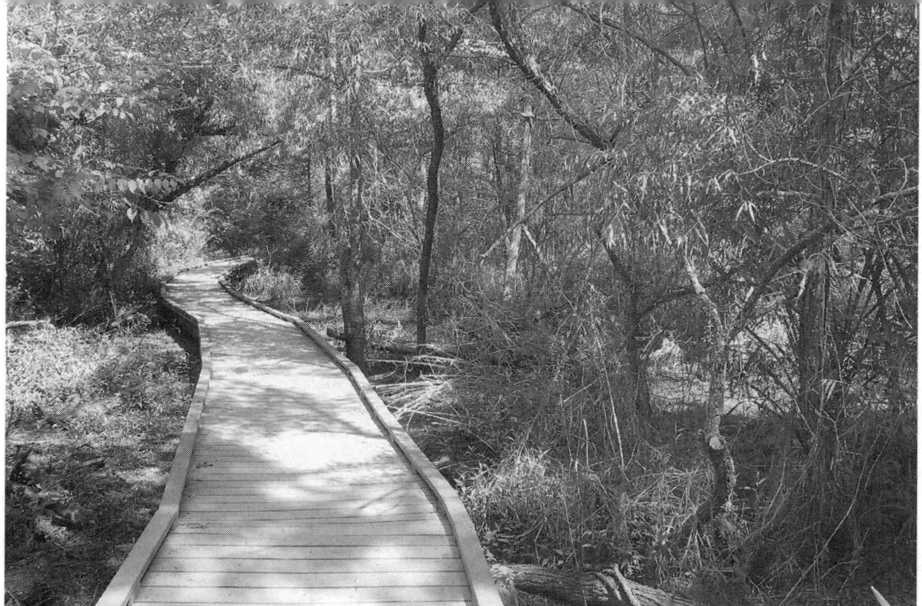

Just off the Fitness Trail is a prime birding spot at Cochran Shoals.

sparrows. This is one of few places near Atlanta you can find these birds, which usually appear in winter. This area also has a good population of the uncommon red-headed woodpecker.

At the trail junction at 2 miles (**Waypoint 5**) you can keep straight (northeast) to hike the Fitness Trail to the Columns Drive Trailhead; turning right accesses restroom facilities. But if you turn left (northwest), a brief loop through the forest takes you by a tranquil creek running through a secluded draw. Take this trail, walking beside the rocky creek to the trail junction at **Waypoint 6.** Turn right to climb the ridge covered in a typical mix of pines and hardwoods. After walking about 0.3 mile on the ridge, look carefully to the left for a faint, narrow path (**Waypoint 7**), which appears just before a major trail junction. Turn left at **Waypoint 7** and take a steep descent to the edge of the stream that slides through a completely forested draw. Here there are no signs of civilization, save a few houses hidden in the trees on the far bluff.

Back at **Waypoint 5**, turn left to continue on the Fitness Trail. At the Columns Drive parking lot bear right to loop back, once again enjoying an easy walk on the wide gravel path along the Chattahoochee River. Just beyond the trail junction at **Waypoint 8**, Gunby Creek spills into the Chattahoochee. This had long been a popular spot for people to play with their dogs, but the bank was denuded by heavy use, and the eroding bank threatened to deposit silt in the river and harm fish species. In 2006, more than 150 volunteers planted native grasses and plants on 1000 square feet of the bank, which recovered within about 7 months.

From **Waypoint 8**, walk about 200 feet farther down the Fitness Trail to reach the restroom on the right. From this point, continue south on the Fitness Trail back to the trailhead.

UTM WAYPOINTS

1. 16S 736247E 3754359N
2. 16S 735875E 3754957N
3. 16S 735169E 3754869N
4. 16S 735158E 3755070N
5. 16S 735876E 3755652N
6. 16S 735595E 3756091N
7. 16S 735590E 3756075N
8. 16S 736031E 3755422N

TRIP 5 Chattahoochee River National Recreation Area: Sope Creek

Distance	3.6 miles (without side trails), loop
Hiking Time	2 hours
Difficulty	Easy to moderate
Elevation Gain/Loss	+/-330 feet
Trail Uses	Leashed dogs, mountain biking, and good for kids
Best Times	Year-round
Agency	National Park Service, Chattahoochee River National Recreation Area
Recommended Maps	A National Park Service map is available online at www.nps.gov/chat. Another map is available online at www.us-parks.com/chattahoochee/maps.html.

HIGHLIGHTS Sope Creek has long been a destination for mountain bikers, but it's popular with hikers and trail runners as well. Hikers can choose from a myriad of loops that snake through rolling forest and trek into deep woods and hide the fact that you're quite close to civilization. The land is cut with ravines, and in the southern portion of this unit an especially peaceful path sidles up to the whispering waters of Fox Creek. The hike detailed below generally makes a large loop through the area, but side trails are worth exploring, and map stands at many trail junctions will help you navigate if you choose to improvise your own route.

DIRECTIONS From Interstate 285 east, take Exit 24, Riverside Drive. Turn left onto Riverside Drive and go 2.3 miles to Johnson Ferry Road. Turn left onto Johnson Ferry Road and go 2.7 miles to the junction with Paper Mill Road. Turn left onto Paper Mill Road and go 2.2 miles. The entrance to the parking area is on the left.

From Interstate 285 west, take Exit 24, Riverside Drive. Go north on Riverside Drive for 2.3 miles to Johnson Ferry Road. Turn onto Johnson Ferry Road and go 2.7 miles to the junction with Paper Mill Road. Turn left onto Paper Mill Road and go 2.2 miles. The entrance to the parking area is on the left.

FACILITIES There are no restroom facilities at the trailhead or along the trails, but there are picnic tables near the parking area. The recreation area charges a $3 parking fee, which you can pay at a kiosk at the trailhead. You can purchase a $25 annual pass for the recreation area by calling (678) 538-1200 or by visiting www.nps.gov/chat/index.htm.

From the east end of the parking lot **(Waypoint 1)** walk down the wide gravel path and continue straight at the first four-way intersection. Circle Sibley Pond and at 940 feet bear right at a Y intersection to continue circling the water and pass beneath magnolias. At 0.3 mile, turn right to cross a bridge, and take the next the left to go northwest and circle through land thick with sweetgum trees, dense brush, and briars.

At 0.8 mile **(Waypoint 2)**, turn right at a T intersection to go southeast. Walk another 300 feet and turn right at a trail junction to continue southwest, following the designated bike path briefly. At 0.9 mile **(Waypoint 3)** turn onto the left-hand trail to go east on a narrow path that descends gradually past holly and a mix of pines and hardwoods. At 1.2 miles, in the heart of the Sope Creek unit **(Waypoint 4)**, make a hard right at a trail junction

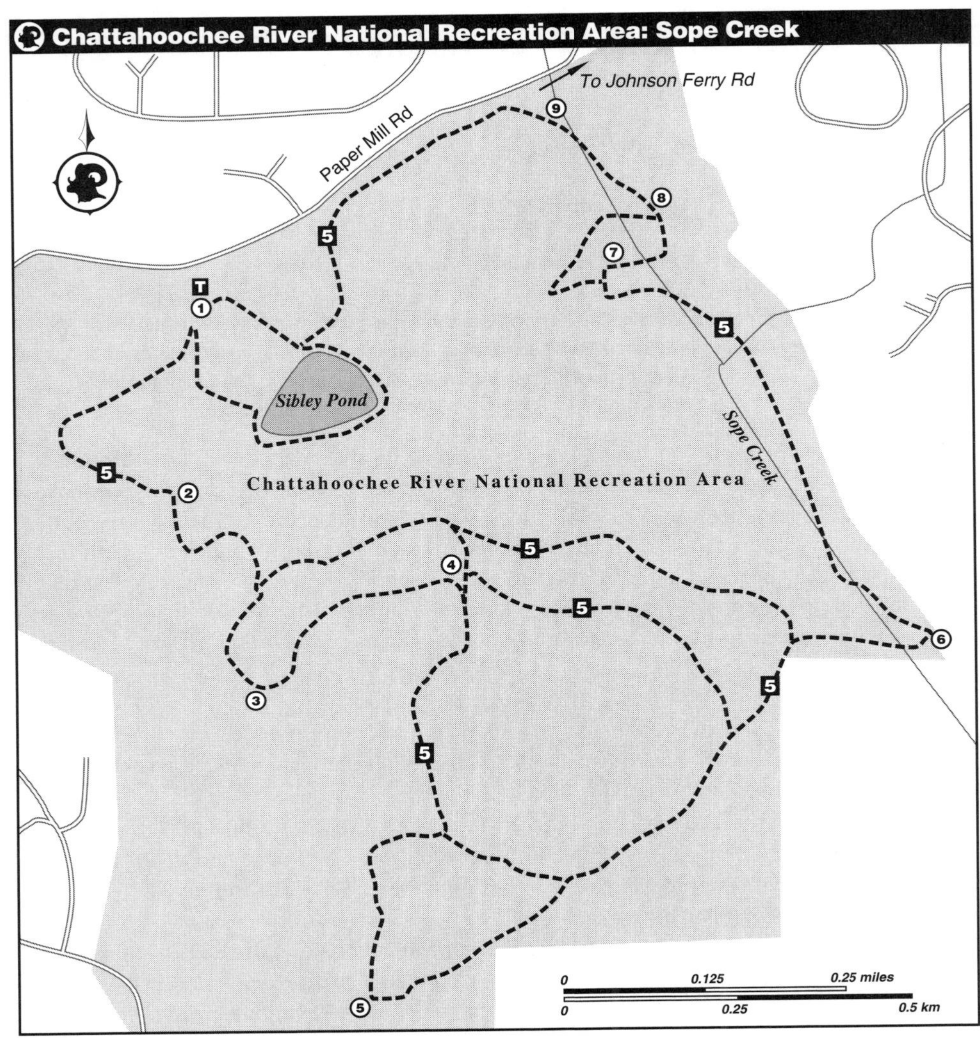

(marked S24 on the map stand) and walk south through high hardwoods dispersed throughout rolling terrain. At 1.5 miles turn right to go west, and then go southbound toward Fox Creek. At 1.7 miles **(Waypoint 5)** turn left to travel northeast into the shaded creek basin. Here among the beech trees, with the creek flowing nearby, you may want to linger a while and take in one of the most pleasant spots in the forest.

Continuing northeast, the trail turns away from the creek. At 2.1 miles (S23 on the map stand) a trail to the left ascends a drainage lorded over by tall oaks—just one of the many side journeys that is certainly worth taking. But you may also continue straight at the junction to head toward Sope Creek. Civilization intrudes for a moment as you pass apartment buildings. At 2.3 miles turn right at the trail junction to travel east, and go another tenth of a mile to the bank of Sope Creek **(Waypoint 6)**.

A curious aspect of this area is the creek's name. According to a 1973 report by the Georgia Historical Commission, the banks of Sope Creek were occupied by Native Americans "prior to the white industrial development of the area in the 19th century." The commission reported that "the Creek is named for a Cherokee Indian called 'Old Sope' who lived in the area perhaps even after the [Indian] Removal" in the 1830s.

From **Waypoint 6**, the path turns left to the northwest, and you begin a sublime walk beside the swift stream chock-full of boulders and stone slabs. The rocky path eventually moves away from the creek and climbs a hill. At 2.8 miles, atop the hill, turn right at the trail junction and descend to the east. At 2.9 miles **(Waypoint 7)** turn left at the trail junction to go southeast, descending to a creek. A rocky stream makes a bold cut through thin forest and open ground. Turn right to cross the creek drainage and hairpin back to the northeast. At the next trail junction, turn right and descend to the east.

At 3 miles **(Waypoint 8)** you approach the creek (marked S9 on the map stand). If you turn right to walk the riverbank, you'll see water flowing in white sheets over beds of rock. To continue from **Waypoint 8**, take the blue blazed trail that climbs steeply to the northeast and tops a hill. Walk about 670 feet to a five-way trail junction **(Waypoint 9)**. Take the blue-blazed trail, which is the flattest of the trails and goes northeast along Paper Mill Road. After going 300 feet, turn left at the T junction and travel west on the well-packed, flat trail.

At 3.3 miles a trail intersects on the left. Keep going straight here (southwest) and pass between two stout pine trees standing shoulder to shoulder. Go a little less than 0.1 mile and turn right at the trail junction. Traveling southwest, cross a hill, and at 3.5 miles turn right to return to the trailhead.

The area around Sope Creek has historic significance because it was the site of a major industrial center in the 1800s. Denmead's Mill, established in the 1840s, was the first major water-powered mill built here, according to a Historic Resource Study by the National Park Service. In the 1850s, the Marietta Paper

The wild, lush banks of Sope Creek

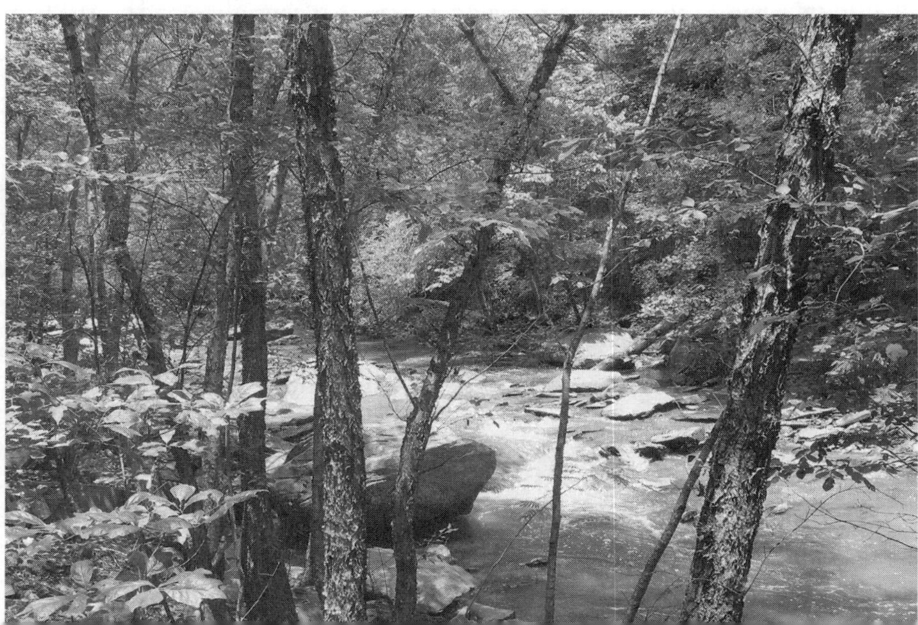

Company harnessed the swift waters of Sope Creek to power a mill that used rags of linen and cotton to make paper. Mill operations were disrupted in July 1864 when Union soldiers marched through Roswell and burned the Marietta Paper Mill as well as Denmead's Mill. By 1868, the Marietta Paper Mill was up and running, and it operated until 1902, when a fire led to its closure.

UTM WAYPOINTS

1. 16S 736356E 3758206N
2. 16S 736365E 3757890N
3. 16S 736404E 3757663N
4. 16S 736682E 3757828N
5. 16S 736537E 3757236N
6. 16S 737316E 3757731N
7. 16S 736860E 3758255N
8. 16S 736920E 3758333N
9. 16S 736797E 3758461N

TRIP 6 Chattahoochee River National Recreation Area: Johnson Ferry

Distance	2.1 miles, semiloop
Hiking Time	1 hour
Difficulty	Easy
Elevation Gain/Loss	+/-75 feet
Trail Uses	Leashed dogs and good for kids
Best Times	Year-round
Agency	National Park Service, Chattahoochee River National Recreation Area
Recommended Maps	A National Park Service map is available online at www.nps.gov/chat. Another map is available online at www.us-parks.com/chattahoochee/maps.html.

HIGHLIGHTS Johnson Ferry is usually buzzing with activity as people walk and bike trails for exercise, or enjoy the wildlife in the emerging wetland on the riverbank. Though the trails lie near heavily traveled Johnson Ferry Road, you can get a sense of escape as you stroll down trails shaded by heavy forest of beech and oak. This riverside wetland also has more birds and greater diversity of wildlife than other wetland habitats along the river. The trail first follows a streambed and moves deeper into quiet woods before looping back to skirt the Chattahoochee River. Here you can sit on a wood bench and watch herons cruising low over the slow-paced river.

DIRECTIONS From Interstate 285 east, take Exit 24 for Riverside Drive. Turn left onto Riverside Drive and continue 2.3 miles to Johnson Ferry Road. Turn left onto Johnson Ferry Road, cross the river, and take an immediate right into the parking area.

From Interstate 285 west, take Exit 24 for Riverside Drive. Turn right onto Riverside Drive and go 2.3 miles to Johnson Ferry Road. Turn left onto Johnson Ferry Road, cross the river, and take an immediate right into the parking area.

FACILITIES/TRAILHEAD There are no restroom facilities at the trailhead or along the trail. The recreation area charges a $3 parking fee, which you can pay at a kiosk at the trailhead. You can purchase a $25 annual pass for the recreation area by calling (678) 538-1200 or by visiting www.nps.gov/chat/index.htm.

The hike begins at the east end of the parking lot **(Waypoint 1)** where a paved path soon becomes gravel and continues through a broad clearing. The old Chattahoochee Outdoor Center building sits to the right. In the 1970s, rafting saw a boom in popularity, and Johnson Ferry became a major launch spot. For years, the Chattahoochee Outdoor Center outfitted thousands of people with boats and gear to raft "The Hooch." But recreation trends shifted by the early 1980s, the boating scene dwindled, and some people avoided Johnson Ferry due to bacteria alerts posted by park officials. Unable to draw enough business, the Chattahoochee Outdoor Center closed.

Chattahoochee River National Recreation Area: Johnson Ferry

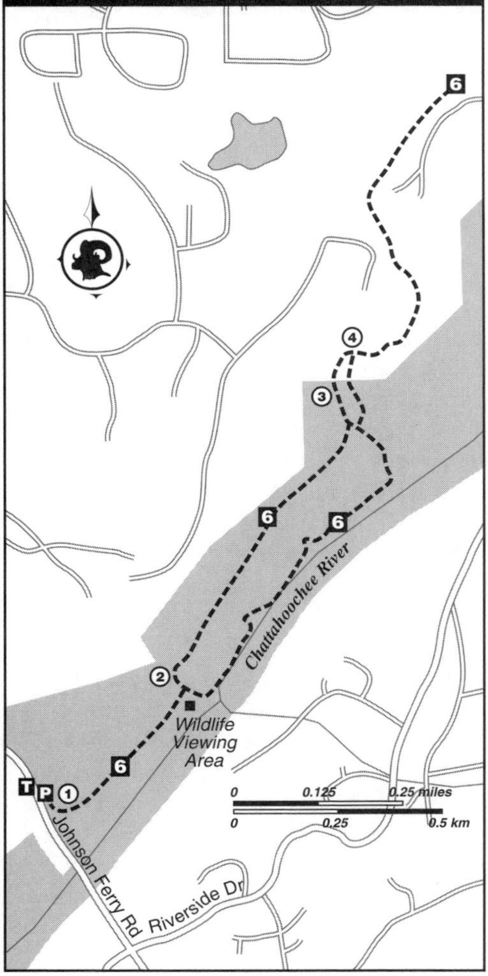

At 0.3 mile you reach a Wildlife Viewing Area sign **(Waypoint 2)**. Turn left and take the wood footbridge, which passes over a vernal pool. This stand of water does not support a constant population of fish, so eggs laid by salamanders and frogs have a chance to survive and even thrive. You soon join a narrow dirt path that remains flat as you trace the base of a ridge. Through history, the land to the right has been used for farming, but it has now transformed into a wetland. Native Americans who lived here dug trenches between the river and inner portions of its bank to create a strip of land suitable for growing crops. Farmers who succeeded the Native Americans planted corn along the river, and they had to continually clear these ditches to prevent flooding. Now that the land is no longer farmed, water has collected in the succession forest, which now provides habitat for owls, hawks, and wood ducks.

At 0.8 mile turn left (northwest) to take the undulating trail along the creek **(Waypoint 3)**. About 45 feet down the trail, the creek bottom is made up of layers of rock, and the shallow stream runs beneath a rocky undercut bank. At a trail junction at the 1-mile mark, you could continue straight to follow the creek **(Waypoint 4)** and access more remote woods, but the trail becomes rutted, overgrown, and largely unattractive. Instead, turn right at the junction to go south and curve around a hill to a trail junction at 1.1 miles. Bear left and take the gently rolling single-track path across a pipeline area.

The trail turns to the southeast and the Chattahoochee appears to the left.

Trees along the bank bow toward the river, and breaks in the foliage allow glimpses of the steady, smooth current. The path twists inland and briefly meets the wide clearing before turning back toward the water for the final stretch back to the junction where you saw the Wildlife Viewing Area sign. Retrace your steps to the parking lot. As you near the closed outdoor center building, a path to the left goes to the river launch ramp used by boaters and floaters.

UTM WAYPOINTS

1. 16S 739733E 3759142N
2. 16S 740081E 3759459N
3. 16S 740523E 3760186N
4. 16S 740534E 3760370N

TRIP 7 Chattahoochee River National Recreation Area: Gold Branch Trail

Distance	3.2 miles, loop
Hiking Time	1½ hours
Difficulty	Moderate
Elevation Gain/Loss	+/-210 feet
Trail Uses	Leashed dogs and good for kids
Best Times	Spring, fall, and winter
Agency	National Park Service, Chattahoochee River National Recreation Area
Recommended Maps	A National Park Service map is available online at www.nps.gov/chat. Another map is available online at www.us-parks.com/chattahoochee/maps.html.

HIGHLIGHTS The Gold Branch Trail takes you along the shores of a section of the Chattahoochee River with an interesting history. In an early effort to bring electricity to the growing city of Atlanta, a dam was constructed in the early 1900s just south of the Gold Branch area where the river was narrow and shallow with a set of falls. Measuring 1031 feet long and 56 feet high, it was the largest dam in the southeastern U.S.

For the most part, the moderate Gold Branch Trail roller coasters along the riverbank and Bull Sluice Lake, the body of water formed behind the dam. The landscape is attractive, primarily composed of hardwoods, and you may see big, beautiful swans trolling across a river inlet.

DIRECTIONS From Interstate 285 west, take Exit 24. Turn left onto Riverside Drive and travel north 2.3 miles. Turn left onto Johnson Ferry Road. Go 2 miles and turn right onto Lower Roswell Road. Go almost 2.5 miles and turn right at the brown GOLD BRANCH sign.

From I-285 east, take Exit 24. Turn right onto Riverside Drive and travel north 2.3 miles. Turn left onto Johnson Ferry Road. Go 2 miles and turn right onto Lower Roswell Road. Go almost 2.5 miles and turn right at the brown GOLD BRANCH sign.

FACILITIES/TRAILHEAD There are no restroom facilities at the trailhead, but there are picnic tables and trash cans. The recreation area charges a $3 parking fee, which you can pay at a kiosk at the trailhead. You can purchase a $25 annual pass by calling (678) 538-1200 or by visiting www.nps.gov/chat/index.htm.

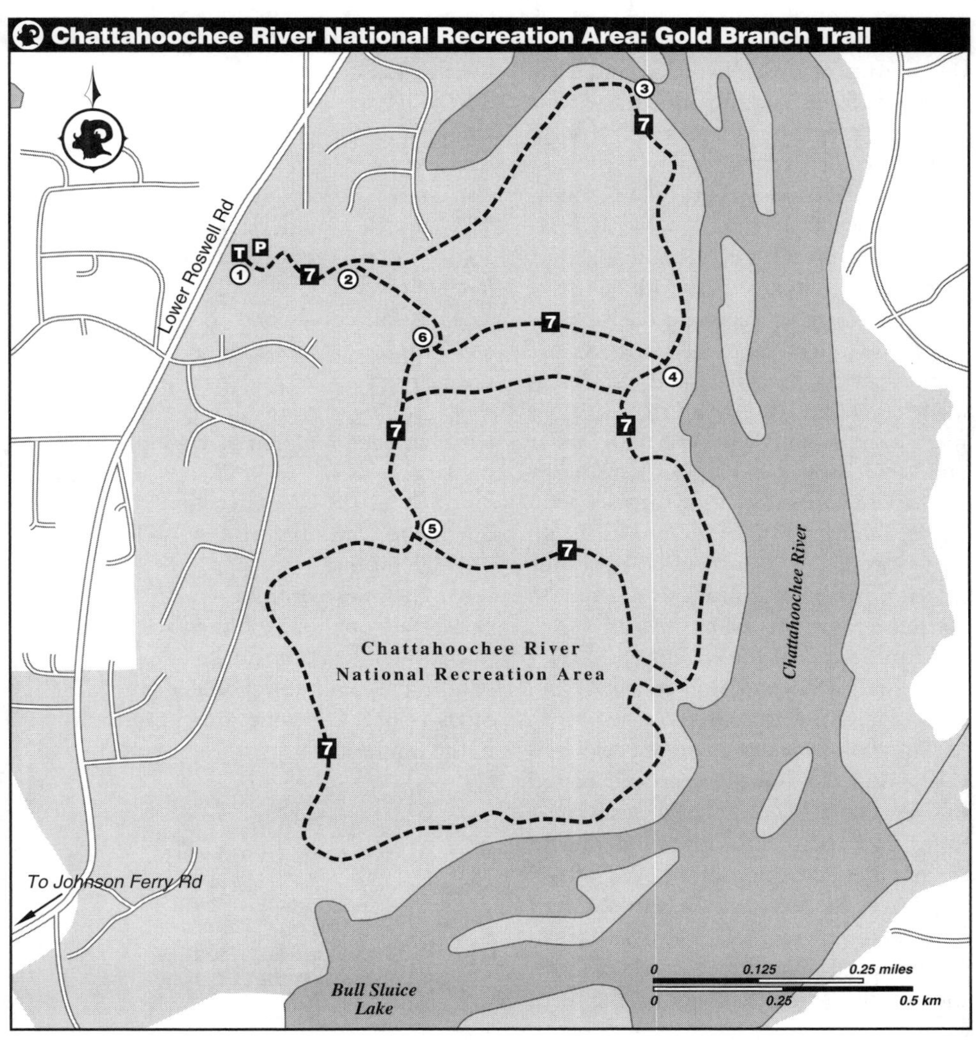

From the parking lot entry, go to the far side of the lot to enter the trail **(Waypoint 1)** and follow blue blazes. The path immediately winds down though a pine and hardwood mix to a wood footbridge that crosses a marshy region, which is actually Gold Branch Creek. At 0.1 mile **(Waypoint 2)** turn left and travel northeast beside the creek, which cuts a thin channel along the forest floor. Plenty of sunshine beams through the open hardwoods to strike rolling, leaf-covered terrain, while smooth beech trees line the path. A river inlet comes into view just ahead, and the path stays near its shore. When I scouted this area, I saw two swans floating and occasionally plunging their long necks beneath the surface, presumably fishing for lunch. At 0.3 mile you reach the first of many intersections with trails that cut across interior hills.

Bend around a point of land, and at 0.5 mile **(Waypoint 3)** turn right on the narrow path and ascend the steep hillside, traveling southwest. (Here, the trail used to run near the water but has been rerouted to climb the hill.) Drop back down near the water's edge and look southeast for a long look down the wide channel of water. As you reach a large water inlet, the trail turns west.

At 1 mile **(Waypoint 4)** turn left (southwest), descend and cross a wood footbridge. Just ahead, tree roots protruding from the hill form steps, which make it much easier to negotiate the slippery slope. A string of short, steep ascents and drops lead you to much flatter ground at a trail junction on a point of land. This nice, low bank puts you close to the water and is free of brush, allowing a full view of the Chattahoochee as it forms a great curve. From the trail junction, the path that ascends to the northwest crosses the interior of the Gold Branch unit. But, to continue your loop, do not take that trail, but instead follow the water's edge, traveling southwest, and immediately bend around another large cove.

The path ahead is at times rocky and rough and flat stones have been placed to even out a few dicey sections. At 2.1 miles you begin a steady, moderate to steep climb as the trail moves inland and leaves Bull Sluice Lake. Just south of here is the Morgan Falls Dam. S. Morgan Smith, inventor and former chaplain in the Union Army for whom the dam is named, was an important figure in the development of hydroelectric power. Smith helped launch the Atlanta Water and Electric Power Company, which constructed the Morgan Falls Dam. He was also known for creating a new type of turbine that would work in low water, according to the Chattahoochee River Recreation Area Historic Resource Study.

The trail crawls onto a large plateau and is more or less level as it traverses open forest of mostly oak trees. Your rocky, rolling scramble along the water's edge has been replaced by a simple stroll in the woods. At 2.5 miles **(Waypoint 5)**, bear left at the Y intersection to travel north and continue the easy walk across the high ground.

At 2.8 miles, continue straight (north) at the trail junction, and then at 2.9 miles **(Waypoint 6)** turn left to take a long gradual descent along the shoulder of the hill to **Waypoint 2**. Continue straight to return to the trailhead.

UTM WAYPOINTS

1. 16S 741541E 3763499N
2. 16S 741707E 3763495N
3. 16S 742140E 3763915N
4. 16S 742230E 3763267N
5. 16S 741843E 3762954N
6. 16S 741910E 3763346N

A swan cruises a sunny inlet at the Chattahoochee's Gold Branch unit.

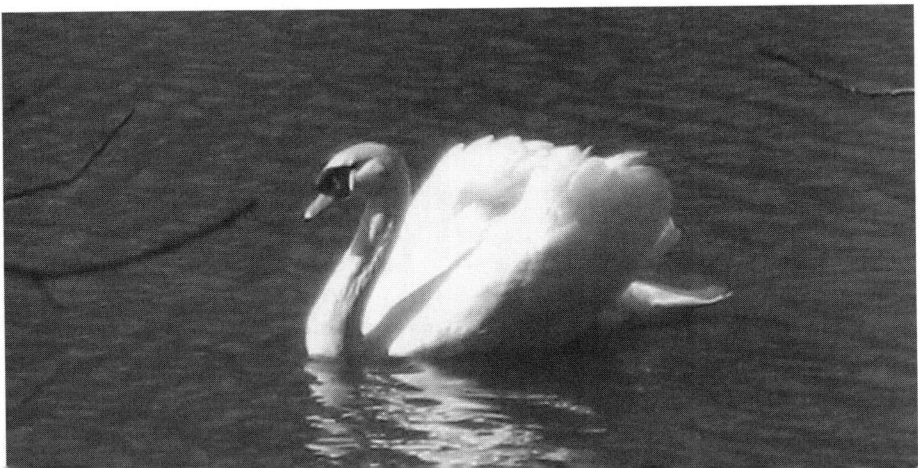

TRIP 8 Chattahoochee River National Recreation Area: Vickery Creek

Distance	3.2 miles, loop
Hiking Time	2 hours
Difficulty	Moderate to strenuous
Elevation Gain/Loss	+300/-305 feet
Trail Use	Leashed dogs
Best Times	Year-round
Agency	National Park Service, Chattahoochee River National Recreation Area
Recommended Map	A National Park Service map is available online at www.nps.gov/chat.
Note	One section of this hike is dangerous, where cables stretch across part of the trail. Avoid this part if you are traveling with children or are unsure of your ability to negotiate rocky, slippery terrain.

HIGHLIGHTS Feeding off the flow of Vickery Creek, the Roswell Mill operated as one of the most important manufacturing facilities in the South from 1838 until the Civil War. One of this hike's highlights is the site of the spillway dam that controlled the flow of water to factory buildings that lay downstream. The Roswell Manufacturing Company operated at times as a gristmill, and at other periods as a sawmill, but it was most noted as a textile producer and supplier of Confederate uniforms during the Civil War. The mill became a primary target for Gen. William Sherman, and Union troops destroyed the mill structures during their devastating Atlanta campaign. This hike not only takes you past the dam but also crosses the prominent knoll that looks over Vickery Creek and hugs a bluff to allow excellent views across the creek gorge.

DIRECTIONS There are three access points for the Vickery Creek area—one off Oxbo Road, one off South Atlanta Street, and one off Riverside Drive. This hike uses the Riverside Drive entrance. From Interstate 285, take Exit 25 for Roswell Road. Travel north on Roswell Road 7 miles to the intersection with Riverside Road. Turn right onto Riverside Road, cross Vickery Creek, and turn left into the road to the parking area.

FACILITIES/TRAILHEAD There are no facilities at the trailhead. Bring enough water for a day of hiking.

At the west end of the parking area, enter the marked trail **(Waypoint 1)**, and walk 160 feet to a trail junction. *A dangerous section of trail lies 0.2 mile ahead, so you may want to turn right at this junction and ascend if you are unsure of your balance or if you are traveling with kids.* Otherwise, keep straight at the junction to skirt Vickery Creek. I walked this section during a summer of drought and the lazy river stood still and brown. But at 0.2 mile things get interesting as you encounter a cable stretched across the path **(Waypoint 2)**. Beyond it is a precarious, rocky stretch where you must step carefully to avoid a nasty fall.

At 0.3 mile, a trail to the left leads to a large pipe that crosses the creek. If you're feeling really adventurous, you can walk across the pipe, turn right and walk 280 feet upstream to a large boulder formation that climbers frequent. If you don't want to cross the pipe, continue straight and keep along the stream between walls of dense brush. At 0.4 mile **(Waypoint 3)** there is a Y junction. (The trail on the left

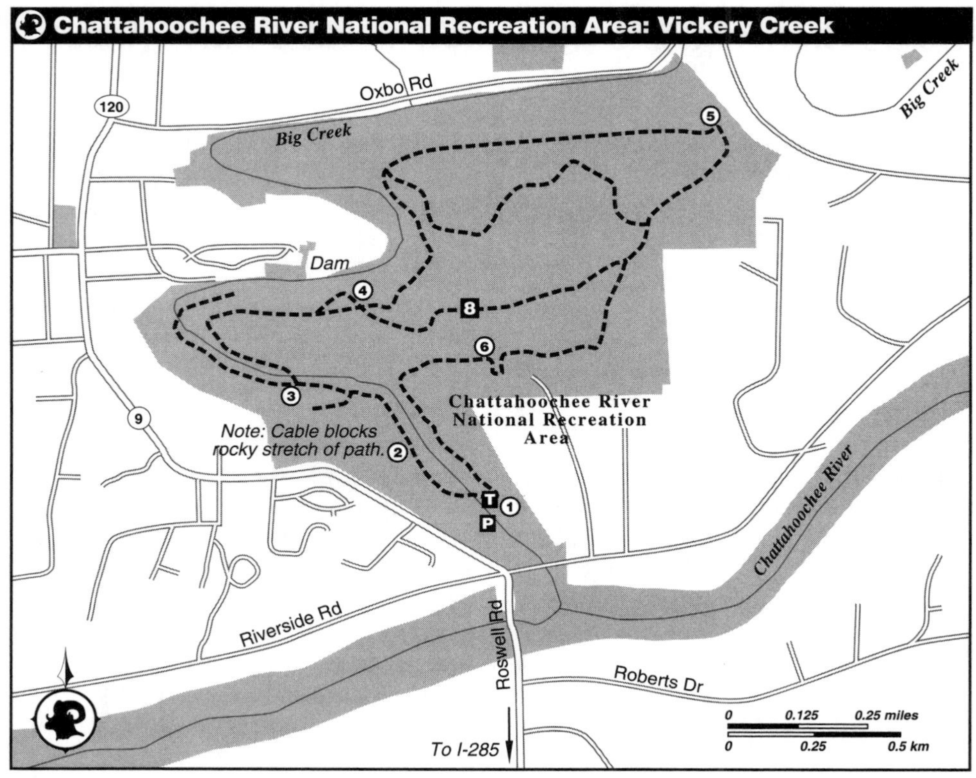

runs beside a series of rapids and extends about 0.3 mile until it peters out just beyond the large wood footbridge that leads to the Roswell Mill ruins. Trail mileages below do not include this walk.)

From **Waypoint 3**, ascend the knoll that towers over Vickery Creek. At 0.6 mile, turn left at the trail junction and walk northwest. The trail bends to the east as a dramatic scene unfolds to your left. At eye level are the tops of towering trees that rise from the creek ravine, and through a canopy of broad leaves you have views across the wide river gorge. At 0.8 mile, continue straight at the trail junction and descend 400 feet to the dam. The thunderous sound of rushing water swells as you approach the great spillway dam, which powered the Roswell Mill **(Waypoint 4)**.

To continue, retrace your steps back up the trail you descended and turn left to go east. At 1.0 mile, turn left at the trail junction to continue the loop. (The path to the right cuts across the interior of the knoll.) The next section has a decidedly different feel from the forest you walked through earlier. Winding along the flank of the hill, the rocky, single-track path is bordered by mountain laurel, and the views across the gorge give the illusion that you're exploring some great mountain in a much wilder northern part of Georgia.

At 1.3 miles, continue straight at the trail junction. The path bends right and heads east. At a trail junction in about 530 feet, the path to the left crosses the bridge that leads to Oxbo Road. To continue your loop hike, go straight (east) and take a long trek through oak-dominated forest that deteriorates into a tangle as you approach Grimes Bridge Road. At 2 miles **(Waypoint 5)**, turn right and go south.

At 2.2 miles and 2.3 miles, you encounter trails to the right that traverse the interior of the area. Because these paths are generally less attractive and choked with pine and underbrush, bypass them and keep going southwest. At 2.5 miles, turn right onto the yellow-blazed trail and travel west, passing through ample deadfall. The trail tops a hill and then drops steeply through tall poplars on a trail of red earth. Turn right at the next trail junction to go northwest, and then at 2.7 miles **(Waypoint 6)**, turn left at the trail junction and travel southwest.

A winding descent takes you past a garden of mature hardwoods that fills a ravine. Near the 2.9-mile mark, turn left at the trail junction and begin a gradual climb. Noise from the road opposite the river rises up the bluff, and the river comes into view below and to the right. A series of switchbacks pass trees wrapped in curious-looking vines that resemble spiderwebs, and the trail drops to a trail junction. Turn left to return to the parking area.

UTM WAYPOINTS

1. 16S 744652E 3766162N
2. 16S 744396E 3766371N
3. 16S 744122E 3766522N
4. 16S 744252E 3766769N
5. 16S 745264E 3767236N
6. 16S 744623E 3766588N

TRIP 9 Chattahoochee River National Recreation Area: Island Ford

Distance	2–3 miles (depending on side trips), semiloop
Hiking Time	1–2 hours
Difficulty	Easy
Elevation Gain/Loss	+115/-110 feet
Trail Uses	Leashed dogs and good for kids
Best Times	Year-round
Agency	National Park Service, Chattahoochee River National Recreation Area
Recommended Maps	A National Park Service map is available online at www.nps.gov/chat. Another map is also available online at www.us-parks.com/chattahoochee/maps.html.

HIGHLIGHTS Before Europeans settled in the Island Ford area, Native Americans had established a major trail that they used as a trade route. In those days, this section of the Chattahoochee River sometimes dropped low enough that people could wade across. As you hike the Island Ford Trail, you will see natural rock alcoves that were used by prehistoric Native Americans as far back as 8000 years ago. It's also likely that you'll see anglers in the river shoals, as this is a popular spot for trout fishing. Much of the trail moves easily along the riverbank, but if you want a little more exercise you can take a path that loops through the hills west of the river.

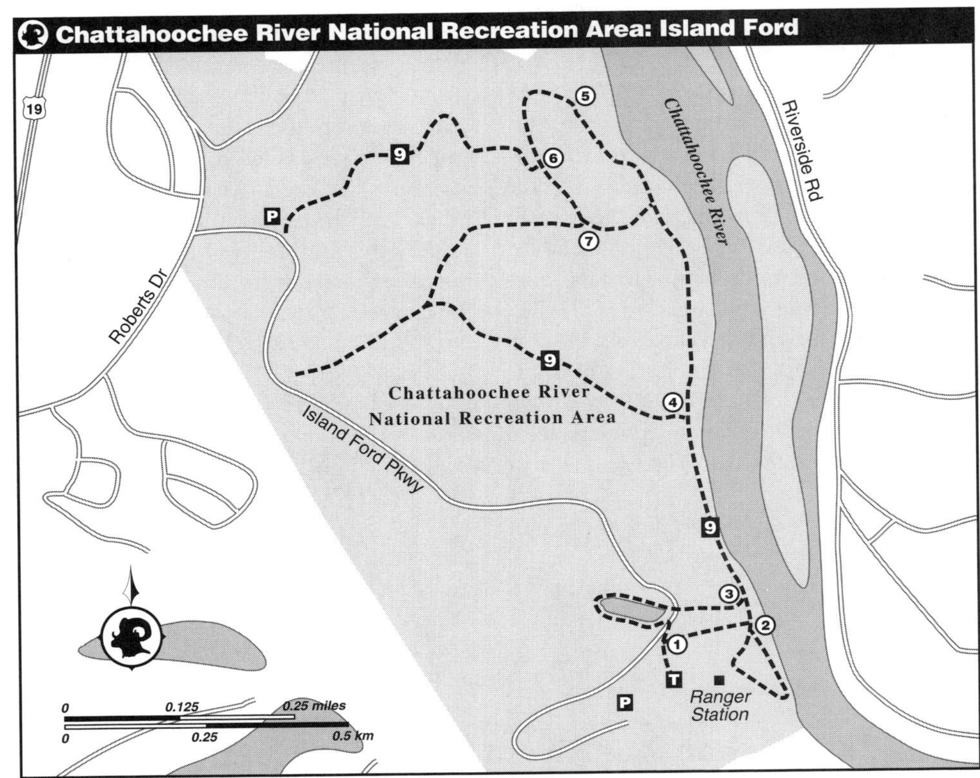

DIRECTIONS From Atlanta travel north on GA Highway 400 and take Exit 6 for Northridge Road. Stay in the middle lane, go straight through the light, and take an immediate right onto Dunwoody Place. Go 0.5 mile and turn right onto Roberts Drive. Go 0.7 mile to the Island Ford entrance on the right. Continue 1.2 miles to a parking area at the end of the road.

FACILITIES/TRAILHEAD The park headquarters and visitors center at the parking area has restrooms and picnic tables. The recreation area charges a $3 parking fee, which you can pay at a kiosk in the parking area. You can purchase a $25 annual pass by calling (678) 538-1200 or by visiting www.nps.gov/chat/index.htm.

The hike begins at the north side of the parking area, the left parking lot when facing headquarters **(Waypoint 1)**. Walk about 70 feet down the path covered with pine needles, and bear right at the first trail junction. Within about 700 feet there is a trail intersection with a footbridge to the left **(Waypoint 2)**. To the right, a path shaded by oaks and pines runs south with clear views of the river, and you may hear geese trading honks back and forth, their calls echoing up and down the Chattahoochee. The path continues down the bank for another tenth of a mile to a boat launch, picnic tables, and wide, grassy area great for tossing a Frisbee around. From here you go west to ascend a paved path back to the visitors center. From the rear of the center, bear right at a Y intersection to head north back toward the river and the footbridge at **Waypoint 2**.

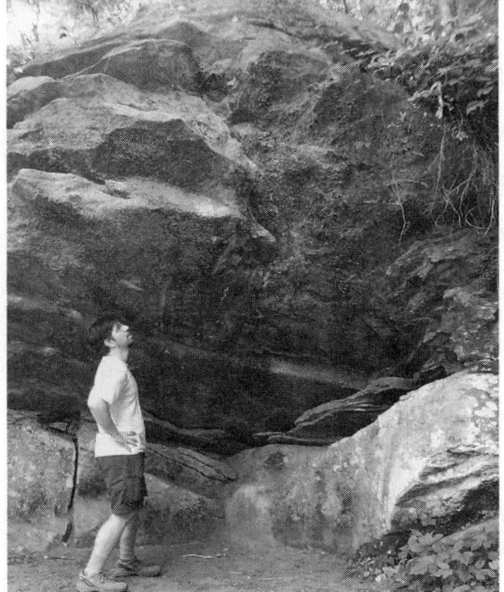

Island Ford rock alcove

From **Waypoint 2**, cross the footbridge, going northwest, and you quickly reach a trail junction **(Waypoint 3)**. The path to the left goes southwest to Island Ford Road and a small pond where you might find parents and children fishing together. A trail circles the pond, but it's not particularly attractive, and I'd say it's more of a simple diversion than a must-see feature.

If you continue straight to go north at **Waypoint 3**, the wide river is on full display, and the easy, flat, and wide path nears its bank. The section of the Chattahoochee at Island Ford is interesting because the water was radically altered by dam construction at the turn of the century. To provide power for Atlanta's streetcars, the Morgan Falls Dam was constructed downstream of Island Ford in 1904. In late 1950s, Buford Dam was constructed upstream at Buford to not only provide power but also control flooding and contribute to Atlanta's water supply. An unintended consequence was that the Chattahoochee at Island Ford transformed from a typical, southern warm-water river to a flow of cold water, leading to the development of trout fishing.

At 0.6 mile a trail enters on the left, but you continue straight and look for rock alcoves on the left **(Waypoint 4)**. Continuing along the river, at 0.8 mile look for large boulders resting in the water near the bank. These make great spots to stretch out and catch some rays. Continuing north, switchbacks lead away from the river and climb a bluff with more interesting boulder formations.

At the 1-mile point **(Waypoint 5)**, turn left and travel west. (Disregard the unmarked trail that goes straight, or northwest.) Next, you will reach a trail junction **(Waypoint 6)**. If you go west, the trail proceeds 0.3 mile, dropping to cross a creek and end at a parking lot. If you turn left at the junction, the trail turns to the southeast and climbs moderately to steeply through magnolia. At 1.3 miles there is a trail junction **(Waypoint 7)**. The path to the left leads to steep steps that descend to the river. If you want to lengthen your hike, turn right at **Waypoint 7** to travel west and loop through the hills. If you ascend this periodically steep section on a blue-sky day, sunlight will pour through the hardwood canopy, lending a very different feel from the shaded corridors along the river. At 1.5 miles, the trail to the right descends to the southwest to meet Island Ford Parkway. Rather than take this trail, turn left at the junction and pass significant blowdown and stands of small cedar trees. Dropping into the Mulberry Creek drainage, you're greeted by stout oaks, and at 1.8 miles turn right at the T junction to travel south. At 2.0 miles, cross the footbridge and turn right to return to the parking area.

UTM WAYPOINTS

1. 16S 747050E 3763987N
2. 16S 747161E 3764083N
3. 16S 747163E 3764118N
4. 16S 747081E 3764525N
5. 16S 746916E 3764988N
6. 16S 746813E 3764900N
7. 16S 746887E 3764797N

TRIP 10 Chattahoochee River National Recreation Area: Medlock Bridge

Distance	1.6 miles, semiloop
Hiking Time	1 hour
Difficulty	Easy
Elevation Gain/Loss	+80/-95 feet
Trail Uses	Leashed dogs and good for kids
Best Times	Year-round
Agency	National Park Service, Chattahoochee River National Recreation Area
Recommended Maps	A National Park Service map is available online at www.nps.gov/chat. Another map is available online at www.us-parks.com/chattahoochee/maps.html.

HIGHLIGHTS The Medlock Bridge unit of the Chatthoochee River National Recreation Area is really a place for a brief escape from the suburban sprawl north of Atlanta. A boat launch gives paddlers and other boaters easy access to the Chattahoochee River, and the riverbank has lots of spots to cast a fishing line and while away a few hours. The Medlock Bridge Trail winds along the twisting waterway, and then climbs a hill where you'll find a rock outcrop. Pack a lunch and sit in this high perch among the tree canopy with an open view of the forest floor below.

DIRECTIONS From Atlanta take Interstate 85 north and take Exit 99 for Jimmy Carter Boulevard. Turn right onto GA Highway 141 and get into lane for GA 141 north. Go 3 miles, and then turn right onto Peachtree Industrial Boulevard. Turn left onto Holcomb Bridge Road, and then turn right onto GA 141/Peachtree Parkway. Go 3.6 miles on GA 141 (Medlock Bridge Road), and turn right into the parking area before crossing the river.

FACILITIES/TRAILHEAD There are no restroom facilities at the trailhead parking area, but there are picnic tables near the boat ramp. The recreation area charges a $3 parking fee, which you can pay at a kiosk in the parking area. You can purchase a $25 annual pass by calling (678) 538-1200 or by visiting www.nps.gov/chat/index.htm.

From the pay station in the parking lot, walk east toward the boat launch. At the first trail intersection **(Waypoint 1)**, you can go left or right along the river. The best option is to turn right and go south, as the path to the left ends at the Medlock Bridge after less than 400 feet.

After turning south, the flat path is lined with thick brush and deep green Christmas ferns. Along here, look for May-apples, a short, squat plant whose leaves fan and droop to form an umbrella shape.

At 0.3 mile **(Waypoint 2)**, bear left at the trail junction to go southwest and climb through beech and oak trees as the river comes into view. At 0.4 mile bear left at a Y junction **(Waypoint 3)** to continue south and cross a wood footbridge over a drainage gully. A steep set of wood and earth steps ascends through rhododendron and pines, and the trail then drops to another drainage as the forest grows more dense, and the river appears intermittently. At 0.6 mile the trail bends to the right at a spot where a NO TRESPASSING sign is posted on a tree **(Waypoint 4)**. Turn around here and retrace your steps to **Waypoint 3**. Bear left for a steep climb to a hilltop where the path levels out. Continue

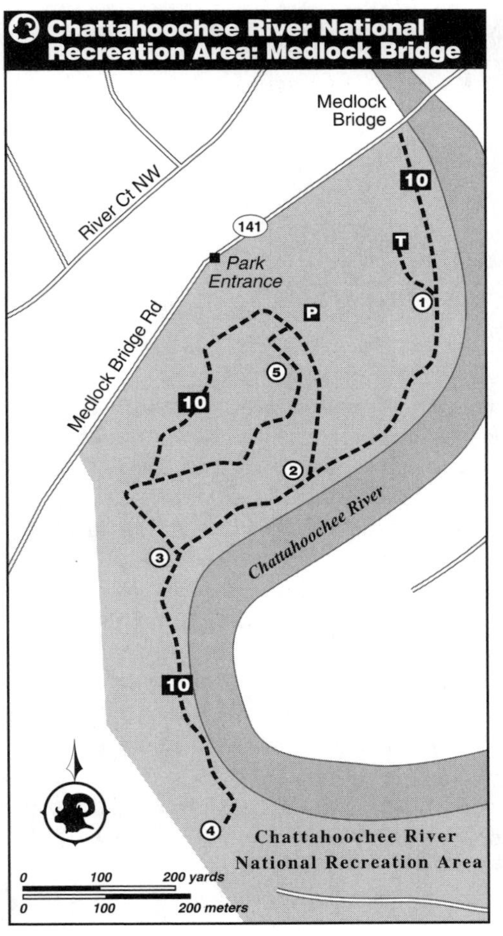

walking through pines and hardwoods to another trail junction at 0.9 mile. Bear right and travel southeast 0.2 mile to the rock outcrop that lies to the right, a few feet below the trail **(Waypoint 5)**. Watch your footing; should you fall . . . well, that first step's a doozy.

As you relax on the rock, eye level with the high boughs of an oak, it's easy to imagine that you're seeing the forest from the point of view of a bird on the hunt. On the leaf-covered ground below, somewhere in the thin underbrush, dinner may scamper by.

After leaving the rock, descend to a trail junction at 1.2 miles, near the entrance road. The path to the left climbs west back up the hill, but you turn right and go south on a wide, well-worn path to make your way back to the parking area. When you return to **Waypoint 2**, turn left to travel northeast and return to the trailhead.

UTM WAYPOINTS

1. 16S 758419E 3765225N
2. 16S 758296E 3764910N
3. 16S 758131E 3764805N
4. 16S 758190E 3764494N
5. 16S 758285E 3765021N

TRIP 11 Stone Mountain Park: Walk-Up Trail

Distance	2.0 miles, out-and-back
Hiking Time	1 hour
Difficulty	Moderate
Elevation Gain/Loss	+/-645 feet
Trail Use	Good for kids
Best Times	Year-round
Agency	Stone Mountain Park
Recommended Map	A Stone Mountain Park hiking trail map is available online at www.stonemountainpark.com.
Note	Pets are prohibited.

HIGHLIGHTS From the summit of Stone Mountain you can see 60 miles in every direction, and on fair-weather days, throngs of people hike to the top via the Walk-Up Trail, which climbs about 650 feet in elevation. From the base to the summit, the trail follows wide, clear expanses of granite bordered by a forest of mostly oaks and pines. Mostly moderate, with short, steep sections near the top, the trail is not difficult if you are fit, and doable for most others. Once you've reached the top and soaked in the view, you can visit the building that serves the Skylift gondola and has good interpretive displays detailing the wildlife and plants in the area. Walk outside the south side of the building onto the balcony for a 180-degree view of the landscape from east to west.

DIRECTIONS From Atlanta take Interstate 285 to Exit 39B for U.S. Hwy 78 east (Snellville/Athens). Travel 7.7 miles and take Exit 8 for the Stone Mountain Park Main Entrance. Follow the exit ramp to the East Gate entrance of Stone Mountain Park. Travel 2.1 miles to the parking lot on the left beside Confederate Hall.

FACILITIES/TRAILHEAD There are restrooms near the trailhead and in Confederate Hall. Also, the Skylift building at the summit has a restroom, water fountain, and snack bar. The park charges an $8 parking fee.

At the east side of Confederate Hall **(Waypoint 1)**, cross the railroad tracks and ascend the wide bed of rock. If you walk this lower portion of the mountain in March you will see patches of wooly ragwort, with its golden petals. The trail up is easy to discern, but there are also yellow lines on the rock to mark the way. The smell of pine grows stronger as you stroll upward, and in spring you can survey the granite outcrops for blooming plants such as St.-John's-wort. Later in the summer, pineweed and the beautiful, blue dayflower rise from small plots of soil. (A brochure available at Confederate Hall highlights several plant species on the trail.) At 0.3 mile, the rock surface is

Stone Mountain Walk-Up Trail

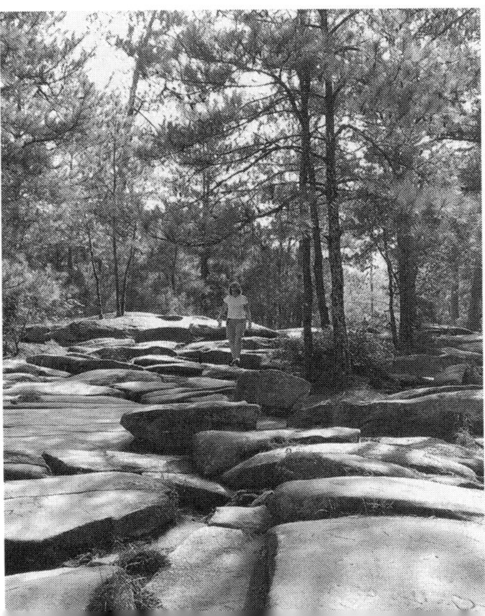

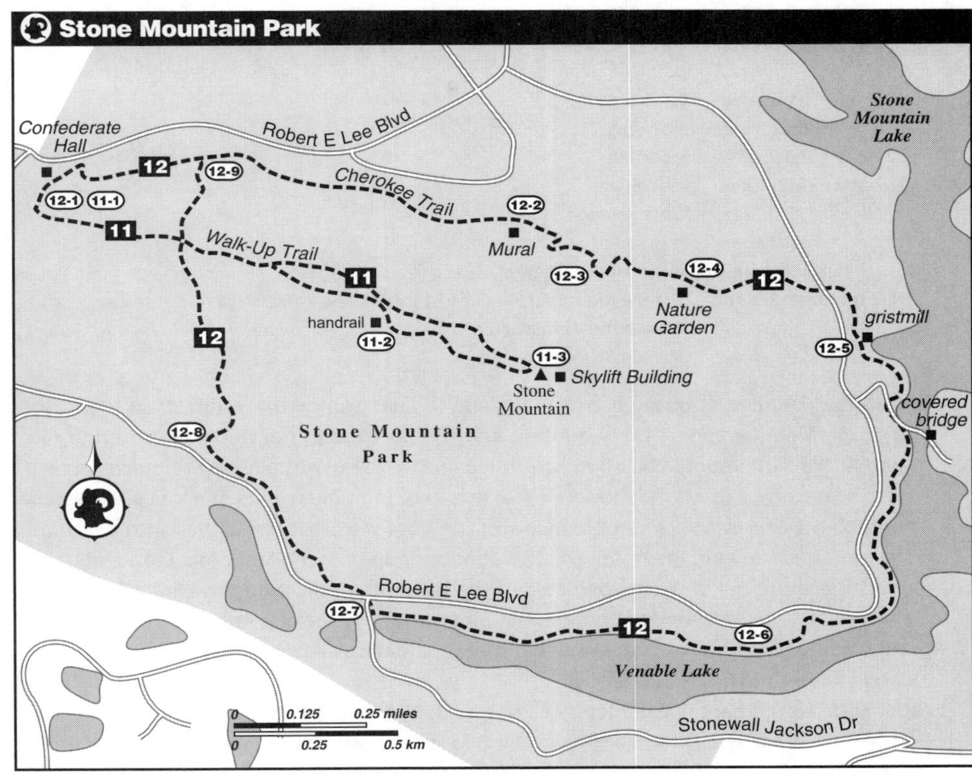

a broken patchwork of stone dotted with pines. As you leave this boulder field, look right for the forest opening with views of low hills to the south and the pale blue band of hills on the horizon.

At 0.8 mile **(Waypoint 2)** a handrail is set into the stone, making it easier to negotiate this steep section of the trail. Take caution if hiking during or after a rainstorm as the rocky trail surface gets slippery. Beyond the rail is another sea of exposed rock and a clear line of sight to the northwest and northeast. At 0.9 mile you have one final steep but brief climb, and the trail ends at the summit at approximately 1 mile **(Waypoint 3)**.

After you visit the building for the Skylift, return to **Waypoint 3** and follow the white line back down the mountain. As you descend you intersect with a gravel path, which eventually bends to meet the yellow path you took up the mountain. Continue down the yellow trail to return to the trailhead.

UTM WAYPOINTS

1. 16S 762748E 3744808N
2. 16S 763815E 3744444N
3. 16S 764232E 3744313N

TRIP 12 Stone Mountain Park: Cherokee Trail

Distance	5.2 miles, loop
Hiking Time	2½ hours
Difficulty	Moderate
Elevation Gain/Loss	+/-375 feet
Trail Use	Leashed dogs
Best Times	Year-round
Agency	Stone Mountain Park
Recommended Map	A Stone Mountain Park hiking trail map is available online at www.stonemountainpark.com.
Note	Pets are prohibited.

see map on p. 229

HIGHLIGHTS Thousands of years ago, Woodland Indians explored the forests at the base of Stone Mountain, most likely hunting and fishing, though not necessarily setting up permanent settlements. The Cherokee Trail encircles the mountain, covering diverse terrain, from stony slabs at the mountain's base to oak and pine woods. The trail also passes through a clearing with a stunning view of the Confederate mural carved into a face of the mountain. Beyond the mural, the trail continues on to Stone Mountain Lake and then skirts the shore in a less-crowded area of the park. After following the bank of Venable Lake, you'll ascend the slopes of Stone Mountain with views of a forested valley spread out below. The path bisects the Walk-Up Trail and finally dives down the mountainside to carry you back to Confederate Hall.

DIRECTIONS From Atlanta take Interstate 285 to Exit 39B for U.S. Highway 78 East (Snellville/Athens) exit. Travel 7.7 miles and take Exit 8 for the Stone Mountain Park Main Entrance. Follow the exit ramp to the East Gate entrance of Stone Mountain Park. Travel 2.1 miles to the parking lot on the left beside Confederate Hall.

FACILITIES/TRAILHEAD There are restrooms near the trailhead and in the Confederate Hall building. Be sure to pack water. There is an $8 vehicle fee for the park.

The hike begins in the same general area where the Walk-Up Trail starts. From the northeast side of Confederate Hall (**Waypoint 1**), take the paved walkway north. After about 700 feet, turn right and ascend the paved path to an orange trail maker on the left. Turn left onto the trail and go east through a pine forest, occasionally breaking into open sunshine to traverse a forest floor of stone.

At 0.6 mile, you walk beneath a high canopy of hardwoods and dip to cross a stream drainage. Shouts and laughter mix with a howling whistle as you approach the station for the passenger train that circles the mountain. Just past a miniature golf course, the trail turns right and goes southeast.

At 1 mile, the trail exits the tree line, and you can turn left to cross open ground where the great stone wall and Confederate mural looms above (**Waypoint 2**). Continue to the statue at the far end of the clearing (**Waypoint 3**). Turn right to go around the backside of the statue and descend to a gravel trail. Turn left onto the gravel trail, traveling northeast. At 1.3 miles, turn right onto the narrower trail where a stone is marked with a red arrow. A creek feeds the poplars and rich understory in this bottomland forest, and the clamor of trains and tourists fades into the background.

A Nature Garden lies to the right of the trail at 1.5 miles **(Waypoint 4)**. Turn right here and continue through the garden to the base of the mountain. Scramble up some rocks, crawl onto a great slope of granite, and crane your neck upward to take in the high reach of the stone wall. From the base of the mountain wall, return to the main trail, turn right, and go southeast. Cross railroad tracks and then a road, descend a hill, and turn right to skirt a series of small stone canals.

The path runs to the edge of Stone Mountain Lake, and a gristmill building lies below and to the left at 1.9 miles **(Waypoint 5)**. This building was moved to this location from Ellijay, Georgia, in 1965 to demonstrate the types of structures built in the South to take advantage of the natural resources. The stream that rushes beneath the building does not power any mill wheel, but rather makes a great watery playground for kids and parents. Take the boardwalk that goes to the left (lakeside) of the building, and once across the boardwalk turn left to continue on the Cherokee Trail. The path here runs right next to the water.

At 2.2 miles you reach a covered bridge that was moved here from the Athens area in the 1890s. To continue, bear right and take the single-track path, traveling southwest, for a very peaceful section. Lake coves lie just below to the left, and rock outcrops form forest openings where you can soak up the sun and look for great blue herons gliding over the water.

At 2.9 miles **(Waypoint 6)**, bear right at the Y intersection (no trail sign here) to begin a quiet walk through a typical pine and hardwood forest along the north bank of Venable Lake. You pass the remains of an old chimney from a homestead dating from the late 1800s to early 1900s. At 3.2 miles cross a stream that is wide and deep enough to soak your shoes.

At 3.7 miles **(Waypoint 7)**, leave the forest and turn right to walk north to Robert E. Lee Boulevard. (The official red trail continues east of this point, but it's overgrown and difficult to navigate.) Turn left onto Robert E. Lee Boulevard. At 3.8 miles turn right, leaving the road and following the red-blazed Cherokee Trail.

The trail visits another chimney from a long-gone homestead and comes to a Y junction. Bear right to continue on the Cherokee Trail and cross the railroad tracks **(Waypoint 8)**. The next leg of the hike is a bit more challenging, as the trail crawls up the smooth stone slope of the

Robert E. Lee, Stonewall Jackson, and Jefferson Davis gallop across granite at Stone Mountain.

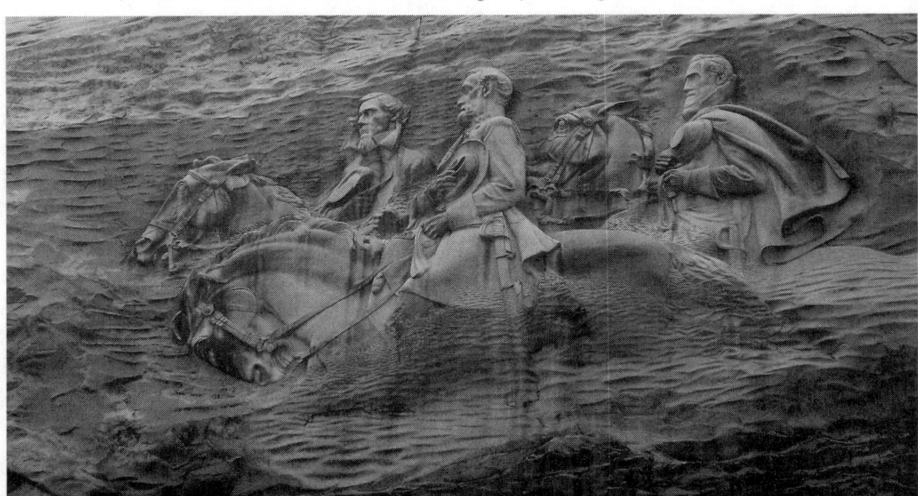

mountain. Proceed with caution because the occasional stream of water flowing down the slabs can be extremely slippery. To navigate, keep a sharp eye out for white lines painted on the rock, and be sure to look over your left shoulder to enjoy the panorama of green forest below. After climbing this steep section (which climbs from 850 to 1170 feet of elevation), cross over the Walk-Up Trail to continue on the Cherokee Trail. Follow the white blazes on the ground and travel north.

The trail then descends the north slope of Stone Mountain, but the white lines marking the trail can be difficult to see. At **Waypoint 9** (4.7 miles), turn left and make your way down, traveling north. At 4.8 miles the path joins another portion of the Cherokee Trail at a T junction. Turn left and travel southwest to return to the trailhead.

UTM WAYPOINTS

1. 16S 762751E 3744844N
2. 16S 764178E 3744789N
3. 16S 764432E 3744647N
4. 16S 764709E 3744595N
5. 16S 765239E 3744384N
6. 16S 764865E 3743413N
7. 16S 763751E 3743531N
8. 16S 763260E 3744117N
9. 16S 763225E 3744841N

TRIP 13 Panola Mountain State Park: Microwatershed, Rock Outcrop, & Fitness Trails

Distance	2.5 miles, semiloop
Hiking Time	1½ hours
Difficulty	Easy
Elevation Gain/Loss	+/-105 feet
Trail Use	Good for kids
Best Times	Spring
Agency	Panola Mountain State Park
Recommended Map	A *Panola Mountain State Park Trail Map* is available in the visitors center.

HIGHLIGHTS Beginning in the visitors center, you might want to spend some time viewing the displays that highlight the plants and animals found on Panola Mountain. The forest around the visitors center is a mixture of mockernut hickory trees, black cherry trees, and loblolly pines, and markers identify the different species. The hike detailed here begins on the Microwatershed Trail, which roams through maples, sweetgum trees, and sassafras trees on its way to a creek bottom. After returning to the visitors center, you take the Rock Outcrop Trail to slabs of exposed granite. One unusual aspect of the park is its Fitness Trail, which lies south of the visitors center. A sort of a gym set completely in the woods, this trail sports a series of exercise stations designed to improve strength, balance, and flexibility.

DIRECTIONS From Atlanta take Interstate 285 to its junctions with Interstate 20 east of downtown. Take I-20 east 2.9 miles to Exit 68 for Wesley Chapel Road. Turn right onto Wesley Chapel Road, and travel south 0.4 mile to Snapfinger Road. Turn left onto Snapfinger Road and travel south 7.2 miles to the entrance of Panola Mountain State Park on the left.

FACILITIES/TRAILHEAD There are restrooms at the visitors center. Pack all the water you will need for the hike. The park charges a $3 parking fee, or you can purchase an Annual ParkPass for $30 by calling (770) 389-7401.

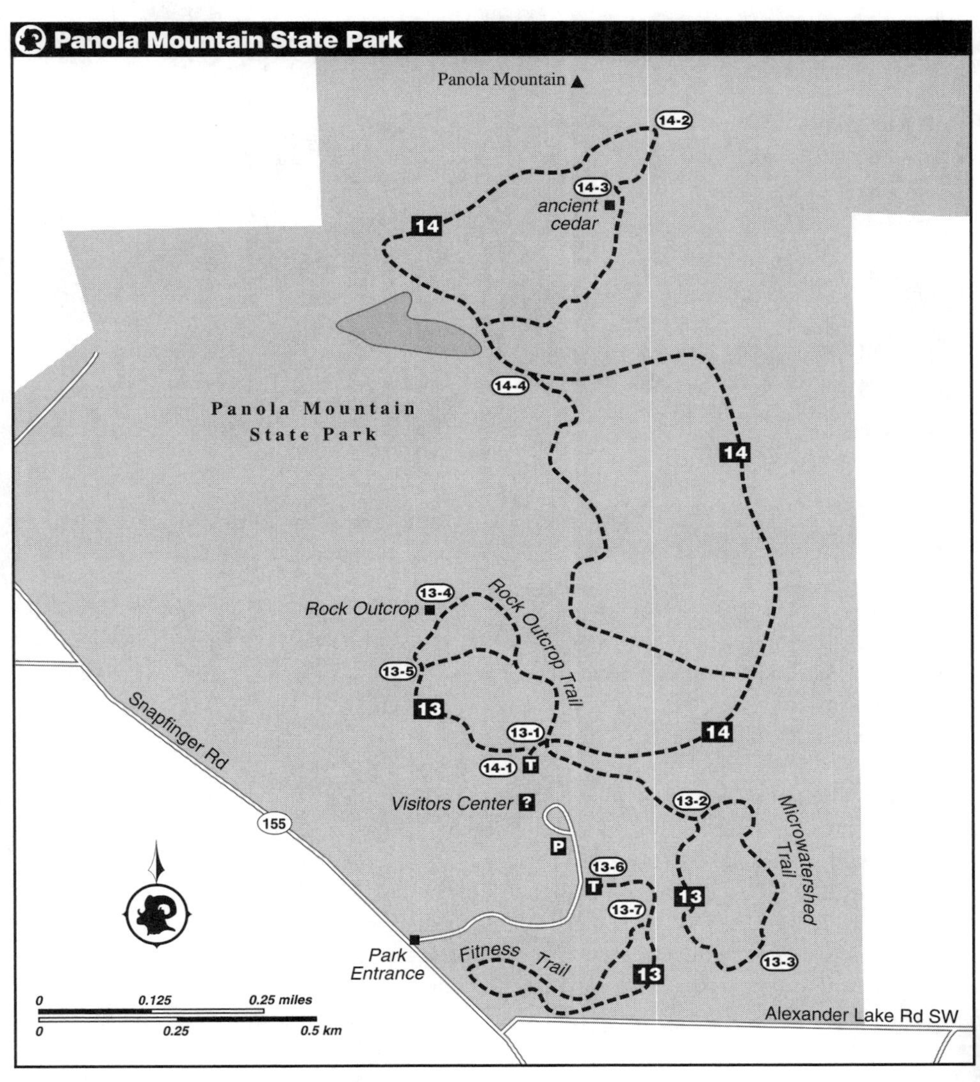

From the rear of the visitors center begin at the trailhead for the Rock Outcrop and Microwatershed Trails **(Waypoint 1)**. Turn right to take the mile-long Microwatershed Trail and descend through the pines. At 0.2 mile an interpretive sign explains how the creek bottom you're headed toward is part of a larger watershed system.

A little father ahead is a Y junction **(Waypoint 2)**. From here you can walk left or right on the Microwatershed loop. Continuing on, you'll walk among young poplars and dogwoods as well as sweetgum.

A footbridge takes you across the creek at **Waypoint 3**, where Christmas ferns thrive as well as oaks and other hardwoods. The creek is fed by the many visible erosion cuts as well as springs. Finish the loop, ascending moderately back to the trailhead at **Waypoint 1**.

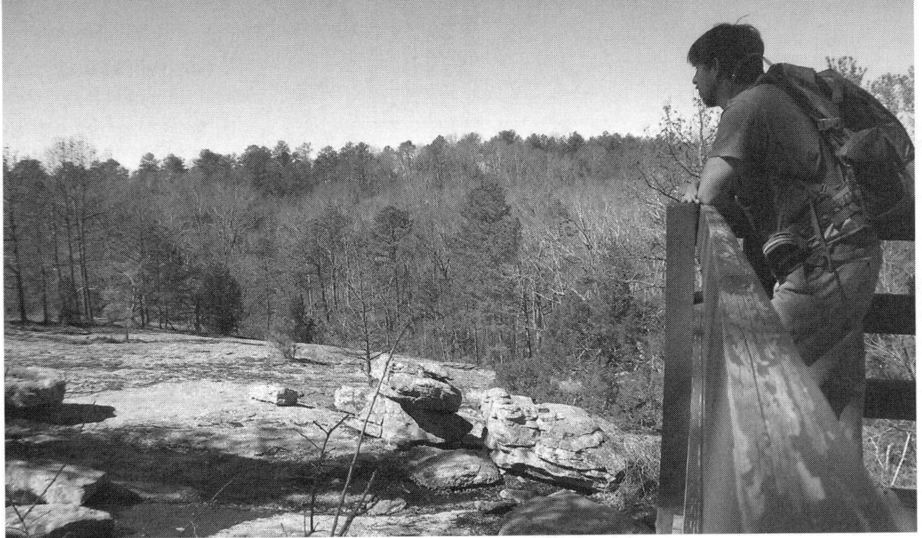

Panola Mountain's Rock Outcrop Trail

Enter the Rock Outcrop Trail and travel north, looking for "Station" markers that indicate interesting tree and plant species along the trail. You first see loblolly pines and black cherry trees, and ahead at a Y junction at Station 2, there's a white oak tree. Bear right and descend, soon arriving at a side trail that leads to Station 3, home of a mockernut hickory tree.

Back at the main trail, turn right and travel northwest, watching for monarch butterflies flitting about or vultures soaring overhead. The trail passes through sloping boulders covered with lichen; an interpretive sign explains how this blend of fungus and algae have formed an unusual partnership. As you continue, look for wildflowers such as lavender beardtongue and fire pink flowers, which show their colors from May to June.

At **Waypoint 4** you reach a wood platform that provides a good view of the granite outcrop, which was a mass of underground molten rock 325 million years ago. An interpretive sign explains that, through erosion, the rock was exposed about 15 million years ago. Scan the stony ground to see the "solution pits" where soil has developed to support the fragile plant life. You might also see yellow sun drop blooms on the stone surface.

Continue on the loop and at **Waypoint 5** a path cuts across to Station 2 and the marked white oak. Or, from **Waypoint 5** you can continue to travel southwest on the loop, which swings back to the east, passes through poplars, and ends at the visitors center.

Fitness Trail

While a walk in the woods can be relaxing, it can also be an opportunity to improve your fitness level. The park's Fitness Trail has a series of clever stations with diagrams that demonstrate exercise procedures for flexibility, strength, and balance.

The trailhead lies about 300 feet south of the parking area near the visitors center **(Waypoint 6)**. The chipped bark path first passes a station with warm-up routines. At a Y junction **(Waypoint 7)** bear right to a series of low balance beams. Next, a series of short, vertical logs form a natural stair-climber.

Down the trail, a set of parallel bars are good for doing dips or handwalking to work your upper body. Farther on, inclined wood platforms are perfect for sit-ups (there's even a bar to hold your feet in place). How many chin-ups can you do? You can find out at the next stop where high bars run between wood posts. If you do each station, you'll notice your heart rate rising, and you can take it up a notch at the side vault beam station, springing from one side to the other.

You can cool down at a series of stretching stations. Then, back at **Waypoint 7**, turn right to return to the trailhead.

UTM WAYPOINTS

1. 16S 762378E 3724278N
2. 16S 762610E 3724178N
3. 16S 762728E 3723971N
4. 16S 762188E 3724550N
5. 16S 762157E 3724440N
6. 16S 762470E 3724069N
7. 16S 762536E 3724006N

TRIP 14 Panola Mountain State Park: Panola Mountain Guided Hike

Distance	3.0 miles, loop
Hiking Time	2 hours
Difficulty	Moderate
Elevation Gain/Loss	+/-375 feet
Trail Uses	Guided hiking and good for kids ages 10 and up
Best Times	Spring
Agency	Panola Mountain State Park
Recommended Map	The route for this hike does not appear on the park's trail map.

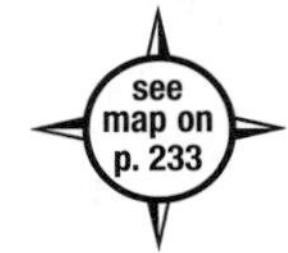
see map on p. 233

HIGHLIGHTS To protect the fragile ecology of Panola Mountain, the park limits public access to certain areas in Panola Mountain State Park, including the summit, but park rangers frequently lead public hikes that allow you a close look at the plant life on the wide tracts of exposed granite. It certainly helps to have an informed guide with a trained eye point out the minute diamorpha that grows on the rocky slopes. The broad, open space at the summit has a great view of Atlanta, and you get to visit one of the mountain's oldest inhabitants—a 250-year-old cedar tree. Your guide will also familiarize you with the plants and animals inhabiting the lower mountain forest. While the hike involves some moderate climbing, it's not especially rigorous.

DIRECTIONS From Atlanta take Interstate 285 to its junctions with Interstate 20 east of the city. Take I-20 east 2.9 miles to Exit 68 for Wesley Chapel Road. Turn right onto Wesley Chapel Road, and travel south 0.4 mile to Snapfinger Road. Turn left onto Snapfinger Road and travel south 7.2 miles to the entrance of Panola Mountain State Park on the left.

FACILITIES/TRAILHEAD There are restrooms at the visitors center. Pack all the water you will need for the hike. The park charges a $3 parking fee. You can purchase an Annual ParkPass for $30 by calling (770) 389-7401.

Park rangers lead hikes to Panola Mountain every third Saturday of the month (every month), and fall, winter, and spring are the best seasons for wildflower blooms. (Call the park office for reservations: $5 per person plus $3 for parking.) The following is a description of the hike a guide led my group on one June day.

From the visitors center **(Waypoint 1)**, the group headed northeast for 0.3 mile and turned left at a Y junction. Not far ahead we paused at an erosion gully to see an example of how poor farming techniques lead to destructive erosion. We then rolled through open forest and at 0.5 mile looked left at a rock that was likely split during an ice age 10,000 years ago. We took a footbridge across a streambed, and our sharp-eyed guide spied the den of a wolf spider in the bank. A bit farther on, he picked out a well-camouflaged eastern box turtle, one of the few turtles that can shut its shell completely for protection. From here the trail is lined with an invasive plant that has many names, one of which is silverberry. On the list of most-unwelcome invasive plants in Georgia, it ranks in the top 10 with kudzu and Chinese privet.

Passing another trail junction, we reached the shore of a mountain lake at 0.9 mile. After swinging to the northwest, the trail turned sharply to the east, and we began climbing the mountain. On the walk up you must step carefully to avoid damaging fragile plants such as lichen, which appears green until it loses its water and becomes black.

As we climbed we examined "solution pits," or small patches on earth, sand, and gravel where tiny diamorpha plants grow on the granite slab. In the wide, clear sky, we saw turkey vultures circling. Just beyond the crest of the mountain **(Waypoint 2)**, you have clear views of Atlanta and Stone Mountain to the north.

Pausing on the mountaintop, we examined one of the creatures that thrives here—the large, yellow and black lubber grasshopper. It reportedly has no natural predators because it tastes so bad—I'll take the guide's word on that.

After we turned south to circle the mountaintop, an ancient cedar tree came into view **(Waypoint 3)**. Appropriately named Methuselah, it is thought to be about 250 years old. We then descended quickly from the mountain to enter the trees and cross a boulder field.

Back at the lake, we turned left, and at the next junction **(Waypoint 4)** took another left, climbing to level ground. The final leg was an easy walk through pine-hardwood forest that brought us back to the visitors center.

UTM WAYPOINTS

1. 16S 762355E 3724271N
2. 16S 762525E 3725387N
3. 16S 762475E 3725296N
4. 16S 762336E 3724958N

TRIP 15 Reynolds Nature Preserve

Distance	1.7 miles, loop
Hiking Time	1 hour
Difficulty	Easy
Elevation Gain/Loss	+/-115 feet
Trail Uses	Leashed dogs and good for kids
Best Times	Year-round
Agency	William H. Reynolds Memorial Nature Preserve
Recommended Map	A trail map is available at the Nature Center and online at http://web.co.clayton.ga.us/reynolds/about.htm.

HIGHLIGHTS With 146 acres of forest and wetlands, including five ponds, the William H. Reynolds Memorial Nature Preserve supports a great variety of wildlife, including turtles, salamanders, toads, and beavers. Many bird species, such as Canada geese, green herons,

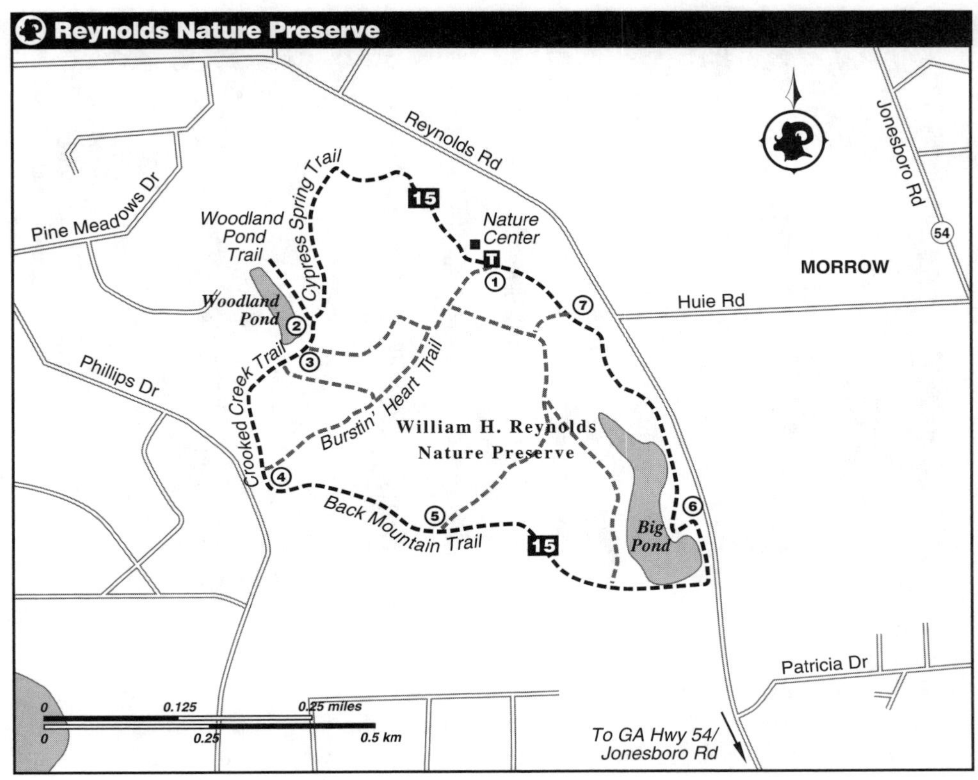

and Kentucky warblers, live here, as well as numerous wildflowers, including American beauty berry, red trillium, and lizards' tail. The preserve has 4.5 miles of easy trails with several loops that you can link for long or short walks. The preserve is named for William Huie Reynolds, a county judge and naturalist who acquired the land in the 1920s and donated it to Clayton County in 1976. Each year about 35,000 people visit the preserve, and 4000 schoolchildren participate in its nature education programs.

DIRECTIONS From Atlanta take Interstate 75 south to Exit 233 for GA Highway 54/Jonesboro Road. Turn left onto GA 54 and travel 0.9 mile to Reynolds Road. Turn left onto Reynolds Road and travel 1.1 miles to the Nature Center parking area.

FACILITIES/TRAILHEAD There are restrooms at the Nature Center. The trails are open daily from 8 AM to dusk.

Begin your hike at the rear of the Nature Center **(Waypoint 1)**. Turn right onto the bark chip path and walk northwest with Azalea Pond to your left. The trail passes an outdoor classroom as well as a barn and reaches a small spring at 0.1 mile. Take the wood footbridge across the spring, and then turn left to go southwest on the Cypress Spring Trail.

The path descends through oaks to a junction with the Woodland Pond Trail at 0.3 mile **(Waypoint 2)**. Turn right to walk along this long, narrow pool, which attracts queen snakes and midland snakes because it's an especially secluded and undisturbed spot.

Return to the Cypress Spring Trail and turn right to travel south. At the

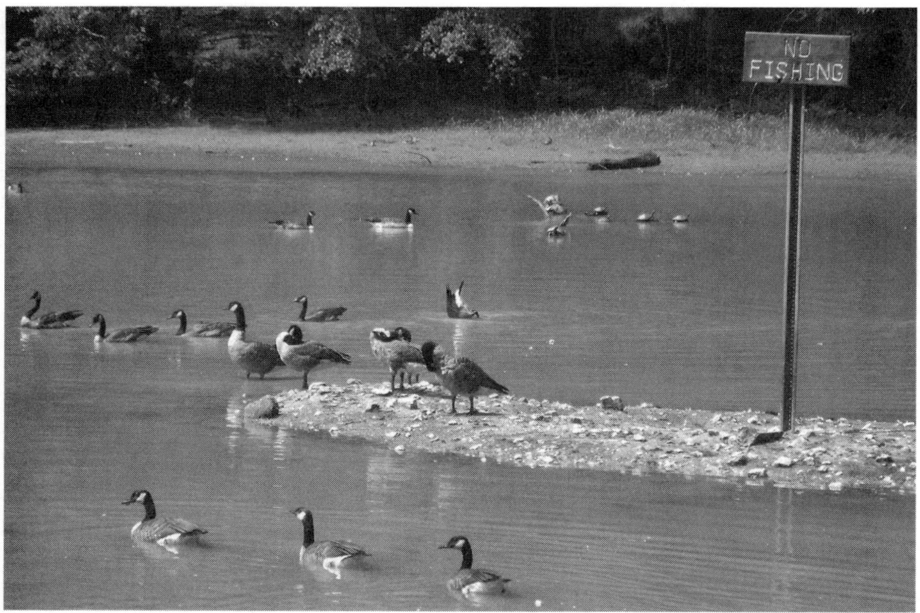

The Big Pond in Reynolds Nature Preserve

next junction **(Waypoint 3)** you can go left (east) or right (west). The path to the left is adorned with purple American beauty berries and large poplars. To continue to loop around the preserve, turn right at **Waypoint 3** and take the Crooked Creek Trail, which climbs through sweetgums along a deep creek drainage.

At 0.7 mile **(Waypoint 4)** the Burstin' Heart Trail enters on the left. This path cuts across the preserve's interior, topping a hill of hardwoods and descending toward Azalea Pond. To continue the long loop, go straight at **Waypoint 4**, taking the Back Mountain Trail, which soon turns to the east. The trail stays on high ground in a forest of sourwood, hickory, and oak trees. At 0.9 mile bear right at a trail junction **(Waypoint 5)** to take the Back Mountain Trail to the Big Pond.

At about the 1-mile mark, a trail enters on the left. Continue straight to walk along the southern end of Big Pond. The path takes a sharp left turn at the southeast corner of the pond to run north. At 1.2 miles **(Waypoint 6)** a wood observation deck to the left gives you a good view of the pond where you might see wood ducks and geese. Big Pond is also home to a group of very large snapping turtles.

From the observation platform, return to the trail and turn left to walk north beside Dry Pond, a good place to spot a great blue heron or green heron. Continue past Island Pond on a shaded trail that is eventually covered in pine needles. At 1.5 miles **(Waypoint 7)** continue straight at a trail junction, traveling northwest to walk toward the Nature Center. At the next Y junction, bear right to return to the center.

UTM WAYPOINTS

1. 16S 746131E 3720990N
2. 16S 745905E 3720882N
3. 16S 745917E 3720840N
4. 16S 745837E 3720667N
5. 16S 746101E 3720564N
6. 16S 746465E 3720575N
7. 16S 746277E 3720895N

Chapter 6
East of Atlanta

The land east of Atlanta is home to popular state parks, such as Fort Yargo and Watson Mill Bridge, which offer plenty of activities for a family camping trip, including hiking, biking, swimming, and fishing. A bit farther south, Hard Labor Creek State Park is situated on former farmland, though you wouldn't know it when walking the trails that roll through hardwood forest and pass a beaver pond popular with birders. Another good destination for observing birds and other animals is the Charlie Elliott Wildlife Center near Mansfield, Georgia. With 6500 acres of fields, bottomland woods, and pine and hardwood forest, this land was designated as an Important Birding Area by the Atlanta Audubon Society in 2002. In Auburn, Georgia, you'll find Little Mulberry Park, a quality county-owned recreation area with trails that visit old-growth forest. It also has wheelchair-accessible trails that visit meadows and a lake with fishing piers.

Fort Yargo State Park

Fort Yargo is one of Georgia's most-visited state parks, drawing hikers, mountain bikers, and campers from Atlanta and Athens. With 260-acre Marbury Creek Reservoir at its center, the park includes a beach and swimming area, plus boat ramps and fishing spots. In the 1700s white settlers considered this land the edge of the frontier, and in 1792 a fort was built here to provide protection from Creek Indians. Part of the old fort still stands, and a park trail passes by the old structure. On the western side of the park, you can stroll along the paved Bird Berry Trail, which crosses a wetland and skirts the lakeshore. At the lower end of the reservoir, a patchwork of trails allows you to link a lake walk with a moderate trek through the park's southern hills. There are also long paths that twist through the eastern portion of the park, and though these woods can offer solitude, the dry pine environment provides little scenery and can be quite hot.

Watson Mill Bridge

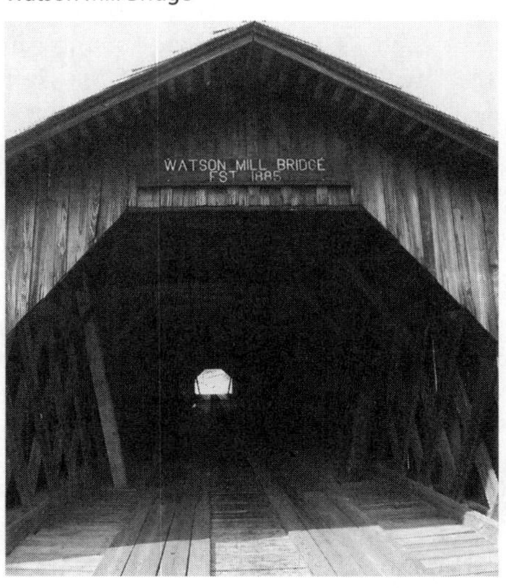

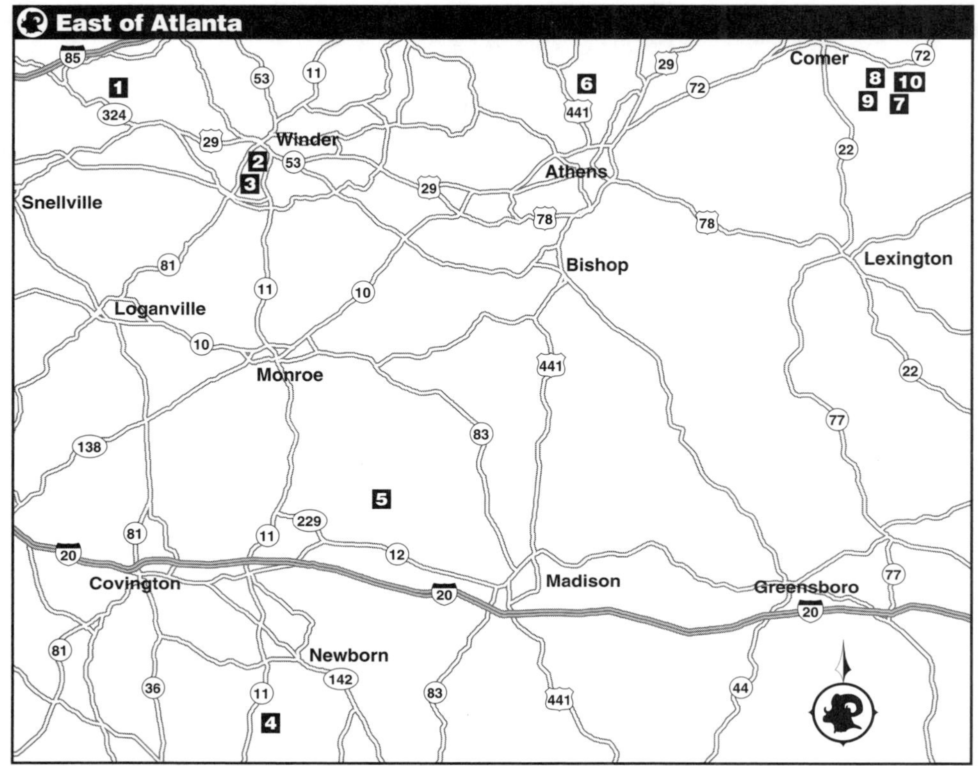

Watson Mill Bridge State Park

This park is notable, not only for its quaint covered bridge spanning the South Fork of the Broad River, but also as the site of a sawmill and gristmill in the late 1800s. This stretch of the river was also used to power a hydroelectric facility that opened in 1905 and operated for almost 50 years. These days, one of the park's main attractions, particularly in summer, is a natural waterslide just downstream from where the river runs beneath the Watson Mill Bridge. Here the shallow water flows down a broad base of rock, and on warm days this becomes a big playground for kids and adults.

The park has a diverse system of trails. The Walking Trail runs along an old canal to the hydroelectric powerhouse ruins. On the opposite side of the river a 2.5-mile hiking and biking trail loops through a shady, pine-hardwood forest—arguably the best dayhike in the park. Two other short hiking trails loop through the forest on the western side of the park road. The Beaver Creek Trail enters a wetland that provides a good spot for birding or simply a quiet walk. The 0.75-mile Ridge Loop Trail climbs to a hilltop that is now heavily forested, though cotton was grown here in the 1800s.

At some point in your trip you'll probably want to pull out your camera and get some shots of the 229-foot covered bridge. According to park literature, Georgia once had more than 200 covered bridges, and the Watson Mill Bridge, constructed in 1885, is one of only 20 that remain.

TRIP 1 Little Mulberry Park

Distance	9.6 miles, loop
Hiking Time	4–5 hours
Difficulty	Moderate
Elevation Gain/Loss	+/-1090 feet
Trail Uses	Leashed dogs, road biking, and horseback riding
Best Times	Year-round
Agency	Gwinnett County Parks and Recreation
Recommended Map	The *Little Mulberry Park Trail Guide* is available at www.gwinnettcounty.com.

HIGHLIGHTS Since the late 1990s, Gwinnett County has been one of the fastest-growing counties in Georgia with a population exceeding 700,000. Fortunately, the county's parks and recreation department has a robust program to preserve green space, and Little Mulberry, located in Auburn, is one of more than 30 parks in Gwinnett County. Opened in 2004, Little Mulberry Park covers 485 acres and includes more than 12 miles of trails, including footpaths through old-growth forest. Within the park lies the 405-acre Karina Miller Nature Preserve, which includes a 2.2-mile wheelchair-accessible trail around a lake with fishing piers, as well as 4 miles of equestrian trails. Additional paved paths circling high meadows are ideal for walking or jogging. The paths in the forest are clear and well-maintained, and a system of seven different trails allows you to tailor your route.

DIRECTIONS From Atlanta travel north on Interstate 85 and take Exit 120 (Hamilton Mill Road/Hamilton Mill Parkway). Turn right onto Hamilton Mill Parkway and travel southwest 0.1 mile. Bear right onto Braselton Highway/GA Highway 124, travel 1.8 miles, and turn left onto Auburn Road/GA Highway 324. Travel 3.3 miles, and turn left onto Fence Road, traveling northeast. Go 0.6 mile and turn left into the Little Mulberry Park entrance.

FACILITIES/TRAILHEAD There are restroom facilities at the trailhead.

From the large kiosk beside the restroom **(Waypoint 1)**, walk up the paved path to the junction with the West Meadow Trail. As you rise into a broad clearing, the path bends left and goes west. At 0.2 mile enter the Ravine Loop Trail, passing beneath the wood trellis **(Waypoint 2)**.

The wide, well-groomed gravel path descends into a mix of pines and hardwoods dominated by white oaks. At 0.5 mile, bear left at the Y intersection and descend gradually on the gravel trail that remains wide, and you'll likely encounter trail runners taking advantage of the smooth path. At 1.1 miles look for mounds of rocks lining the trail **(Waypoint 3)**. An interpretive sign explains that the exact age and purpose of the rock mounds is not known, but archaeologists believe that Native Americans constructed them.

The path becomes stepped as it drops to a small creek, and then turns to the northeast and follows a curved wood bridge with thick beech trees at the opposite end. At 1.8 miles you reach the

Ravine Loop Trailhead

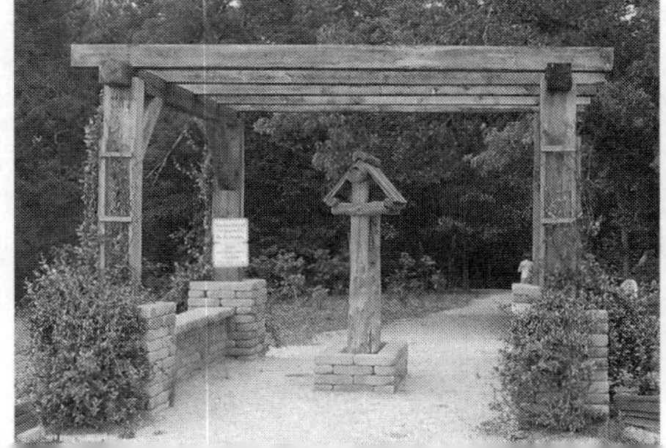

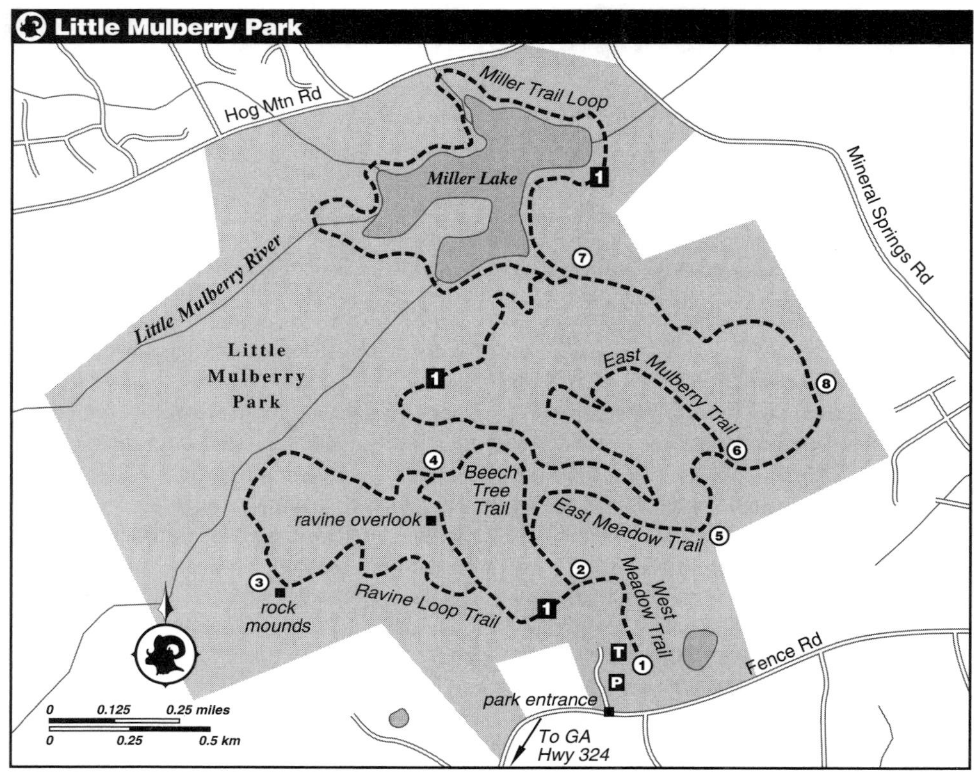

intersection with the Beech Tree Trail **(Waypoint 4)**. Stay on the Ravine Loop, traveling southwest, and walk 900 feet to the Ravine Overlook on the right. The ravine overlook path goes left and right, and a short walk in either direction takes you to benches overlooking the forested cut. The overlook to the left is the better of the two as the woods are more open, but each gives you a chance to slip away for a moment of solitude.

From the overlook, return to **Waypoint 4** and turn onto the Beech Tree Trail, traveling northeast. Blackberry bushes and dense brush line the path as you rise and fall, eventually climbing to the intersection with the West Meadow Trail. Turn left onto the paved West Meadow Trail and continue west across the hill.

At 2.9 miles the West Meadow and East Meadow trails intersect **(Waypoint 5)**. Turn left onto the East Meadow Trail and go north. At 3.2 miles **(Waypoint 6)** turn off the paved path onto the East Mulberry Trail, which drops into hardwood forest. I descended this in a driving rain, skating down the slick, red earth. But even in a downpour, the next 2 miles lifted my spirits because I was greeted by open forest with high oaks, lush ravines, and a feeling that I was not so much in a "park" but remote woodlands.

At 5.4 miles, the trail nears the bank of Miller Lake **(Waypoint 7)**. Turn left and then bear left to travel clockwise on the Miller Trail Loop. The paved path makes for an easy walk. Just past the second fishing pier you pass along the way, look for a tall bird feeder with gourds dangling from the limbs of a skinny tree. At 6.9 miles you will have a view of the lake that could easily be a painting, with a pier framing the right side of the canvas, a small island perched in the water, and rolling green hills beyond.

Continue around the lake and to the left you will see an alternate park entry point off of Hog Mountain Road. At 7.7 miles you complete the Miller Trail Loop and rejoin the East Mulberry Trail, traveling southeast through rolling terrain. The path winds as it ascends through sky-high hickory trees and poplars, and your long, gradual climb ends as you exit the forest.

Once again on the edge of high, open ground, you reach an intersection with the East Meadow Trail **(Waypoint 8)**. Continue straight on the narrow dirt and bark path that traverses the meadow and descend to **Waypoint 6**. Turn left to take the East Meadow Trail, and then join the West Meadow Trail to walk back to the trailhead.

UTM WAYPOINTS

1. 17S 234360E 3770209N
2. 17S 234169E 3770428N
3. 17S 233245E 3770512N
4. 17S 233756E 3770801N
5. 17S 234601E 3770581N
6. 17S 234670E 3770820N
7. 17S 234206E 3771441N
8. 17S 234952E 3771054N

TRIP 2 Fort Yargo State Park: Bird Berry Trail & Trails West of the Lake

Distance	6.0 miles, loop
Hiking Time	3 hours
Difficulty	Easy
Elevation Gain/Loss	+/-265 feet
Trail Uses	Leashed dogs and good for kids (Bird Berry Trail)
Best Times	Year-round
Agency	Fort Yargo State Park
Recommended Map	A trail map is available at the park office and online at www.gastateparks.org.

HIGHLIGHTS Fort Yargo's paved Bird Berry Trail is easy, convenient, and a prime spot to observe birds and other wildlife that inhabit the wetland area on the north shore of the Marbury Creek Reservoir. After enjoying this trail, you can take a short walk on the park road to join another path that passes the old fort and climbs into the pine and hardwood forest west of the lake. You can then visit the park's southwestern corner and walk along the shoreline to maybe glimpse an osprey or great blue heron. From there, an easy walk through the pines along the water returns you north to retrace your steps to the parking lot.

DIRECTIONS From Atlanta take Interstate 85 north, and take Exit 106 for GA Highway 316 toward Lawrenceville/Athens. Travel east on GA 316 for 21.2 miles and bear left onto GA Highway 81. Travel north on GA 81 about 3 miles to the entrance for Fort Yargo State Park on the right.

FACILITIES/TRAILHEAD There are restroom facilities near the trailhead in the Will-A-Way Recreation Area. The park has 40 tent, trailer, and RV sites, as well as seven walk-in tent sites. The park charges a $3 parking fee, or you can purchase an Annual ParkPass for $30 by calling (770) 389-7401.

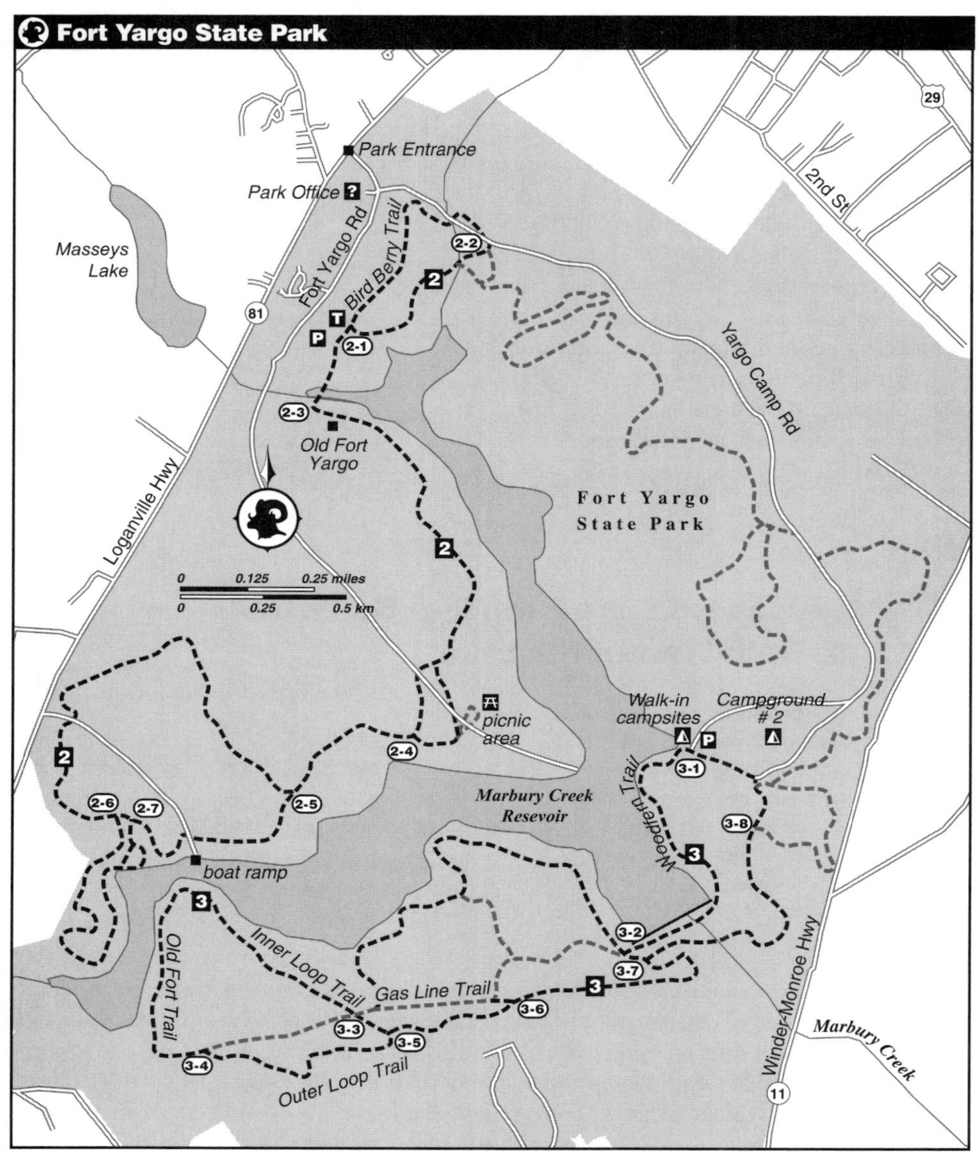

This hike begins at the Will-A-Way Recreation Area parking lot. At the northeast side of the parking area, enter the asphalt trail at the COTTAGE GUESTS ONLY sign **(Waypoint 1)**. You start high on a cleared slope, and then descend into a thicket and parallel a road. At 0.5 mile bear right at a Y junction **(Waypoint 2)**, and then bear right again to travel southwest on the paved Bird Berry Trail. This walk can be quite entertaining as you can hear rustling in the brush to your left and right as birds dart from one side of the path to the other. The trail then proceeds through a wetland habitat along the north side of the lake where you might see the belted kingfisher plucking a fish from the water or hear the croak of an American bullfrog. A pavilion that overlooks the water is a comfortable, shaded spot to enjoy the lake and try to spot birds.

Pass beneath the cottages and then walk back up to the parking area. Turn left and walk down the park road a little more than 0.1 mile and turn left of off the road **(Waypoint 3)**. As you walk southeast on a narrow dirt path you'll pass the historic old fort. After walking about 0.1 mile the trail diverges. Turn left to take the Rock Garden Trail, which is interesting as it rolls through boulders along the lakeshore and soon reconnects with the main trail. Or bear right to stay on the main path. Either way, you then climb steeply through pines and hardwoods with a good view of the lake ahead.

Cross Fort Yargo Road, continue straight, and descend to a trail junction at the lakeshore **(Waypoint 4)**. Turn right and travel west and cross another road.

At 2.2 miles **(Waypoint 5)**, bear right at the Y junction to walk northwest. The next mile is a twisting route through more pine-hardwood mix. At 3.3 miles **(Waypoint 6)** bear right at the Y junction and travel southeast on the Outer Loop to one of the most attractive parts of the hike—the trail runs near the shore of the lake, which is ringed by forest. The trail then turns back to the north, stays near the water for a bit, and then climbs a slope where you will have a view of a long stretch of the water in late fall and throughout winter.

At the next trail junction, turn right onto the Root Garden Trail. Appropriately named, this knobby path is heavily rooted and runs within 5 feet of the waterline. At the next T junction, turn right to walk north, and then turn right at the next junction **(Waypoint 7)** to go southeast back toward the lake. As you approach the shore of the lake, the trail can be a bit difficult to pick out. Just continue to walk near the water, traveling east to pass the boat ramp and stay near the shore. Enter the pine forest to continue on the trail, and at 4.6 miles you will reach a trail junction **(Waypoint 4)**. Continue straight, traveling northeast, and at the next trail junction **(Waypoint 3)**, bear left and retrace your steps to the Will-A-Way Recreation Area parking lot.

UTM WAYPOINTS

1. 17S 247426E 3763278N
2. 17S 247821E 3763475N
3. 17S 247278E 3763004N
4. 17S 247510E 3761930N
5. 17S 247149E 3761781N
6. 17S 246593E 3761734N
7. 17S 248169E 3761201N

TRIP 3 Fort Yargo State Park: Woodfern & Outer Loop Trails

Distance	4.5 miles, loop
Hiking Time	2 hours
Difficulty	Easy
Elevation Gain/Loss	+/-310 feet
Trail Uses	Leashed dogs, mountain biking, and good for kids
Best Times	Year-round
Agency	Fort Yargo State Park
Recommended Map	A trail is available at the park office and online at www.gastateparks.org.

see map on p. 244

HIGHLIGHTS Half of this long loop tours the southern shore of the Marbury Creek Reservoir, occasionally turning inland to wander the lower flanks of two hills that rise to more than 900 feet of elevation. At 2.2 miles, you briefly follow the Gas Line Trail, which heads straight through a wide forest break. Then a trail snakes across the hills populated with dense stands of pines and oaks. Proceeding east, you descend into the shaded pine forest below the Marbury Creek dam and then top a small hill. The ascents along this loop are gradual, and the total amount of elevation gained and lost is modest. If there is any challenge to this hike, it's that you must remain alert for mountain bikers who may come whirring down the Gas Line Trail and zip through the woods below the dam.

DIRECTIONS From Atlanta take Interstate 85 north and take Exit 106 for GA Highway 316 toward Lawrenceville/Athens. Travel east on GA 316 for 21.2 miles and bear left onto GA Highway 81. Travel north on GA 81 about 3 miles to the entrance for Fort Yargo State Park on the right. Park on the right. Once inside the park, take Yargo Camp Road past Campground #2 to the parking area near the walk-in campsites.

FACILITIES/TRAILHEAD There are tent walk-in campsites near the trailhead ($15 per night) as well as a bathhouse and central water spigot. The park charges a $3 parking fee, or you can purchase an Annual ParkPass for $30 by calling (770) 389-7401.

This hike begins from the parking area for the walk-in campsites, in the southeast corner of the park. From the parking area, walk southwest 220 feet to the trailhead for the Woodfern Trail **(Waypoint 1)**. The wide, packed-dirt path remains flat at is runs along the lake, and it's a popular area to run for exercise.

At 0.4 mile continue southwest on the grassy path across the lake dam to a junction of several trails **(Waypoint 2)**. Turn right onto the far right trail for hiking and biking and walk northwest with the lake to your right and tall pines to the left. Soon, oaks surround you, and the trail stays low, near the water. At 1.1 miles you'll climb through pines, and then alternate between walking the slope and the lakeshore.

At 1.7 miles **(Waypoint 3)** there is a four-way trail junction. Turn right onto the Inner Loop path and travel northwest on an old roadbed. At 2.2 miles you will reach a bridge that spans the lake and leads to the boat ramp. Rather than crossing the bridge, bear left onto the blue-blazed Old Fort Trail to go south. This is a nice environment, with pines shading a path that hugs the lakeshore.

At 2.5 miles turn left onto the Gas Line Trail, which goes through a wide break in the forest. Because this corridor is completely exposed to the sun, you might want to leave it to walk through more-shaded forest. At the next Y junction **(Waypoint 4)** bear right, leaving the Gas Line to take the Outer Loop Trail. Though you'll initially encounter dense forest, the woods quickly transition to nice mix of pines and hardwoods. Cross a power line break, and descend moderately to a trail junction **(Waypoint 5)**. Bear right, traveling east, to climb back up into the forest on a winding, undulating trail. Near the top of a hill, you will reach an intersection with the Gas Line Trail **(Waypoint 6)**. Go straight, traveling east on the Gas Line Trail, which takes a long downhill run to woods below the lake dam, and then loops back to the west. On your walk through here stay alert for bikers who can really pick up speed on this hill.

At 3.7 miles bear right at the Y junction **(Waypoint 7)** and go east to cross Marbury Creek and take switchbacks up onto a pine-covered hill. At **Waypoint 8**, turn left to go northeast, and bear left at the next two junctions to head northwest and back to the parking area.

UTM WAYPOINTS

1. 17S 248288E 3761805N
2. 17S 248113E 3761211N
3. 17S 247316E 3761041N
4. 17S 246829E 3760982N
5. 17S 247389E 3761004N
6. 17S 247793E 3761096N
7. 17S 248170E 3761202N
8. 17S 248565E 3761585N

TRIP 4 Charlie Elliott Wildlife Center Loop

Distance	3.4 miles, loop
Hiking Time	2–3 hours
Difficulty	Easy
Elevation Gain/Loss	+125/-130 feet
Trail Uses	Leashed dogs and good for kids
Best Times	Year-round
Agency	Charlie Elliott Wildlife Center
Recommended Map	A trail map is available in the park office and online at http://georgiawildlife.dnr.state.ga.us.

HIGHLIGHTS A writer, conservationist, and the first director of Georgia's Game & Fish Commission, Charlie Elliott (1906–2000) devoted his life to sharing his passion for the state's wildlands. It's fitting that the 6400-acre wildlife center bearing his name serves as an outdoor classroom and promotes hiking and birding, as well as fishing, hunting, and horseback riding. The center's hiking trails explore a granite outcrop, the rushing waters of Murder Creek and the banks of three lakes, which provide habitat for geese, herons, and a variety of other birds. This hike combines four trails into one loop that can be walked in a few hours.

DIRECTIONS From Atlanta take Interstate 20 east to Exit 89 for GA Highway 11/Monroe-Monticello. Turn right onto GA 11, travel south 9.5 miles, and then turn left onto Marben Farm Road at the entrance for the Charlie Elliott Wildlife Center. Go 1.2 miles and turn right onto Elliott Trail. Go 0.6 mile and turn left at the CHARLIE ELLIOTT VISITORS CENTER sign.

FACILITIES/TRAILHEAD There are restrooms at the visitors center. The area is always open and accessible, but the visitors center and its facilities are open Tuesday–Saturday 9 AM– 4:30 PM (closed Sunday, Monday, and state holidays).

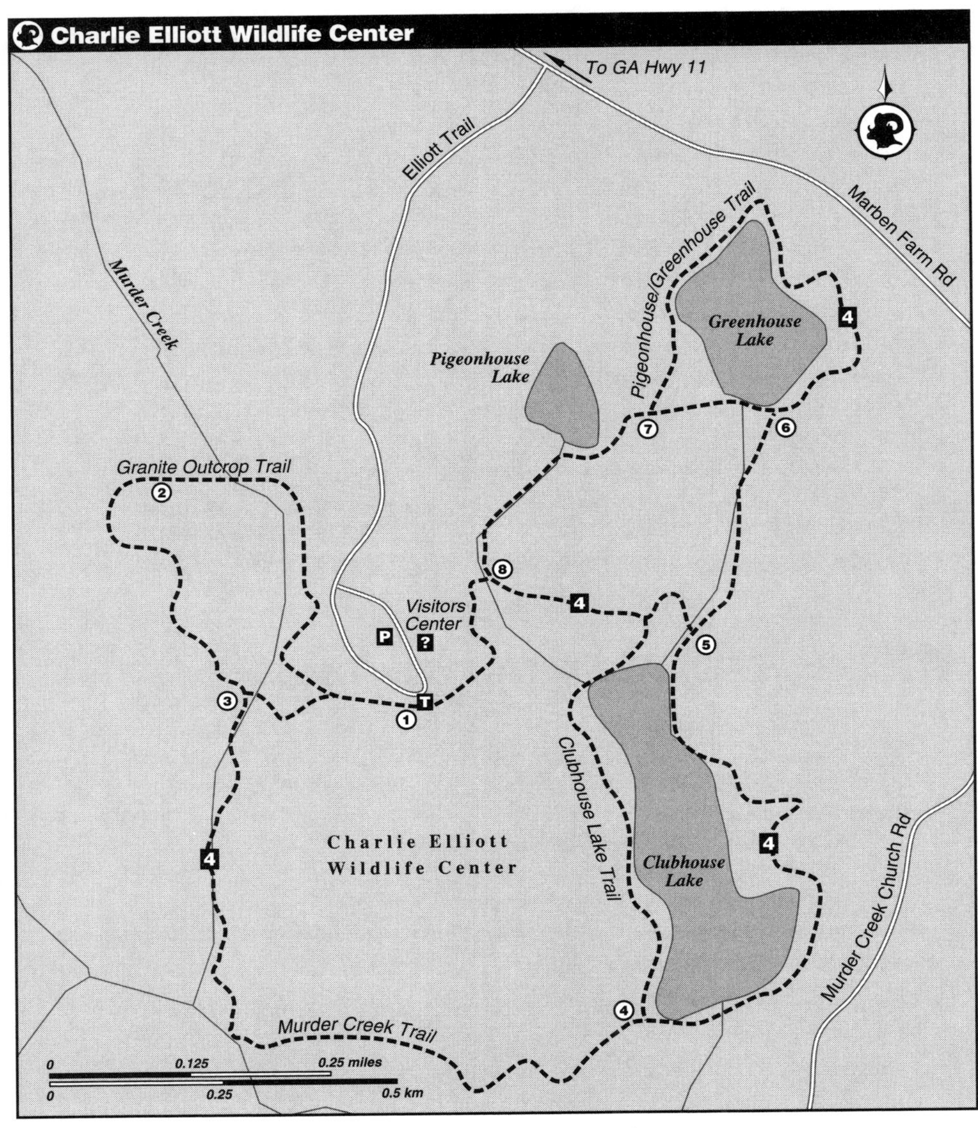

Your hike begins with the Granite Outcrop Trail. From the visitors center parking lot, walk southeast on the road about 360 feet to the trailhead on the right **(Waypoint 1)**. Climb on the dirt path through young hardwoods and pines and descend to a Y junction at 0.1 mile. Turn right and travel northwest along a creek that has dredged deeply into the land.

At a 5-acre granite outcrop at about 0.4 mile **(Waypoint 2)**, notice the lichen growing on the rock slab. This combination of fungus and algae emits acids that, over time, break the rock down into sand particles, leading to the formation of soil. From this soil, plants begin to grow on the otherwise inhospitable rock surface.

Circle the outcrop and then take an easy descent on a trail blanketed with

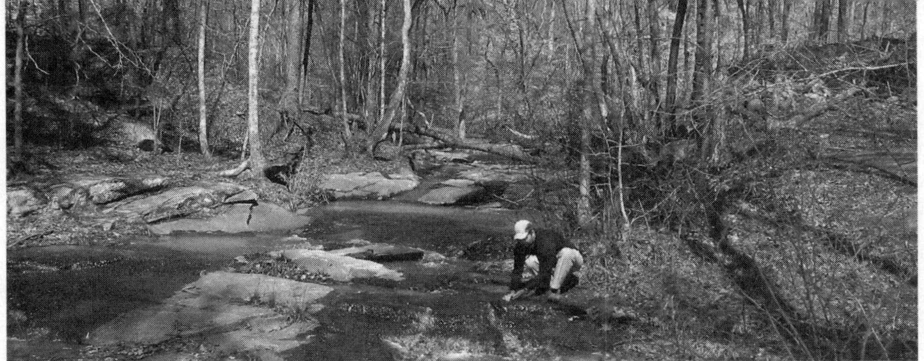

Washing off the evidence in Murder Creek

pine needles. At the next trail junction, the Granite Outcrop Trail intersects with the Murder Creek Trail **(Waypoint 3)**. Turn right onto the yellow-blazed Murder Creek Trail and travel southwest to skirt Murder Creek, which appears at first as a thin, shallow stream and then becomes a wider flow through boulders. Linda May, the center's wildlife interpretive specialist, said the creek most likely was named for deaths that occurred in this area when settlers battled the Creek Indians in the early 1800s.

As you round a bend, Margery Lake lies to the right, and you'll likely hear the honking of Canada geese, which live here year-round. Also be on the lookout for herons, egrets, and white ibis.

At 1.6 miles **(Waypoint 4)** you can bear left or right at the Y junction to take the red-blazed Clubhouse Trail, which circles Clubhouse Lake. Bearing right, travel east among oaks and beeches with the southern end of Clubhouse Lake to your left. At the lake's southeast corner, ascend wood steps, and walk to the left of the Brook Ager Discovery Building. Walk just beyond a trailhead bulletin board and look right to see a red blaze on a tall pine. The Clubhouse Trail proceeds northeast through pines, and not far ahead there is an abrupt shift to hardwoods.

At 2 miles **(Waypoint 5)** the Clubhouse Trail intersects with the Pigeonhouse/Greenhouse Trail. These trails are named for structures that stood when this was still farmland in the late 1800s and early 1900s. Turn right onto the Pigeonhouse/Greenhouse trail, traveling northeast toward Greenhouse Lake, climbing gradually through a beech grove.

At 2.3 miles, you reach a trail junction at Greenhouse Lake **(Waypoint 6)**. To the left, the berm running along the south bank of the lake is a good place to look for wood ducks or the other bird species that wander from lake to lake. You can also turn right to travel east on the wide trail that has been cut through the tall brush, which obscures your view of the lake as you walk around its eastern side.

After circling the lake you will reach a trail junction **(Waypoint 7)** at 2.8 miles. Turn right to continue toward the visitors center. (The path to the left returns to Greenhouse Lake.) Pass through dense forest, and at the next Y junction (3.3 miles), the Pigeonhouse/Greenhouse Trail ends at a junction with the red-blazed Clubhouse Trail **(Waypoint 8)**. Bear right onto the Clubhouse Trail, descend briefly, and then make a final climb to reach the visitors center.

UTM WAYPOINTS

1. 17S 245900E 3705839N
2. 17S 245529E 3706189N
3. 17S 245624E 3705886N
4. 17S 246198E 3705384N
5. 17S 246262E 3705937N
6. 17S 246417E 3706266N
7. 17S 246226E 3706241N
8. 17S 245967E 3706022N

TRIP 5 Hard Labor Creek State Park: Beaver Pond & Brantley Trails

Distance	2.0 miles, loop
Hiking Time	1½ hours
Difficulty	Easy to moderate
Elevation Gain/Loss	+/-165 feet
Trail Uses	Leashed dogs and good for kids
Best Times	Year-round
Agency	Hard Labor Creek State Park
Recommended Map	A Hard Labor Creek State Park trail map is available at the park's Trading Post and online at http://gastateparks.org/info/hardlabor.

HIGHLIGHTS Plantations and small farms once occupied the 5805 acres of land that now make up Hard Labor Creek State Park, but efforts to grow cotton and corn were tedious, as plantation slaves had to clear stones from fields to prepare the land. This strenuous work may be the source of the park's name, or it could have come from Native Americans who lived in the area and found it difficult to cross Hard Labor Creek when the water ran high. Two hiking trails wind through the pines and hardwoods west of the creek, and these connect, allowing you to make a loop. The Brantley Trail rolls through mature oak and hickory trees along the ravines formed by farming, and the Beaver Pond Trail takes you to mature forest with large poplars and a wetland that's good for birding.

DIRECTIONS From Atlanta take Interstate 20 east to Exit 105. Turn left onto Newbord Road and take it 2 miles to Rutledge. Turn left on West Dixie Highway, and then right onto Fairplay Road. Take Fairplay Street and then Fairplay Road 2.6 miles to Knox Chapel Road. Turn left onto Knox Chapel Road, go 0.4 mile, and then turn right onto Campground Road. Proceed to the parking lot just beyond the Trading Post. To reach the trailhead, walk northeast on the road to the campground for 230 feet to the trailhead on the left.

FACILITIES/TRAILHEAD There is a restroom north of the trailhead, down the road to the campground. The park charges a $3 parking fee, or you can purchase an Annual ParkPass for $30 by calling (770) 389-7401.

Enter the Brantley Trail **(Waypoint 1)** and follow yellow blazes through forest that becomes increasingly attractive as you move west. The Hard Labor Creek area is rich with oak, hickory, and poplar, as well as beech, sourwood, and dogwood.

At 0.1 mile **(Waypoint 2)** bear right at the Y junction and descend earth and wood steps. After another 0.1 mile there will be a wood bridge on the left. Continue straight here, traveling northeast, and take the trail to low ground and skirt the creek.

At 0.4 mile bear left at a Y junction (the path to the right leads to campsites 20–49). Not far ahead, the Brantley Trail intersects with the Beaver Pond Trail. At this Y junction **(Waypoint 3)** bear right to take the red-blazed Beaver Pond Trail northwest, and bear right again at the next junction to continue. After walking among older-growth poplars, you'll look out over rolling terrain and see the pond below and to the right. Passing large oaks and tall pines, the trail drops down toward the pond. At **Waypoint 4**, standing slightly above the water, you'll have a good vantage point to observe breeding wood ducks, green herons, and

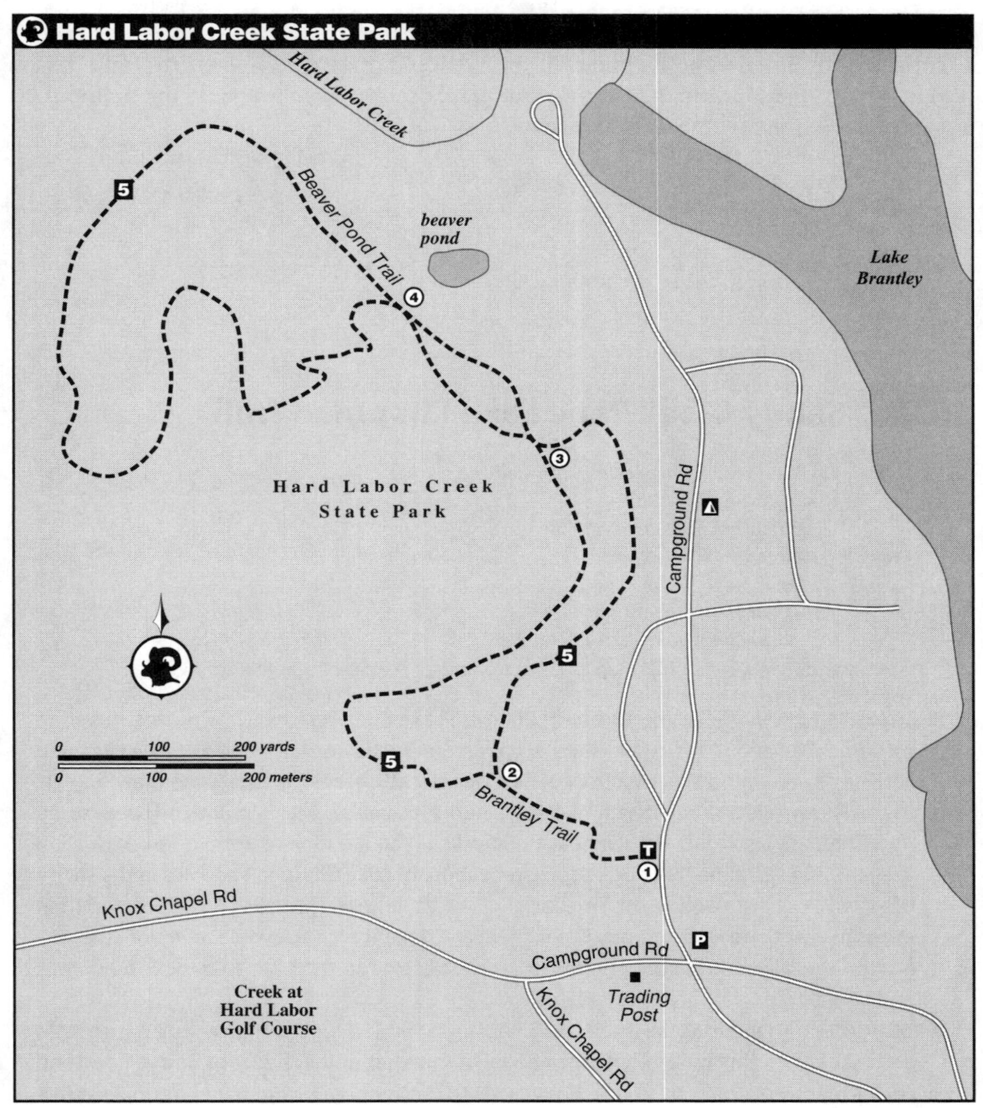

red-winged blackbirds. During summer, look for swallows feeding on insects over the water, and you might spy a pair of Eastern kingbirds.

Just ahead are trees that bear permanent scars from people carving their initials (which is not a good idea as it can kill the trees), and the path veers away from the pond. The trail climbs and then crosses wood bridges over gullies, proceeding toward a hilltop where pine saplings give way to large oaks. In the 1930s, farming ended in the area that is now the park, though gullies throughout the hardwood forest remain as evidence of the poor farming techniques that eroded the land.

After topping the hill, the trail steadily loses elevation as it turns south to drop and swing northeast. Wind down a series of switchbacks and turn southeast to reach a trail junction at 1.4 miles. Bear right at the junction, and then at the next junction (**Waypoint 3**) bear right to take the yellow-blazed Brantley Trail.

After skirting the west side of the creek, the path gains elevation in a pine-hardwood area with dense undergrowth and drainage cuts that slice through land. Take a footbridge across the creek and descend to **Waypoint 2**. Turn right and walk southeast to return to the trailhead.

UTM WAYPOINTS

1. 17S 258379E 3728042N
2. 17S 258220E 3728220N
3. 17S 258292E 3728479N
4. 17S 258161E 3728627N

TRIP 6 Sandy Creek Park: Lake Chapman Trail

Distance	5.9 miles, out-and-back
Hiking Time	3 hours
Difficulty	Easy to moderate
Elevation Gain/Loss	+/-95 feet
Trail Use	Leashed dogs
Best Times	Year-round
Agency	Sandy Creek Park
Recommended Maps	A trail map is available in the park office; USGS 7.5-min. *Nicholson*

HIGHLIGHTS Sandy Creek Park surrounds 260-acre Lake Chapman, which was constructed to preserve the Sandy Creek watershed, act as an emergency water reservoir for Athens, and serve as a recreation site. Healthy populations of catfish, bass, and crappie draw anglers to the lake, while a sandy beach make this park a popular place to swim and catch some rays. The park also rents out canoes and kayaks. If you are looking for a good dayhike in the park, the Lakeside Trail hugs the eastern shore of Lake Chapman and lies in the shade of a pleasant hardwood forest. The trail climbs to hilltops with views of the lake, and then drops to a wetland where Sandy Creek meets the lake. It is not possible to hike all the way around the lake, but the park hopes to eventually extend the path to cross Sandy Creek and connect the east and west shores.

DIRECTIONS From Atlanta take Interstate 85 north to Exit 137 for U.S. Highway 129. Turn right and take U.S. Highway 129 south for 11.6 miles. Turn left onto New Kings Bridge Road and go 5.3 miles. Bear right onto U.S. Highway 441/GA Highway 15 and travel south 3.4 miles. Turn left onto Bob Holman Road, go 0.7 mile, and turn right into Sandy Creek Park. Go 0.1 mile to reach the park office. To reach the trailhead from the park office, travel south 0.2 mile on Sandy Park Drive and then turn right onto Campsite Drive. Go 0.5 mile to the trail parking area.

FACILITIES/TRAILHEAD There is a restroom near the trailhead. The park charges a $2 fee.

At the southwest corner of the parking area, enter the wide path at the CAMPGROUND sign (**Waypoint 1**). Walk down to a prominent LAKESIDE TRAIL sign (**Waypoint 2**), and turn right onto the wide dirt path covered in leaves. Beneath a canopy of oak and hickory trees, the trail passes primitive campsites, and the laughter and shouts from the park beach echo across the water.

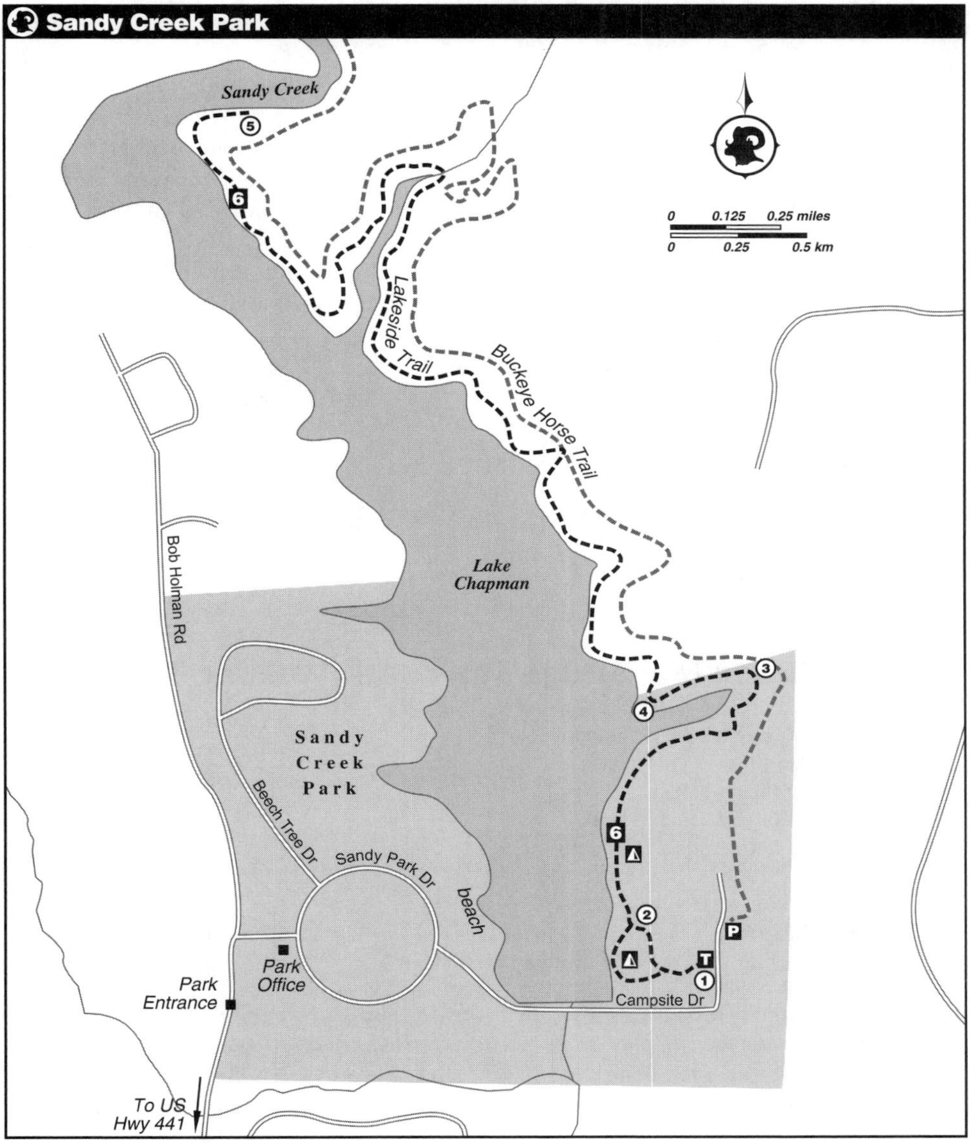

Sandy Creek Park

As the trail swings to the east, the noise from the beach fades, and the trail cuts across a drainage. At 0.7 mile, you'll cross a small stream and then turn north. At the junction with the Buckeye Horse Trail **(Waypoint 3)**, turn left to travel southwest on the Lakeside Trail. After a brief climb, the trail descends to a spot where you can sit in the shade of a tree on the lakeshore **(Waypoint 4)**.

A gradual ascent leads to another intersection with the Buckeye Horse Trail. Bear left to stay on the Lakeside Trail, and look to the right for the ruins of an old cabin built in the 1800s. Crumbling stone walls and portions of the brick fireplace and chimney remain standing.

The trail rises into more hickory and oak trees, with the lake visible beyond. At 1.3 miles bear left at a junction with the horse trail. The path returns to the lake, and then takes an uphill turn. At 1.5 miles, cross a stream drainage and bear left at another junction with the horse trail.

The forest here is quiet, with the park noise replaced by the wind in the pines and much larger hardwoods. At 2.1 miles, bear left at the Y junction, cross a tributary of Sandy Creek and climb through dense forest. Turn left at the next junction with the horse trail and walk downhill on a finger of land with a clear forest of hickory and oak, and the lake nearby. The trail then roller coasters and rises to a rock outcrop above the water.

The hike continues with a moderate descent, and the trail bends right to run east, ending abruptly in dense forest beside Sandy Creek **(Waypoint 5)**. Retrace your steps to **Waypoint 2** where you can turn left to return to the parking area. Or from **Waypoint 2**, you can go straight to take the Lakeside Trail on a quick swing through campsites and rejoin the path that leads to the parking area.

UTM WAYPOINTS

1. 17S 280676E 3767561N
2. 17S 280438E 3767669N
3. 17S 280767E 3768285N
4. 17S 280520E 3768199N
5. 17S 279660E 3769723N

TRIP 7 Watson Mill Bridge State Park: Walking Trail

Distance	1.0 mile, loop
Hiking Time	30 minutes
Difficulty	Easy
Elevation Gain/Loss	+/-85 feet
Trail Uses	Leashed dogs and good for kids
Best Times	Year-round
Agency	Watson Mill Bridge State Park
Recommended Map	A *Watson Mill Bridge State Park Trail Map* is available in the park office and online at www.gastateparks.org.

HIGHLIGHTS The hike begins with a good view of the shoals beneath the bridge, which serves as a natural water park for visitors. You can then descend to the bottomland forest along the river, or walk along the 300-yard stone canal to reach the powerhouse ruins. From the ruins, walk southeast on the upper slope where a wood platform provides a good view of the river. You then reach an intersection with the Holly Tree Loop Trail. From here you can continue to explore the river and a nearby tributary, but only a very brief stretch of this is worth checking out. I recommend you take the Holly Tree Loop Trail, which rolls through beeches, oaks, and sweetgum trees and provides another good view of the hydroelectric powerhouse.

DIRECTIONS From Atlanta take Interstate 85 to Exit 106 for GA Highway 316 east. Take GA 316 east for 39.6 miles, and exit at the GA Highway 10 Loop North. Take the loop 0.4 mile and merge onto U.S. Highway 29 north. Take U.S. 29 north 10.3 miles and bear right onto GA Highway 72 East. Take GA 72 east for 17.3 miles, turn right onto New Town Road, and then turn immediately left onto GA Highway 426 (Old Fork Cemetery Road). Take GA 426

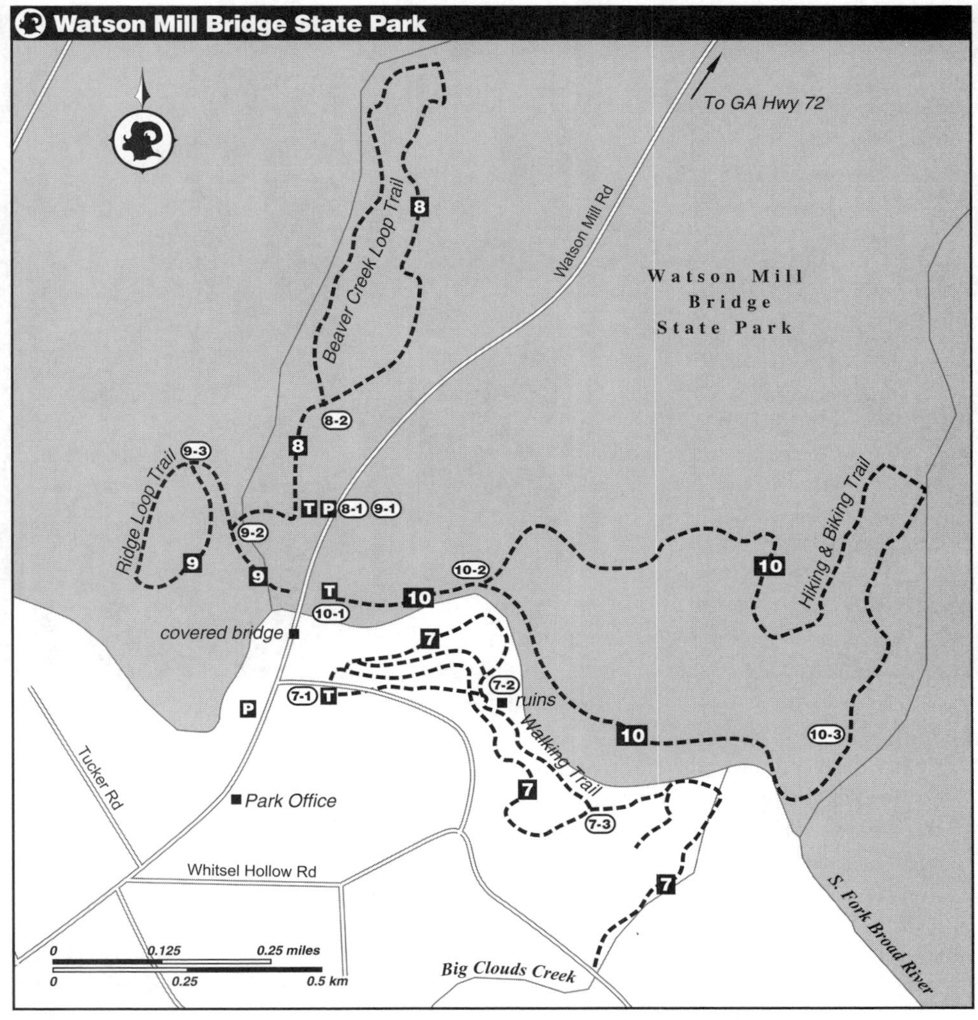

about 0.4 mile and turn right onto Covered Bridge Road, which leads to the park. To reach the park office, go through the covered bridge, pass Whitsel Hollow Road and take the next left.

FACILITIES/TRAILHEAD There are no facilities at the trailhead. The nearest restrooms are at the park office or the campground. The park charges a $3 parking fee, or you can purchase an Annual ParkPass for $30 by calling (770) 389-7401. The park has 32 tent, trailer, and RV sites ($22–$24).

The Walking Trail begins on the north side of Whitsel Hollow Road (**Waypoint 1**). Take the wood and metal stairs down to a bridge, which stands at the site of the former mill facilities, which not only produced flour and cornmeal but also included a sawmill, wool factory, furniture shop, and cotton gin. Now all

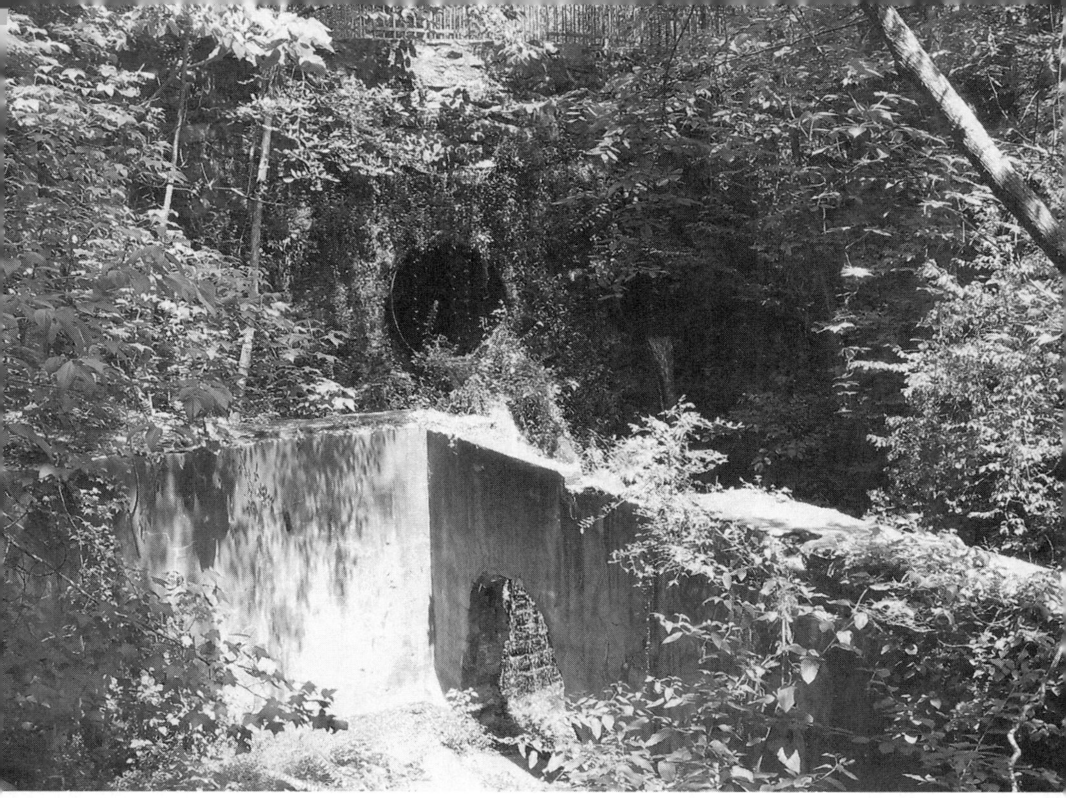

Dense forest envelops the ruins of the hydroelectric powerhouse.

signs of the mill have disappeared. From the bridge, a trail to the left descends to the dense bottomland forest of ferns, beeches, sweetgums, and river cane along the creek bank. If you don't wish to visit the bottomland, from **Waypoint 1** go straight to take the Powerhouse Raceway Trail. Walk along the levee that forms one side of the canal to reach the ruins of the powerhouse **(Waypoint 2)**. From the bridge over the canal, look down through the trees to see the stone walls and foundation covered in foliage, as if they are slowly being consumed by the forest. This is all that remains of the plant that fed electricity to a textile mill 10 miles away in Crawford.

From the bridge over the canal, turn left to take the South Fork River Trail southeast. The flat path traverses the side of the slope, and at 0.3 mile a wood platform surrounded by beech trees overlooks the river. At the next trail junction **(Waypoint 3)**, bear right to take the Holly Tree Loop Trail. (The path to the left continues along the river, turns southwest along a silted, unattractive tributary, and ends at campsites.) The Holly Tree Loop rises, dips, and winds through a decent if not particularly impressive forest of pines, hardwoods, holly, and sweetgums. One plus is the bird's-eye view of the powerhouse below.

The trail leads back to a junction near the powerhouse ruins **(Waypoint 2)**. Bear right and travel northeast to walk along the south side of the canal and return to the trailhead. From **Waypoint 2**, a path to the left also leads you there.

UTM WAYPOINTS

1. 17S 308482E 3766951N
2. 17S 308735E 3766924N
3. 17S 308949E 3766696N

TRIP 8 Watson Mill Bridge State Park: Beaver Creek Loop Trail

see map on p. 255

Distance	1.4 miles, loop
Hiking Time	1 hour
Difficulty	Easy
Elevation Gain/Loss	+/-55 feet
Trail Uses	Good for kids
Best Times	Spring and fall
Agency	Watson Mill Bridge State Park
Recommended Map	A *Watson Mill Bridge State Park Trail Map* is available in the park office and online at www.gastateparks.org.

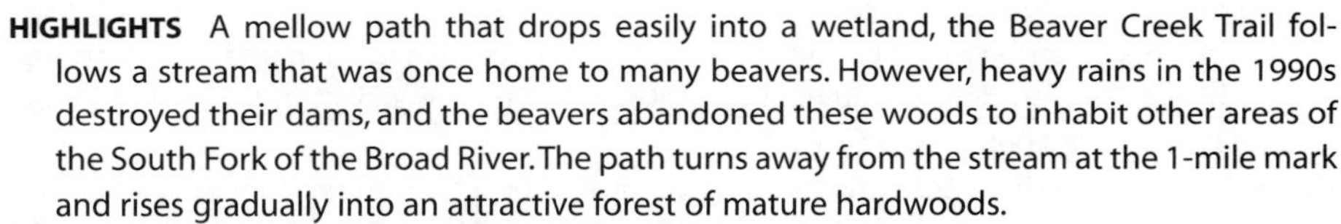

HIGHLIGHTS A mellow path that drops easily into a wetland, the Beaver Creek Trail follows a stream that was once home to many beavers. However, heavy rains in the 1990s destroyed their dams, and the beavers abandoned these woods to inhabit other areas of the South Fork of the Broad River. The path turns away from the stream at the 1-mile mark and rises gradually into an attractive forest of mature hardwoods.

DIRECTIONS From Atlanta take Interstate 85 to Exit 106 for GA Highway 316 east. Take GA 316 east for 39.6 miles, and exit at the GA Highway 10 Loop North. Take the loop 0.4 mile and merge onto U.S. Highway 29 north. Take U.S. 29 north 10.3 miles and bear right onto GA Highway 72 East. Take GA 72 east for 17.3 miles, turn right onto New Town Road, and then turn immediately left onto GA Highway 426 (Old Fork Cemetery Road). Take GA 426 about 0.4 mile and turn right onto Covered Bridge Road, which leads to the park. To reach the park office, go through the covered bridge, pass Whitsel Hollow Road, and take the next left.

FACILITIES/TRAILHEAD There are no facilities at the trailhead. The nearest restrooms are at the park office or the campground. The park charges a $3 parking fee, or you can purchase an Annual ParkPass for $30 by calling (770) 389-7401. The park has 32 tent, trailer, and RV sites ($22–$24).

To reach the trailhead, cross the covered bridge going northeast (as if you were leaving the park) and enter the second parking area on the left. At the northwest side of the parking area enter a paved path at the sign marked BEAVER CREEK LOOP TRAIL (**Waypoint 1**). Walk 28 feet and turn right onto the Beaver Creek Loop Trail, traveling north through the pines. At 0.1 mile (**Waypoint 2**) bear left at the Y junction and go north. You rise gradually into oaks with the creek on the left cutting a deep channel across the forest floor.

At 0.6 mile the path turns away from the creek and swings to the south where pines mix with the older maples and poplars. As you leave the high ground and descend toward the creek, sweetgum and holly trees join the mix. At 1.2 miles you return to **Waypoint 2** and complete the loop. Turn left to return to the trailhead.

UTM WAYPOINTS

1. 17S 308449E 3767287N
2. 17S 308500E 3767499N

TRIP 9 Watson Mill Bridge State Park: Ridge Loop Trail

Distance	0.8 mile, loop
Hiking Time	30 minutes
Difficulty	Easy
Elevation Gain/Loss	+80/-65 feet
Trail Use	Good for kids
Best Times	Spring and fall
Agency	Watson Mill Bridge State Park
Recommended Map	A *Watson Mill Bridge State Park Trail Map* is available at the park office and online at www.gastateparks.org.

see map on p. 255

HIGHLIGHTS While the Ridge Loop Trail makes for a very brief hike, it takes you to one of the more attractive spots in the park. From a picnic area, the path climbs gradually, leaving the more dense woods to gain a hilltop with more open ground and widely spaced hardwoods. The summit of the hill sits at about 600 feet of elevation, where holly trees and cedars grow beneath tall oaks.

DIRECTIONS From Atlanta take Interstate 85 to Exit 106 for GA Highway 316 east. Take GA 316 east for 39.6 miles, and exit at the GA Highway 10 Loop North. Take the loop 0.4 mile and merge onto U.S. Highway 29 north. Take U.S. 29 north 10.3 miles and bear right onto GA Highway 72 East. Take GA 72 east for 17.3 miles, turn right onto New Town Road, and then turn immediately left onto GA Highway 426 (Old Fork Cemetery Road). Take GA 426 about 0.4 mile and turn right onto Covered Bridge Road, which leads to the park. To reach the park office, go through the covered bridge, pass Whitsel Hollow Road, and take the next left.

FACILITIES/TRAILHEAD There are no facilities at the trailhead. The nearest restrooms are at the park office or the campground. The park charges a $3 parking fee, or you can purchase an Annual ParkPass for $30 by calling (770) 389-7401. The park has 32 tent, trailer, and RV sites ($22–$24).

To reach the trailhead, cross the covered bridge going northeast (as if you were leaving the park) and enter the second parking area on the left. At the northwest side of the parking area, enter a paved path at the sign marked Beaver Creek Loop Trail **(Waypoint 1)**. Continue on the paved path to a sign marked PICNIC AREA/TO RIDGE LOOP TRAIL and go straight. The paved path ends and a dirt trail begins.

Descend and cross the silted stream to reach a trail junction **(Waypoint 2)**. Turn right to travel northwest, gaining elevation gradually. At 0.2 mile a holly tree stands at a trail junction **(Waypoint 3)**. Bear right and go west. Now close to the top of the hill, you walk beneath white oaks, characterized by their upper limbs that spread to form a crown. You will also see cedars as you continue along the hilltop.

At 0.4 mile make a horseshoe to swing north, still crossing the hill in a pretty hardwood forest. After returning to **Waypoint 3**, turn right to retrace your steps to the junction at **Waypoint 2**. From here you can turn left to return to the parking area, or continue straight to walk 0.1 mile to the parking area that is immediately north of the covered bridge.

UTM WAYPOINTS

1. 17S 308449E 3767287N
2. 17S 308316E 3767261N
3. 17S 308242E 3767385N

TRIP 10 Watson Mill Bridge State Park: Hiking & Biking Trail

Distance	2.3 miles, loop
Hiking Time	1½ hours
Difficulty	Moderate
Elevation Gain/Loss	+/-100 feet
Trail Uses	Mountain biking and good for kids
Best Times	Spring, summer (for playing in the river), fall
Agency	Watson Mill Bridge State Park
Recommended Map	A *Watson Mill Bridge State Park Trail Map* is available in the park office and online at www.gastateparks.org.

HIGHLIGHTS This 2.3-mile Hiking and Biking Trail begins on the north bank of the river and then loops through an open forest of pines and hardwoods. Multiple canopy layers cloak the majority of the trail in shade, and there are no long, steep grades, making this a pretty comfortable path. As you walk, be alert and prepared to give way to bikers. And if you're a beginner mountain biker, you might enjoy this trail as it has few technical sections.

DIRECTIONS From Atlanta take Interstate 85 to Exit 106 for GA Highway 316 east. Take GA 316 east for 39.6 miles, and exit at the GA Highway 10 Loop North. Take the loop 0.4 mile and merge onto U.S. Highway 29 north. Take U.S. 29 north 10.3 miles and bear right onto GA Highway 72 East. Take GA 72 east for 17.3 miles, turn right onto New Town Road, and then turn immediately left onto GA Highway 426 (Old Fork Cemetery Road). Take GA 426 about 0.4 mile and turn right onto Covered Bridge Road, which leads to the park. To reach the park office, go through the covered bridge, pass Whitsel Hollow Road, and take the next left.

FACILITIES/TRAILHEAD There are no facilities at the trailhead. The nearest restrooms are at the park office or the campground. The park charges a $3 parking fee, or you can purchase an Annual ParkPass for $30 by calling (770) 389-7401. The park has 32 tent, trailer, and RV sites ($22–$24).

The Hiking and Biking Trail begins just north of the covered bridge, on the east side of the road, at a sign marked HIKING AND BICYCLING TRAIL **(Waypoint 1)**. The beginning of the hike is interesting as you descend through cedar trees on a bed of rock with a stream rushing on the right. You'll cross a covered wood footbridge, get a good look at the river, and then reach the beginning of the trail loop at 0.2 mile **(Waypoint 2)**. If you bear left, you will have a long, sustained climb, so I recommend that you bear right and travel southeast.

The clear hardwood forest is open and inviting, while the swish of South Fork River creeps in, soft and steady. You'll climb to a more dry forest of pine and the drop to a trail junction at 0.8 mile **(Waypoint 3)** where a path on the right goes to the location of a former beaver pond. You can take this short path to a wood platform that stands over low ground covered in grass and brush. Though this wetland was once flooded, the water has receded, transforming the plot of land into a meadow.

From the platform, return to the main trail and turn right to proceed to the northeast. The trail rolls moderately and visits a creek at 1.1 miles. The next gradual

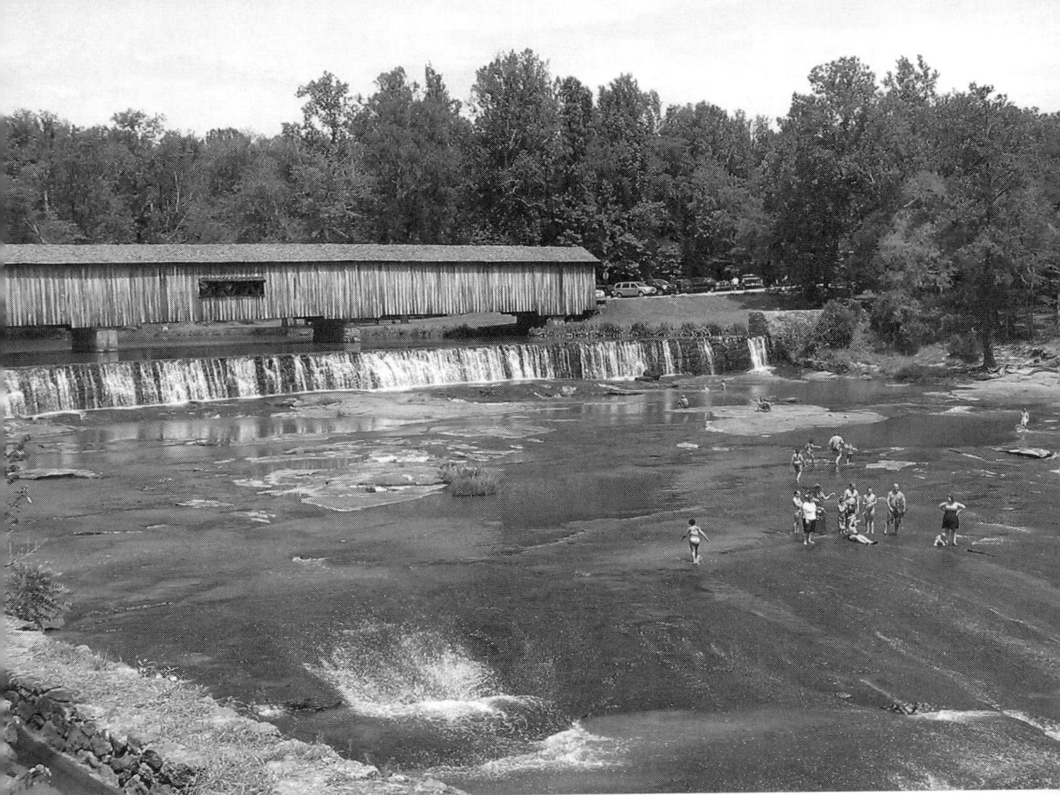

The shallow waters below Watson Mill Bridge make a great natural slide.

climb runs through a carved landscape of drainages, cuts, and trenches that snake through holly, pines, and hardwoods. A series of brief ups and downs through similar woods brings you to the final, moderate descent to close the loop at 2.1 miles **(Waypoint 2)**. Turn right and head west to return to the trailhead.

UTM WAYPOINTS

1. 17S 308521E 3767109N
2. 17S 308790E 3767126N
3. 17S 309438E 3766803N

Chapter 7
South of Atlanta

Stroll along a wild river, take a trip back in time, or search for an endangered bird species. All of these journeys are available to those who explore the land south of Atlanta. Near Thomaston, Georgia, Sprewell Bluff State Park boasts trails that offer lofty views of the great Flint River and drop to its banks where you might glimpse a great heron in flight. Southwest of Monticello, Georgia, long trails delve deep into the Oconee National Forest, and you can walk for miles in seclusion along the Ocmulgee River. Southeast of the Oconee National Forest, the Piedmont National Wildlife Refuge holds stands of tall pines that provide habitat for the red-cockaded woodpecker, which nearly faded away with the destruction of Georgia's longleaf pines. Travelers interested in Georgia history should definitely venture to Ocmulgee National Monument in Macon, Georgia, where easy paths wind among earth mounds constructed a thousand years ago by Mississippian Native Americans.

Ocmulgee National Monument

Whether it was meant to demonstrate their pride or trumpet their social authority, the Mississippian people made a lasting mark on human history when they constructed the mounds at Ocmulgee. Though people have inhabited the Ocmulgee area for 10,000 years, from 900 to 1100 BCE the Mississippians developed a society that was especially impressive and successful. They not only built great earth mounds and lodges to serve

Native American mounds at Ocmulgee National Monument (Trip 3)

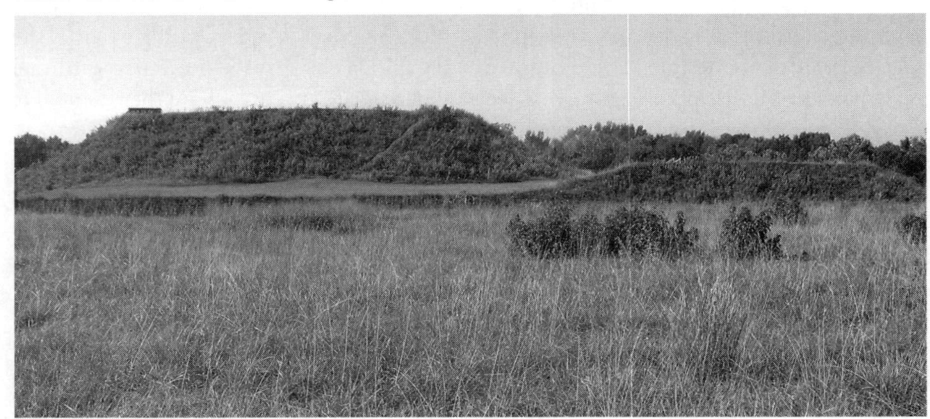

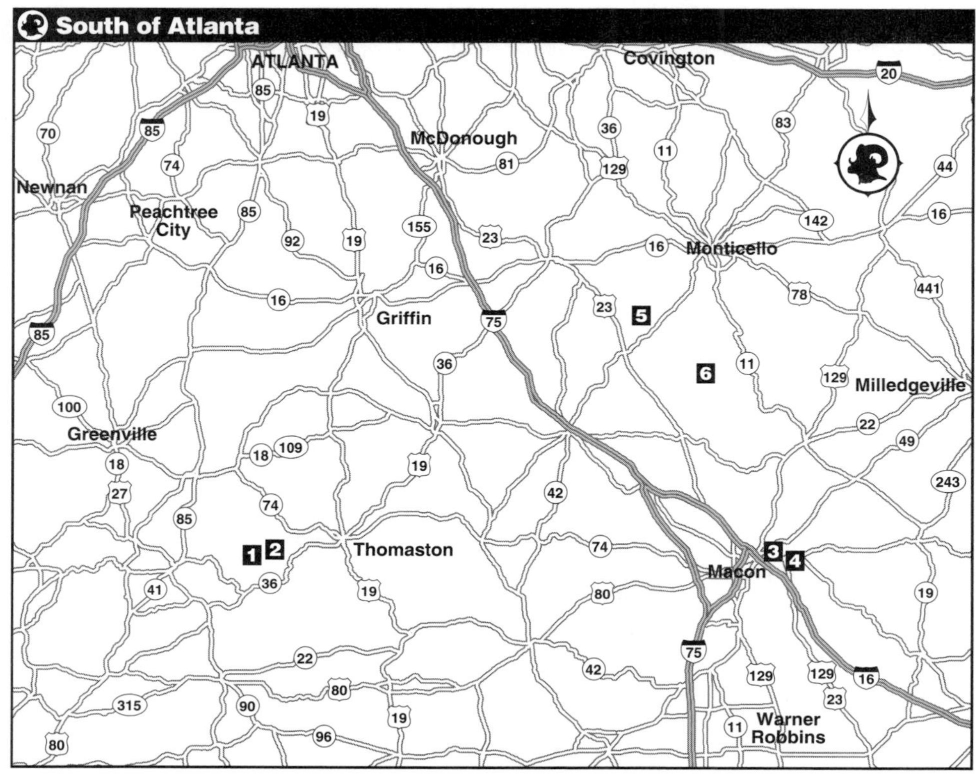

religious and political purposes but also developed a sophisticated society. Raising large crops of corn, beans, and tobacco, they expanded the concept of farming in the area and established sizeable villages. About 1000 Mississippians lived at Ocmulgee, which was an important center for trade. They also demonstrated an appreciation for art, etching their pottery with intricate designs. For unknown reasons, the Mississippian culture faded away after 1100 BCE, and the Lamar culture arose, carrying on the practices of mound building and farming. Ocmulgee remained a cultural hub into the 1600s when the Creek Indians moved in, and the English established a trading post.

Any visit to Ocmulgee should include plenty of time to visit the monument's excellent museum, which chronicles the complete history of habitation here, going all the way back to the Clovis people who inhabited the Southeast before 9000 BCE. After you visit the museum, you can walk a series of trails that visit several different types of earth mounds. From the top of the Great Temple Mound you have a great view of the Walnut Creek wetland to the immediate southeast. For an inside look at Mississippian culture, visit the Earthlodge and walk the narrow tunnel that leads to its core where there is a large meeting room.

Ocmulgee is not only noted for its cultural history but it is also emerging as a destination for observing wildlife. The newer River Trail includes a boardwalk that crosses the wetland surrounding Walnut Creek. The Opelofa and Loop trails explore the creek as well, while the Bartram Trail makes for a peaceful walk through the monument's eastern forest.

TRIP 1 Sprewell Bluff State Park: West Trails

Distance	2.9 miles, semiloop
Hiking Time	3 hours
Difficulty	Easy to moderate
Elevation Gain/Loss	+330/-335 feet
Trail Uses	Leashed dogs and good for kids
Best Times	Year-round
Agency	Sprewell Bluff State Park
Recommended Map	USGS 7.5-min. *Roland* and *Sunset Village*

HIGHLIGHTS The Flint River is a broad, beautiful thing as it flows between high rocky bluffs in Sprewell Bluff State Park. Gazing at the Flint from an overlook along the Sprewell Bluff Trail, it's hard to imagine that this natural wonder begins as groundwater beneath Atlanta's Hartsfield-Jackson International Airport. But once the Flint leaves the city to course through the Georgia Piedmont, it turns wild and flows unimpeded for more than 200 miles.

Covering 1372 acres, Sprewell Bluff State Park draws visitors to its day-use area where a slow-flowing stretch of the river makes a great place to swim and fish. From this recreation area, a trail climbs to an overlook and a rock outcrop with great views of a river bend and far cliffs. After climbing higher into hardwoods and shortleaf pines, the trail then descends to the woods near the riverbank, which is rich with hickory trees, birches, and wildflowers.

DIRECTIONS From Atlanta take Interstate 75 south to Exit 235 toward U.S. Highway 19/U.S. Highway 41. Merge onto Tara Boulevard, which in 11.6 miles becomes U.S. Highway 19 south/U.S. Highway 41 south/GA Highway 3 south. Go 16.6 miles and turn right onto U.S. 19 south/GA 3 south. Go 23.6 miles and turn right onto West Main Street/GA Highway 36 west/GA Highway 74 west. Go 0.1 mile and turn left onto South Green Street/GA Highway 36/GA Highway 74. Go 0.1 mile and turn right onto West Gordon Street/GA 74. Take this 5.6 miles and turn left onto South Old Alabama Road at the sign for Sprewell Bluff. Go 6.5 miles to the parking area at the Flint River.

FACILITIES/TRAILHEAD The day-use area near the trailhead has restrooms. The park charges a $3 parking fee, or you can purchase an Annual ParkPass for $30 by calling (770) 389-7401.

The trailhead lies at the north side of the day-use area, to the left of a restroom and trailhead kiosk **(Waypoint 1)**. You immediately ascend a dirt surrounded by oaks, maples, sweetgums, and pine. At 0.1 mile **(Waypoint 2)** the first overlook lies to the left. From the wood platform, you can look down on a wide expanse of the river that forms a great S.

From the overlook, walk another 200 feet and look left for rock outcrops with more good views of the river. Continue a gradual ascent, and at the next Y junction **(Waypoint 3)** bear left to travel north and make a steep descent with the river visible on your left. Hickory trees and river cane grow near the bank, and the trail runs flat for a brief time. On a summer day, this lower forest hums with insects. The path turns away from the water to rise gradually, and at 0.6 mile bear left to walk southwest toward the river again. After a brief walk along the riverbank, take the sandy path back to the northeast.

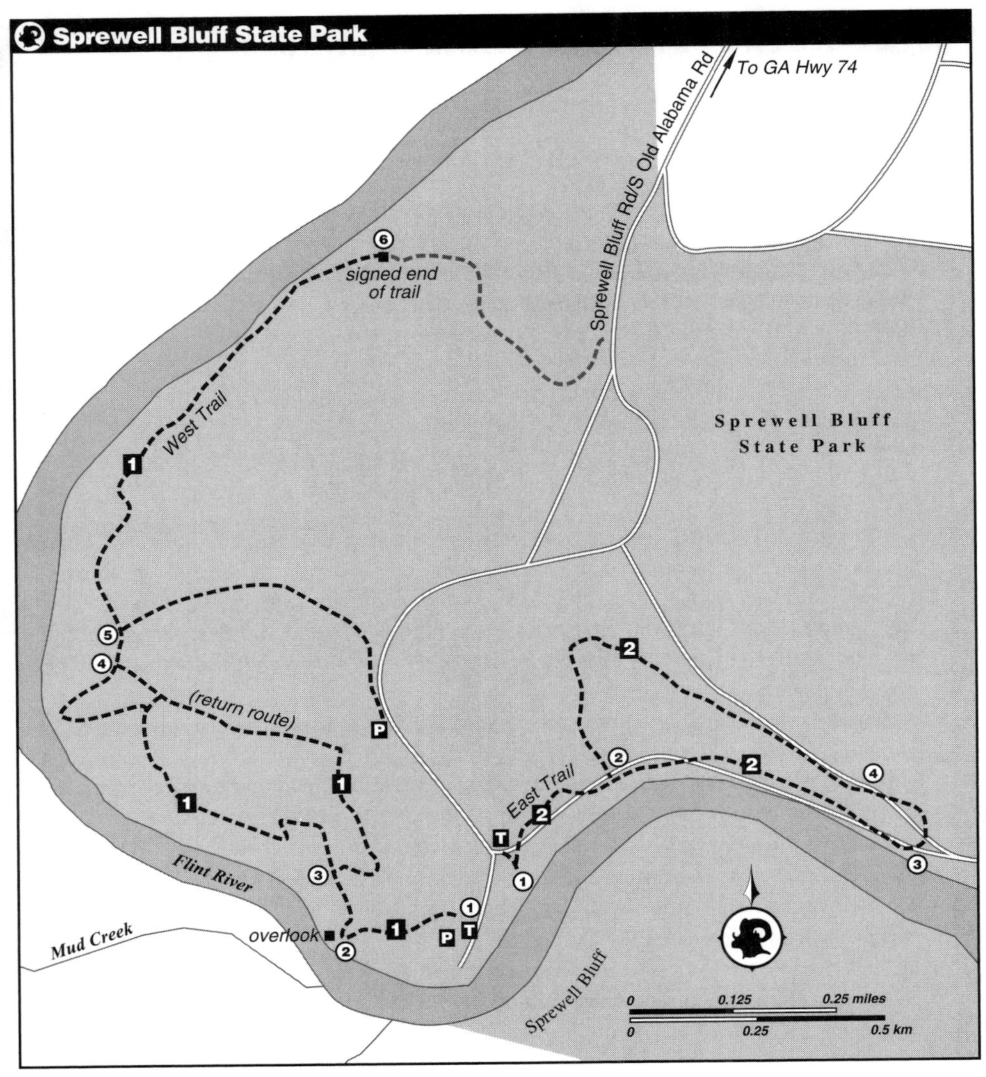

At 0.8 mile **(Waypoint 4)** you reach a creek drainage. Bear left and walk north about 230 feet to another trail junction **(Waypoint 5)**. The trail to the right climbs to an alternate parking area and trailhead. To continue exploring the river from **Waypoint 5**, bear left and go northwest through a shaded forest of hickory and young pines. To the right, a rocky, open slope of oaks provides an interesting contrast to the heavy brush on the river plain.

Ahead is one of the best stretches of the trail; you can look far upstream to see the river disappear into the green hills. On a summer walk, I stopped at one of the breaks in the brush to watch two great blue herons perched on the shoals.

At 1.5 miles **(Waypoint 6)** a marker indicates that this is the end of the trail. (The path to the right makes a steep 0.4-mile climb to Sprewell Bluff Road, though this is a real slog and not scenic.) From

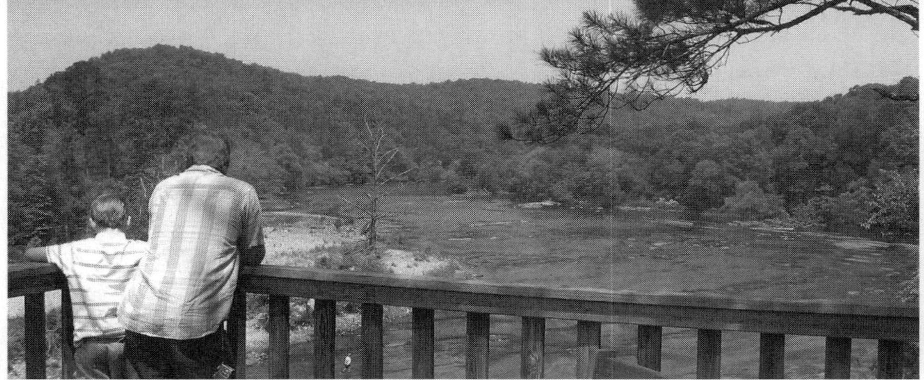

Bluff view of the Flint River

Waypoint 5 retrace your steps to **Waypoint 4** and bear right to travel south. Back at **Waypoint 3** (2.2 miles), turn left and take a long, moderate climb through pines and hardwoods to a hilltop. Compared to all the activity at the riverside parking area, these woods are remote. You might even see a few deer bounding across the open, leaf-covered slope.

At 2.4 miles, the trail tops the hill at the alternate trailhead, and then turns south to pass through a hall of pines. You then steeply descend through hardwoods to **Waypoint 3**. Turn left to retrace your steps to the trailhead.

UTM WAYPOINTS

1. 16S 735669E 3637879N
2. 16S 735469E 3637841N
3. 16S 735461E 3637964N
4. 16S 735015E 3638422N
5. 16S 735028E 3638477N
6. 16S 735556E 3639260N

TRIP 2 Sprewell Bluff State Park: East Trail

Distance	1.5 miles, loop
Hiking Time	1 hour
Difficulty	Moderate
Elevation Gain/Loss	+/-315 feet
Trail Uses	Leashed dogs and good for kids
Best Times	Winter
Agency	Sprewell Bluff State Park
Recommended Map	USGS 7.5-min. *Roland*

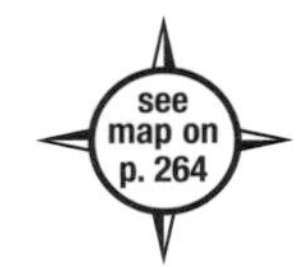

HIGHLIGHTS From the day-use area a trail on the eastern side of the park follows the Flint River and then climbs a ridge with a lofty view of it. Trees obscure the river in spring and summer, so this hike is best in winter. It involves a moderate ascent and descent.

DIRECTIONS From Atlanta take Interstate 75 south to Exit 235 toward U.S. Highway 19/U.S. Highway 41. Merge onto Tara Boulevard, which in 11.6 miles becomes U.S. Highway 19 south/U.S. Highway 41 south/GA Highway 3 south. Go 16.6 miles and turn right onto U.S. 19 south/GA 3 south. Continue another 23.6 miles and turn right onto West Main Street/GA Highway 36 west/GA Highway 74 west. Go 0.1 mile and turn left onto South Green Street/GA Highway 36/GA Highway 74. Go 0.1 mile and turn right onto West Gordon Street/GA 74. Take this road for 5.6 miles and turn left onto South Old Alabama Road at the sign for Sprewell Bluff. Go 6.5 miles to the parking area at the Flint River.

FACILITIES/TRAILHEAD The day-use area near the trailhead has restrooms. The park charges a $3 parking fee, or you can purchase an Annual ParkPass for $30 by calling (770) 389-7401.

To reach the trailhead, cross Sprewell Bluff Road and enter the gravel path near the bank of the river **(Waypoint 1)**. You walk for a bit on a path that hugs the wide river channel, and at 0.2 mile **(Waypoint 2)** a path enters on the left. Continue straight to walk along a slow-flowing bend in the Flint River, turning gradually to the southeast. At 0.6 mile **(Waypoint 3)** turn left, leaving the riverbank, to enter a blue-blazed path. The trail hairpins back to the northwest, rises, and crosses a power line break. Continue to where the path intersects the power line break again. This time, follow the break, traveling northwest on an old roadbed.

At 0.8 mile **(Waypoint 4)** turn left off of the roadbed and enter the blue-blazed path. At a high point on the ridge, to the west you can look straight down a long stretch of the river—a sight that is worth the climb. Continue northwest across the grassy ridge topped with oaks and other hardwoods. Soon, the trail drops quickly from the ridge and turns south to descend through a narrow, shady creek drainage.

At a T junction near the riverbank **(Waypoint 2)**, turn right to return to the trailhead.

UTM WAYPOINTS

1. 16S 735818E 3637978N
2. 16S 736013E 3638156N
3. 16S 736609E 3638012N
4. 16S 736498E 3638139N

TRIP 3 Ocmulgee National Monument: Mound Walk

Distance	2.4 miles, loop
Hiking Time	2 hours
Difficulty	Easy
Elevation Gain/Loss	+/-75 feet
Trail Uses	Leashed dogs and good for kids
Best Times	Spring, fall, and winter
Agency	National Park Service, Ocmulgee National Monument
Recommended Map	An *Ocmulgee National Monument* map is available at the visitors center and online at www.nps.gov/ocmu.

HIGHLIGHTS This hike focuses on Ocmulgee Monument's main attraction, the earth mounds, which were built for a variety of reasons. The first stop along this hike, the Earthlodge, is a reconstructed building that served as a meeting place for village leaders. You can then visit the ceremonial mounds dotting the monument, including the Great Temple Mound, which you can climb via stairs. On the western side of the site you will find the Funeral Mound, which was a burial site.

DIRECTIONS From Atlanta take Interstate 75 south to Interstate 16 east. Take I-16 east to Exit 2 (Coliseum Drive). Turn left onto Coliseum Drive and take this until it ends at Emery Highway. Turn right onto Emery Highway and go to the third traffic light. The entrance to Ocmulgee National Monument is on the right.

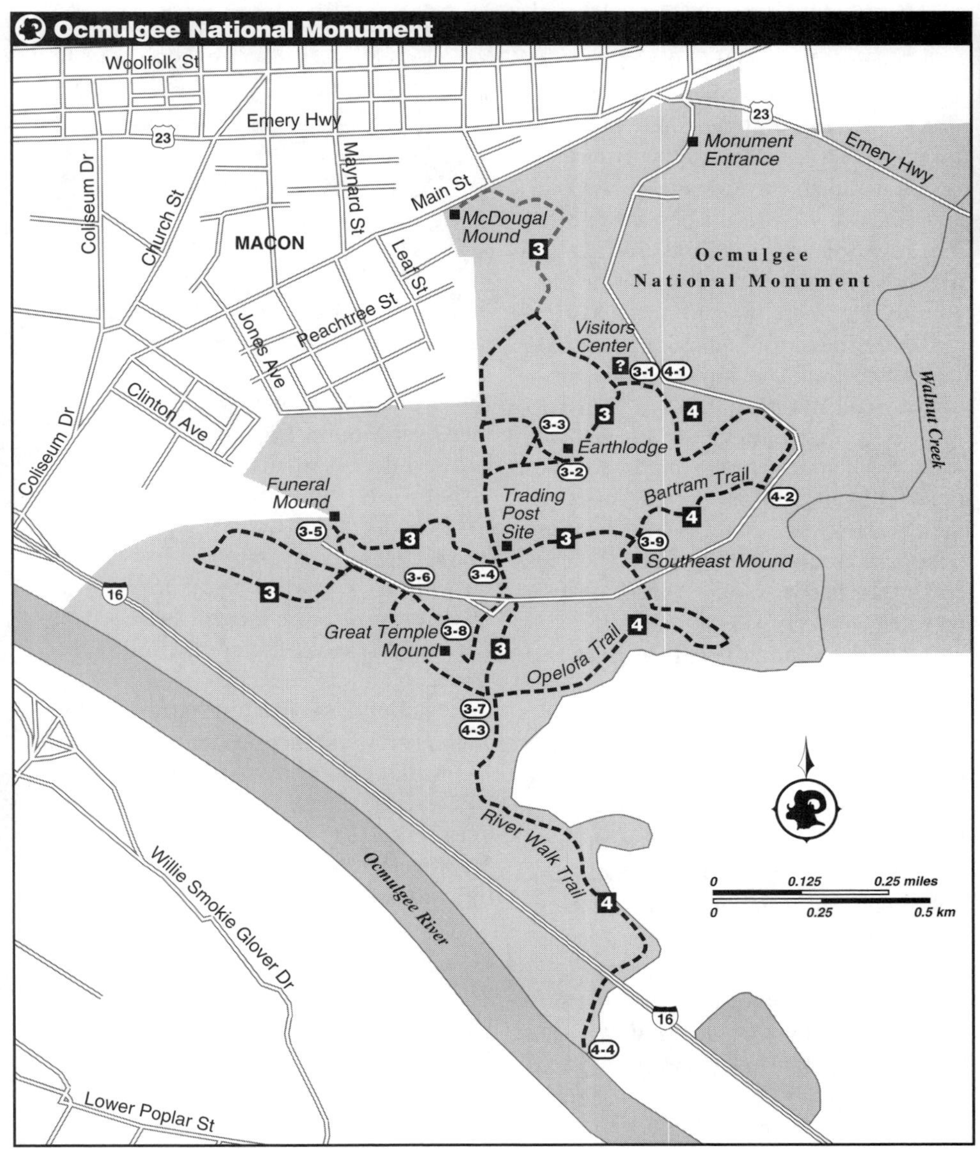

FACILITIES/TRAILHEAD The visitors center has restrooms. Entrance to the monument is free, and it's open 9 AM–5 PM daily except Christmas Day and New Year's Day.

Begin at the rear of the visitors center **(Waypoint 1)** and take the paved path southwest. Cross the wood bridge, and proceed to the Earthlodge straight ahead **(Waypoint 2)**. As you round the Earthlodge, its entrance is on the right. The round meeting room inside has a clay floor with a platform that seats 3, and the benches along the perimeter of the room have scooped-out seats for 47 people.

From the Earthlodge, continue west to a trail junction. Bear right onto a gravel path to visit the Cornfield Mound **(Waypoint 3)**, which once stood about 8 feet high and covers a field the Mississippians farmed. Continue north through the grassy field, and you will see two ditches where earth may have been excavated and used to build mounds. Continue north to a junction with the Heritage Trail and turn left.

At the next trail junction, continue straight to walk south toward the center of the site. You then reach a four-way junction at the Trading Post site **(Waypoint 4)**; British colonists from Charles Town in the colony of Carolina (later Charleston, South Carolina) established a trading post here around 1690 to trade firearms and other goods for deerskins and furs with the Creek Indians in the area.

From the Trading Post turn right and travel west to reach the Funeral Mound **(Waypoint 5)**. Likely built in seven stages, this mound was once about 25 feet high, though railroad construction in the 1870s destroyed much of it. From the Funeral Mound, take the park road east to the base of the Great Temple Mound **(Waypoint 6)**. Turn right onto the path that crawls up the mound's western side (and keep an eye out for deer grazing on the slope).

Continue around the mound to a junction with the Opelofa Trail **(Waypoint 7)**. At this point, turn left and travel north alongside the Great Temple Mound. When you reach the park road, turn left to swing south and take the path toward the Great Temple Mound. A set of steps will carry you to its summit **(Waypoint 8)** where you can look southeast for a sweeping view of the wetlands below. Wood structures once stood on top of this mound, which was likely used for religious ceremonies.

As you retrace your steps and walk back down, a path on the left leads to the Lesser Temple Mound, which sits left of the Great Mound. The exact relationship between the two structures is unknown.

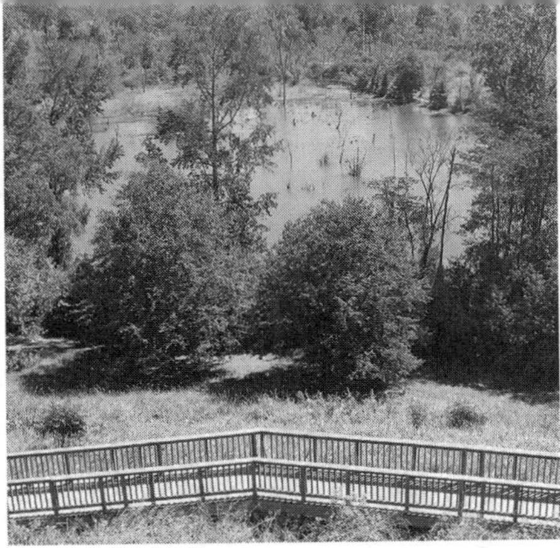

Atop Great Temple Mound overlooking wetlands

Return to the park road and cross it to walk north to the Trading Post Site **(Waypoint 4)**. Turn right to travel east on the flat, grassy path for 0.2 mile to reach the Southeast Mound **(Waypoint 9)**. Located just east of the junction of the Bartram and Opelofa trails, this "platform" mound was likely an early stage for a temple mound or a residential mound.

From the Southeast Mound, there are two ways to return to the visitors center. One option is to retrace your steps to the Trading Post site **(Waypoint 4)** and turn right to walk north. A wood and metal bridge takes you over train tracks to a path junction. Turn right to walk east back to the visitors center. If you prefer, you can instead walk northeast from the Southeast Mound on the Bartram Trail, which goes 0.7 mile to the visitors center parking lot.

UTM WAYPOINTS

1. 17S 256281E 3636800N
2. 17S 256187E 3636685N
3. 17S 256102E 3636687N
4. 17S 255970E 3636416N
5. 17S 255617E 3636508N
6. 17S 255766E 3636359N
7. 17S 255937E 3636094N
8. 17S 255882E 3636204N
9. 17S 256296E 3636450N

TRIP 4 Ocmulgee National Monument: Bartram, Opelofa, & River Walk Trails

see map on p. 267

Distance	4.1 miles, out-and-back
Hiking Time	2 hours
Difficulty	Easy
Elevation Gain/Loss	+35/-30 feet
Trail Use	Leashed dogs
Best Times	Spring, fall, and winter
Agency	National Park Service, Ocmulgee National Monument
Recommended Map	An *Ocmulgee National Monument* map is available at the visitors center and online at www.nps.gov/ocmu.

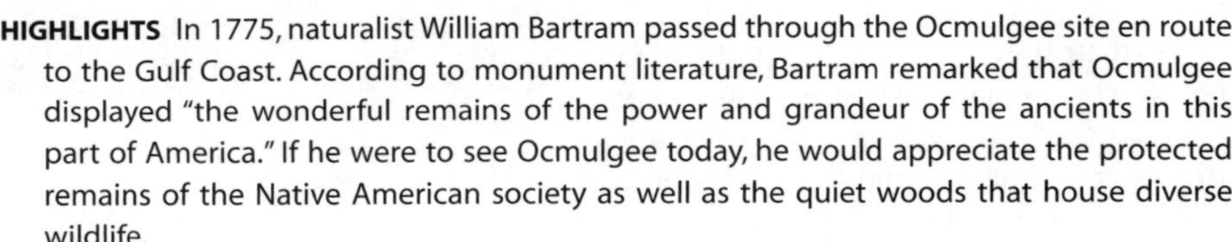

HIGHLIGHTS In 1775, naturalist William Bartram passed through the Ocmulgee site en route to the Gulf Coast. According to monument literature, Bartram remarked that Ocmulgee displayed "the wonderful remains of the power and grandeur of the ancients in this part of America." If he were to see Ocmulgee today, he would appreciate the protected remains of the Native American society as well as the quiet woods that house diverse wildlife.

A trail bearing Bartram's name winds through the pine-hardwood forest in the northeastern section of the site. Just beyond the Southeast Mound it intersects with the Opelofa Trail, which drops from mature hardwoods into the Walnut Creek wetland. The Opelofa Trail connects with a new River Walk Trail that provides a great opportunity to see the many bird species in the wetland. Beyond the boardwalk, the trail continues along Walnut Creek, passes under Interstate 16, and ends at the Ocmulgee River.

DIRECTIONS From Atlanta take Interstate 75 south to Interstate 16 east. Take I-16 east to Exit 2 (Coliseum Drive). Turn left onto Coliseum Drive and take this until it ends at Emery Highway. Turn right onto Emery Highway and go to the third traffic light. The entrance to Ocmulgee National Monument is on the right.

FACILITIES/TRAILHEAD The visitors center has restrooms. Entrance to the monument is free, and it's open 9 AM–5 PM daily except Christmas Day and New Year's Day.

The Bartram Trail begins at the southeast side of the visitors center parking area (**Waypoint 1**). Travel south through oaks and pines, and then turn northeast where fern beds cover the forest floor.

The trail then leaves the trees and passes through a brick railroad tunnel that was constructed soon after the Civil War. The trail follows the park road until **Waypoint 2**, where you turn right to enter the forest and enjoy the best section of this trail—a long corridor of unbroken woods much more wild than the parklike mound region. "There is some wonderful birding on the forest trails along the Ocmulgee River and Walnut Creek, especially during migration," says Georgia birder Giff Beaton. According to Beaton, the area provides habitat for such interesting breeding species as anhinga, Mississippi kite, and the prothonotary warbler.

At 0.7 mile (**Waypoint 3-9**), just past the Southeast Mound, turn left onto the Opelofa Trail and walk south toward Walnut Creek. At 0.8 mile, turn left onto a short loop trail cloaked by tall magnolias, high pines, and large oaks. This path swings by the banks of Walnut Creek and turns northwest to meet the main trail. When you've completed the loop, turn left to travel southwest.

Cross a wood and metal bridge to move through the heart of the Walnut Creek wetland, walking close to a good-sized body of water where locals fish for bass, catfish, and crappie. At 1.4 miles **(Waypoint 3)** turn left onto the 800-foot River Walk Trail boardwalk. This swampy land was a hardwood forest until a flood brought drastic change in 1994, and now more than a third of the monument's 660 acres is wetland. Perhaps in another two hundred years, soils will build up, the water will recede, and the hardwoods will reign again. This cycle occurs a few times every thousand years, and we just happen to be living during the latest flood stage. The boardwalk, completed in 2006, sits a few feet above the water and really immerses you in the environment. It also provides a convenient platform for observing bluebirds, blue herons, ducks, and prothonotary warblers.

Once you cross the boardwalk the trail becomes a dirt path that enters dense forest. As you continue southeast with Walnut Creek close on the left, the rumble of traffic on I-16 grows louder. The trail runs beneath the highway and ends where Walnut Creek meets the Ocmulgee River **(Waypoint 4)**.

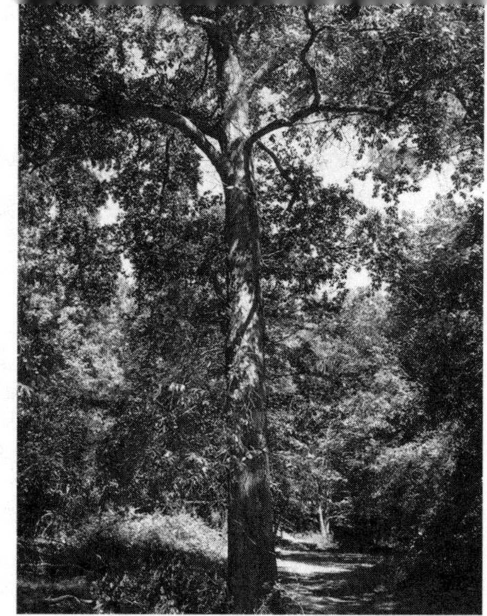

Bartram Trail

From the river, walk back across the boardwalk to **Waypoint 3**. To return to the trailhead, turn right and retrace your steps. Or, from **Waypoint 3** you can turn left and take a right at the next junction to walk through the center of the monument and return to the visitors center.

UTM WAYPOINTS

1. 17S 256323E 3636830N
2. 17S 256602E 3636559N
3. 17S 255953E 3636089N
4. 17S 256115E 3635224N

TRIP 5 Oconee National Forest: Ocmulgee River Trail

Distance	3.7 miles, loop; 12.7 miles, out-and-back
Hiking Time	2 hours for short loop; 6 hours for longer out-and-back
Difficulty	Easy
Elevation Gain/Loss	+/-435 feet
Trail Uses	Horseback riding and backpacking
Best Times	Spring, fall, and winter
Agency	U.S. Forest Service, Oconee District
Recommended Map	*Trails of the Chattahoochee-Oconee National Forests* is available at Forest Service offices, and you can order it online at www.fs.fed.us/conf/.

HIGHLIGHTS Coursing through the Oconee National Forest, the ambling Ocmulgee River is a major drainage for the Piedmont and Coastal Plain regions of Georgia. Once an area of eroded farmland, the Oconee is a recovering forest with hiking and equestrian trails that skirt the Ocmulgee River through bottomland woods. These days, the trails in Oconee National Forest are primarily used for horseback riding, and several hiking paths have become overgrown and difficult to navigate. But the Ocmulgee River Trail makes for a nice walk as it offers occasional views of the water and climbs into the pine and hardwood hills east of the river.

For this book, I have described this as an out-and-back hike. But it's possible to spot cars at both the trailhead and the Ocmulgee Bluff Horse Camp, so you can shuttle back.

DIRECTIONS From Atlanta, travel south on Interstate 75 south and take Exit 187 for GA Highway 83. At the bottom of the ramp, go left and travel east on GA 83 for 12.3 miles to the small parking area on the left. (To reach Ocmulgee Flats Horse Camp, continue east on GA 83 0.5 mile and turn left onto Forest Service Road 1099. Go 0.9 mile. The camp is on the left.)

To reach the Ocmulgee Bluff Horse Camp, from the trailhead parking, continue east on GA 83 3 miles and turn left onto Smith Mill Road. Travel west about 2.7 miles on Smith Mill Road. The Ocmulgee Bluff Horse Camp is on the left.

FACILITIES/TRAILHEAD There are no facilities at the trailhead or at the Ocmulgee Flats and Ocmulgee Bluff horse camps. Water is available at the many tributary streams, but water levels are unpredictable—pack what you'll need.

At the south side of the gravel parking area, enter the narrow path at the trail marker **(Waypoint 1)**. The path is marked with green diamond blazes (and white diamond blazes) but is easy to follow. If you hike this path, you'll likely encounter people on horseback who set out from the Ocmulgee Flats Camp to enjoy a peaceful ride through this secluded tract of wild land. Be alert for riders, and give way as they pass. You'll soon encounter signs of horse travel as you negotiate wide patches of dark, churned earth. Some spots can be quite muddy, so you might want to wear low gaiters. Also, be sure to wear footwear appropriate for trekking through mud and streams.

Much of the Ocmulgee River Trail runs through succession forest with young pines, sweetgums, and hickory and maple trees, which cast the trail in an even blend of sun and shade. While the Creek Indians once inhabited the forest, European settlers moved into the area in the 1800s and used the land primarily for farming. By the time farming ended in 1930s, the landscape had become severely eroded. The 115,000-acre Oconee National Forest

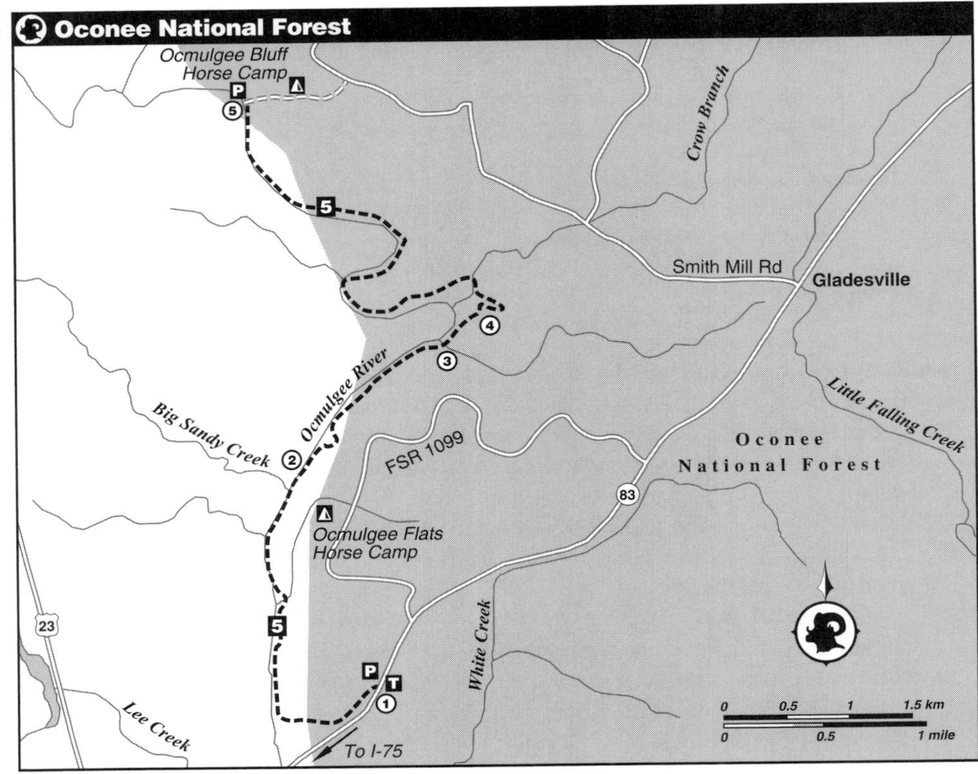

was designated in 1959, and the forest has made a slow, but steady recovery ever since.

At 0.6 mile, the path approaches the bank of the river and turns to the north to parallel the wide, creeping channel of water. Thin stalks of river cane line the path, and to the right the forest floor is broad, even, and fairly attractive with modest undergrowth. Your course north remains mostly level, and the trail stays on a low bluff along the river's eastern shore.

Just beyond the 1-mile mark, take a wood footbridge across the first of several tributary streams. Soon, a berm of earth and crowded trees lies between the trail and the river, blocking your view of the channel. When I hiked the trail in summer, the forest undergrowth was thick through here and crowded the path. Still wet from recent rain, the heavy brush mopped across my knees.

For the next 2 miles, the trail continues to flirt with the river, and you make several mellow creek crossings. The trail cuts through hallways of high river cane, with hickory and other hardwoods providing shade. As I moved through this solitary stretch scouting the area, a deer (presumably visiting the river) burst out of the brush and sprinted across the trail, quickly disappearing.

At 2.1 miles **(Waypoint 2)**, you reach a trail junction. The trail to the right goes 0.3 mile to the Ocmulgee Flats Horse Camp. For a shorter hike, you can proceed to the Ocmulgee Flats Horse Camp, and then walk on gravel Forest Service 1099. This road connects with GA Highway 83. A brief walk down GA 83 returns you to the trailhead.

For a longer hike, bear left at **Waypoint 2** and travel north on the Ocmulgee River Trail, which eventually leads to the Ocmulgee Bluff Horse Camp. The trail runs well away from the river and drops into a gulley to cross a stream at 3.2 miles (**Waypoint 3**). After your scramble up the far bank, the trail enters a markedly different environment as you climb moderately through forest dominated by hardwoods.

Topping a hill, the trail passes a stand of tall, thin pines, and at 3.4 miles (**Waypoint 4**) bear left at a junction with an old roadbed and descend a narrow path to skirt a ravine with hilly terrain surrounding you.

Leaving the hills, you drop into low land and face another muddy creek crossing at 3.9 miles. Walk another tenth of a mile to follow the edge of a large clearcut. The path then drifts back toward the Ocmulgee River, but the water remains out of sight as you follow the narrow, flat path through more bottomland woods.

After a long, quiet stroll on flat ground, faint sounds from the river rise gradually, and shoals come into view at 4.8 miles. The Ocmulgee moves in and out of sight until you reach the Ocmulgee Bluff Horse Camp (**Waypoint 5**) at 6.4 miles.

UTM WAYPOINTS

1. 17S 237417E 3673167N
2. 17S 237066E 3675046N
3. 17S 238191E 3675913N
4. 17S 238413E 3676139N
5. 17S 236760E 3677946N

Ocmulgee River

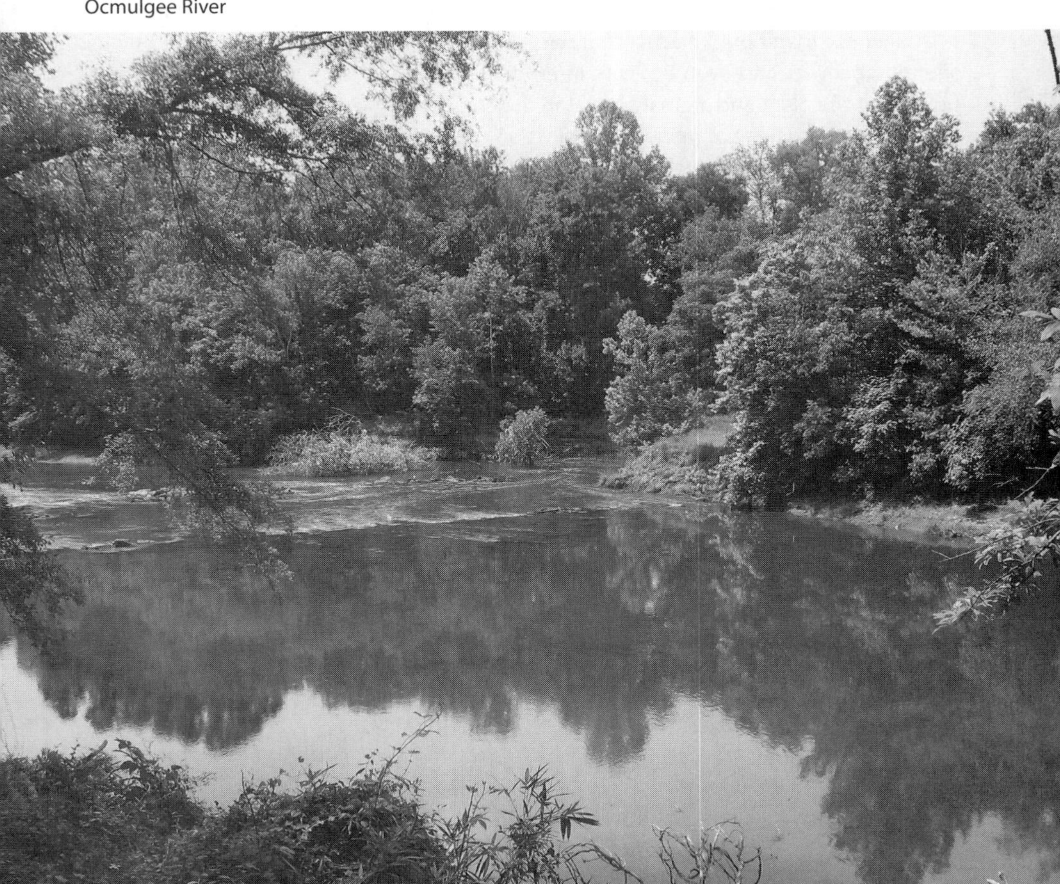

TRIP 6 Piedmont National Wildlife Refuge: Red-Cockaded Woodpecker Trail

Distance	3.0 miles, semiloop
Hiking Time	1½ hours
Difficulty	Easy
Elevation Gain/Loss	+/-270 feet
Trail Uses	Leashed dogs and good for kids
Best Times	Spring, fall, and winter
Agency	Piedmont National Wildlife Refuge
Recommended Map	A Piedmont National Wildlife Refuge trail map is available online at www.fws.gov/piedmont.

HIGHLIGHTS Red-cockaded woodpeckers were once common in the longleaf pine forests of Georgia. Timber harvesting and farming that began in the 1800s, however, destroyed much of the longleaf pine habitat, and in 1970 the red-cockaded woodpecker was declared an endangered species. Fortunately, the population of these birds is recovering thanks to conservation efforts on private and public lands. The 35,000-acre Piedmont National Wildlife Refuge is home to several colonies of red-cockaded woodpeckers that inhabit well-managed tracts of loblolly and shortleaf pines.

The Red-Cockaded Woodpecker Trail passes through a colony site about 1.5 miles into the hike described here. The trail also runs through bottomland forest inhabited by fox squirrels, beavers, and even bobcats. Interpretive signs along the trail provide information about the plant and animal species in the area. At the 0.7-mile mark, you pass an old cemetery, which is one of many burial plots on the refuge.

DIRECTIONS From Atlanta travel south on Interstate 75 and take Exit 186 in Forsyth. Travel east on Juliette Road 18 miles to a Y junction. Bear right to go to the refuge Office and Visitors Center, or bear left to continue 0.4 mile to the paved parking area.

FACILITIES/TRAILHEAD The refuge doesn't charge fees for day use. The trailhead doesn't have facilities; the nearest restrooms are in the refuge visitors center. Be sure to pack all the water you will need. The refuge is open seven days a week during daylight hours, except during scheduled refuge hunts.

From the parking area (**Waypoint 1**), you can either descend the paved road to Allison Lake or you can walk to the entrance of the parking area and enter the trailhead for the Red-Cockaded Woodpecker Trail and Allison Lake Trail behind the roadside kiosk, which holds pamphlets concerning woodpeckers and other birds, plus refuge and hunting and fishing regulations. In either case, proceed to the lake dam at **Waypoint 2**.

From **Waypoint 2** head west across the lake dam on a wide gravel roadbed and then ascend briefly. At 0.2 mile (**Waypoint 3**) turn left off the gravel road to take the marked RED-COCKADED WOODPECKER TRAIL. Cleared land lies to the left, and much of the forest here has been thinned, so the path lies exposed to sunlight. After another tenth of a mile, the trail drops into more shaded forest with a mix of pines and hardwoods, such as poplars and white oaks.

You reach a Y junction at 0.5 mile (**Waypoint 4**). The shortest route to the woodpecker colony lies to the right, but to explore the entire trail, bear left and travel south. The grass-covered trail passes the interpretive sign for bobcats, and then reaches an area where the charred trunks of pines indicate that fire has thinned the forest. At 0.6 mile **(Waypoint 5)** on the left stands a sign for the RED-COCKADED WOODPECKER TRAIL CEMETERY. The cemetery, enclosed in a rectangular 3-foot-high stone wall, lies a few yards away to the left. A stone marker sitting in the cemetery is too weathered to make out a name or dates, but it's believed that this cemetery dates back to the 1800s. From the 1800s to the 1930s, many families occupied and grew cotton and other crops on the land that is now a refuge, and many of them maintained their own cemeteries here.

From the cemetery, return to the trail and descend gradually on the mellow path into hardwood bottomland, and at the 1-mile mark the still, brown waters of Allisons Creek flow below and to the left. An interpretive sign suggests that you might see beavers near the creek banks in this area.

The trail leaves the creek and climbs onto the high, drier land populated by tall loblolly and shortleaf pines. Once again, the parklike forest is awash in sunlight as you approach the woodpecker colony.

At 1.5 miles **(Waypoint 6)** you reach a portion of the woodpecker colony site, indicated by pines painted with white bands. The birds stay in the area year-round, though the best chance of spotting them is during the nesting season from late April to May. Be sure to pack binoculars.

These woodpeckers are unique in that they are the only woodpecker species in North America that nests in living pine trees. To identify an active tree that woodpeckers are excavating, look for holes surrounded by gray color and pitch flowing down the bark. Red-cockaded woodpeckers have black and white bars on their wings, and males have a red patch on their crown, which becomes a full cockade (or 'hat') during fall of their first year of life.

You'll also see an interpretive sign for flying squirrels that points out that these animals don't actually fly (bummer) but glide using flaps of skin between their front and back legs. They nest in cavities previously used by woodpeckers. The colony site continues ahead where you reach a trail junction near a wood bench

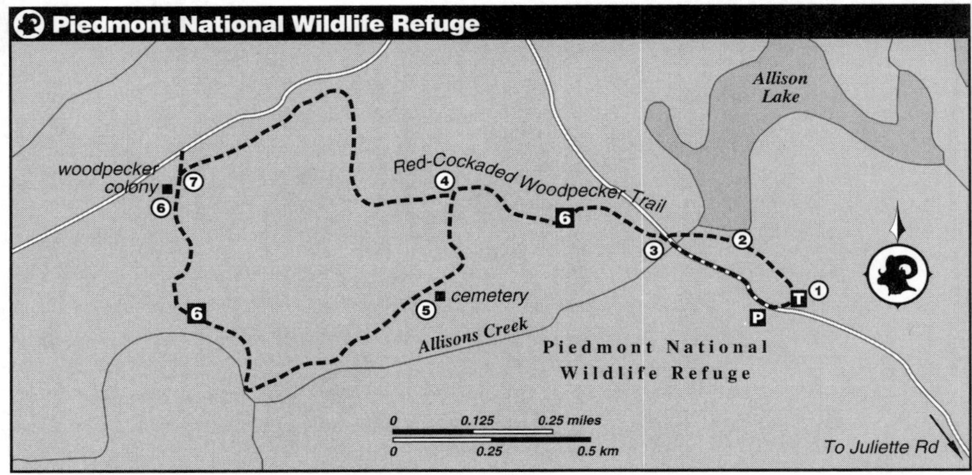

(Waypoint 7), a good place to pull out your binoculars and sit while looking carefully for signs of the woodpeckers. The birds live in family groups that usually include a male, female, and up to four offspring. The male and female form a nesting cavity in the roosting tree chosen by the male. As they form the cavity, they scrape away bark surrounding the hole to release pitch, which provides a chemical and physical defense against predators.

From the Y junction at **Waypoint 7**, bear right to continue on the Red-Cockaded Woodpecker Trail, traveling northeast. (The path to the left ends at a junction with a gravel road.) At 1.7 miles an interpretive sign about the red-tailed hawk sits to the right of the trail, and beyond is clear forest with high pines. Peer above the tops of the trees, and you might see one of these birds circling slowly.

In spring, this trail also makes a good wildflower walk, with trilliums and a variety of other species lining the trail. At 1.8 miles you can look for violet blue flag flowers, yellow-eyed grass, and meadow beauties.

The path descends through oaks and returns to the bottomland forest to cross a small creek. You then climb gradually from the low basin to return to **Waypoint 4** at 2.2 miles. Bear left to return to Allison Lake and ascend the paved road to the parking area.

UTM WAYPOINTS

1. 17S 249466E 3667156N
2. 17S 249412E 3667289N
3. 17S 249154E 3667370N
4. 17S 248661E 3667480N
5. 17S 248648E 3667260N
6. 17S 247986E 3667491N
7. 17S 247998E 3667522N

Appendix 1
Best Hikes by Theme

Backpacking

Cohutta Wilderness: East Cowpen, Hickory Ridge, & Rough Ridge Loop *(Chapter 1: Trip 1)*
Cohutta Wilderness: Jacks River Trail *(Chapter 1: Trip 5)*
Fort Mountain State Park: Gahuti Trail *(Chapter 2: Trip 1)*
Appalachian Approach Trail *(Chapter 2: Trip 12)*
Vogel State Park: Coosa Backcountry Trail *(Chapter 2: Trip 15)*
Appalachian Trail & Benton MacKaye Trail Loop *(Chapter 3: Trip 1)*
Appalachian Trail: Woody Gap to Neels Gap *(Chapter 3: Trip 2)*
Appalachian Trail: Neels Gap to Hog Pen Gap *(Chapter 3: Trip 3)*
Appalachian Trail: Hog Pen Gap to Unicoi Gap *(Chapter 3: Trip 4)*
Appalachian Trail: Unicoi Gap to Dicks Creek Gap *(Chapter 3: Trip 5)*
Black Rock Mountain State Park: James E. Edmonds Backcountry Trail *(Chapter 3: Trip 26)*

Birdwatching

Pocket Recreation Area *(Chapter 1: Trip 12)*
Lake Conasauga Recreation Area: Lake, Songbird, & Tower Trails *(Chapter 2: Trip 3)*
Brasstown Valley Resort: Miller Trek Trail *(Chapter 3: Trip 8)*
Chicopee Woods: West Lake & East Lake Trails *(Chapter 3: Trip 17)*
Warwoman Dell & Becky Branch Falls Trail *(Chapter 3: Trip 27)*
F. D. Roosevelt State Park: Dowdell Loop Trail *(Chapter 4: Trip 8)*
Chattahoochee River National Recreation Area: Cochran Shoals *(Chapter 5: Trip 4)*
Reynolds Nature Preserve *(Chapter 5: Trip 15)*
Fort Yargo State Park: Bird Berry Trail & Trails West of the Lake *(Chapter 6: Trip 2)*
Charlie Elliott Wildlife Center Loop *(Chapter 6: Trip 4)*
Hard Labor Creek State Park: Beaver Pond & Brantley Trails *(Chapter 6: Trip 5)*
Piedmont National Wildlife Refuge: Red-Cockaded Woodpecker Trail *(Chapter 7: Trip 6)*

History

Chickamauga Battlefield Memorial Trail *(Chapter 1: Trip 8)*
Chickamauga Battlefield Hunt Cemetery Loop *(Chapter 1: Trip 9)*
New Echota Cherokee Capital *(Chapter 1: Trip 13)*
Arrowhead Wildlife Interpretive Trail *(Chapter 1: Trip 14)*
Brasstown Valley Resort: Miller Trek Trail *(Chapter 3: Trip 8)*
Smithgall Woods: Martin's Mine & Cathy Ellis Memorial Trails *(Chapter 3: Trip 15)*
Warwoman Dell & Becky Branch Falls Trail *(Chapter 3: Trip 27)*
Pickett's Mill Battlefield: Red, Blue, & Brand House Trails Loop *(Chapter 4: Trip 1)*
Pickett's Mill Battlefield: Blue Trail Loop *(Chapter 4: Trip 2)*
Kennesaw Mountain National Battlefield Park Loop *(Chapter 4: Trip 3)*

Sweetwater Creek State Park: History & Non-Game Wildlife Trails Loop *(Chapter 4: Trip 4)*
Watson Mill Bridge State Park: Walking Trail *(Chapter 6: Trip 7)*
Ocmulgee National Monument: Mound Walk *(Chapter 7: Trip 3)*

Lakes

Lake Conasauga Recreation Area: Lake, Songbird, & Tower Trails *(Chapter 2: Trip 3)*
Carters Lake: Amadahy Trail *(Chapter 2: Trip 6)*
Carters Lake: Oak Ridge Nature Trail *(Chapter 2: Trip 7)*
Red Top Mountain State Park: Homestead Loop, Sweetgum, & White Tail Trails *(Chapter 2: Trip 8)*
Lake Winfield Scott Recreation Area: Slaughter Creek Trail, Appalachian Trail, & Jarrard Gap Loop *(Chapter 3: Trip 6)*
Stone Mountain Park: Cherokee Trail *(Chapter 5: Trip 12)*
Little Mulberry Park *(Chapter 6: Trip 1)*
Fort Yargo State Park: Bird Berry Trail & Trails West of the Lake *(Chapter 6: Trip 2)*
Charlie Elliott Wildlife Center Loop *(Chapter 6: Trip 4)*

Places to Take the Kids

Cloudland Canyon State Park: Overlook, West Rim, & Waterfalls Trails *(Chapter 1: Trip 7)*
Fort Mountain State Park: Stone Wall, Tower, & West Overlook Trails *(Chapter 2: Trip 2)*
Lake Conasauga Recreation Area: Lake, Songbird, & Tower Trails *(Chapter 2: Trip 3)*
Carters Lake: Talking Rock Nature Trail *(Chapter 2: Trip 4)*
Carters Lake: Oak Ridge Nature Trail *(Chapter 2: Trip 7)*
Desoto Falls Recreation Area: Lower & Upper Falls *(Chapter 2: Trip 17)*
Smithgall Woods: Laurel Ridge Trail *(Chapter 3: Trip 13)*
Chicopee Woods: Mathis Trail, Ed Dodd Trail, & Elachee Creek Loop *(Chapter 3: Trip 18)*
Unicoi State Park: Bottoms Loop & Lake Trail *(Chapter 3: Trip 21)*
Moccasin Creek State Park: Non-Game Interpretive Trail *(Chapter 3: Trip 23)*
High Shoals Falls Scenic Area & Falls Trail *(Chapter 3: Trip 25)*
Tallulah Gorge State Park: North Rim, Hurricane Falls, & South Rim Trails *(Chapter 3: Trip 29)*
Sweetwater Creek State Park: History & Non-Game Wildlife Trails Loop *(Chapter 4: Trip 4)*
Stone Mountain Park: Walk-Up Trail *(Chapter 5: Trip 11)*
Panola Mountain State Park: Microwatershed, Rock Outcrop, & Fitness Trails *(Chapter 5: Trip 13)*
Reynolds Nature Preserve *(Chapter 5: Trip 15)*
Fort Yargo State Park: Bird Berry Trail & Trails West of the Lake *(Chapter 6: Trip 2)*
Charlie Elliott Wildlife Center Loop *(Chapter 6: Trip 4)*
Sprewell Bluff State Park: West Trails *(Chapter 7: Trip 1)*
Ocmulgee National Monument: Mound Walk *(Chapter 7: Trip 3)*

Running Trails

Chattahoochee River National Recreation Area: East Palisades Trail *(Chapter 5: Trip 1)*
Chattahoochee River National Recreation Area: Cochran Shoals *(Chapter 5: Trip 4)*
Chattahoochee River National Recreation Area: Sope Creek *(Chapter 5: Trip 5)*
Panola Mountain State Park: Microwatershed, Rock Outcrop, & Fitness Trails *(Chapter 5: Trip 13)*
Little Mulberry Park *(Chapter 6: Trip 1)*

Swimming Holes

Cohutta Wilderness: Jacks River Trail *(Chapter 1: Trip 5)*
High Shoals Falls Scenic Area & Falls Trail *(Chapter 3: Trip 25)*
Watson Mill Bridge State Park: Walking Trail *(Chapter 6: Trip 7)*
Sprewell Bluff State Park: West Trails *(Chapter 7: Trip 1)*

Views

Cloudland Canyon State Park: Overlook, West Rim, & Waterfalls Trails *(Chapter 1: Trip 7)*
Fort Mountain State Park: Gahuti Trail *(Chapter 2: Trip 1)*
Fort Mountain State Park: Stone Wall, Tower, & West Overlook Trails *(Chapter 2: Trip 2)*
Lake Conasauga Recreation Area: Lake, Songbird, & Tower Trails *(Chapter 2: Trip 3)*
Appalachian Trail: Woody Gap to Neels Gap *(Chapter 3: Trip 2)*
Appalachian Trail: Neels Gap to Hog Pen Gap *(Chapter 3: Trip 3)*
Appalachian Trail: Unicoi Gap to Dicks Creek Gap *(Chapter 3: Trip 5)*
Wagon Train Trail *(Chapter 3: Trip 9)*
Arkaquah Trail *(Chapter 3: Trip 10)*
Jacks Knob Trail: North to Brasstown Bald *(Chapter 3: Trip 11)*
Yonah Mountain *(Chapter 3: Trip 16)*
Black Rock Mountain State Park: James E. Edmonds Backcountry Trail *(Chapter 3: Trip 26)*
Tallulah Gorge State Park: North Rim, Hurricane Falls, & South Rim Trails *(Chapter 3: Trip 29)*
Chattahoochee River National Recreation Area: Vickery Creek *(Chapter 5: Trip 8)*
Stone Mountain Park: Walk-Up Trail *(Chapter 5: Trip 11)*
Panola Mountain State Park: Panola Mountain Guided Hike *(Chapter 5: Trip 14)*
Sprewell Bluff State Park: West Trails *(Chapter 7: Trip 1)*

Waterfalls

Cohutta Wilderness: Beech Bottom Trail & Jacks River Falls *(Chapter 1: Trip 2)*
Cloudland Canyon State Park: Overlook, West Rim, & Waterfalls Trails *(Chapter 1: Trip 7)*
Amicalola Falls State Park: Base of Falls Trail *(Chapter 2: Trip 9)*
Desoto Falls Recreation Area: Lower & Upper Falls *(Chapter 2: Trip 17)*
Unicoi State Park: Smith Creek Trail *(Chapter 3: Trip 20)*
Moccasin Creek State Park: Hemlock Falls Trail *(Chapter 3: Trip 24)*
High Shoals Falls Scenic Area & Falls Trail *(Chapter 3: Trip 25)*

Warwoman Dell & Becky Branch Falls Trail *(Chapter 3: Trip 27)*
Rabun Beach Recreation Area: Angel Falls Trail *(Chapter 3: Trip 28)*
Tallulah Gorge State Park: North Rim, Hurricane Falls, & South Rim Trails *(Chapter 3: Trip 29)*
Panther Creek Trail *(Chapter 3: Trip 32)*
Sweetwater Creek State Park: History & Non-Game Wildlife Trails Loop *(Chapter 4: Trip 4)*
F. D. Roosevelt State Park: Wolfden Loop, White Candle, & Beaver Pond Trails *(Chapter 4: Trip 7)*
Chattahoochee River National Recreation Area: Vickery Creek *(Chapter 5: Trip 8)*

Wildflowers

Pocket Recreation Area *(Chapter 1: Trip 12)*
Fort Mountain State Park: Gahuti Trail *(Chapter 2: Trip 1)*
Lake Conasauga Recreation Area: Lake, Songbird, & Tower Trails *(Chapter 2: Trip 3)*
Red Top Mountain State Park: Homestead Loop, Sweetgum, & White Tail Trails *(Chapter 2: Trip 8)*
Len Foote Hike Inn Trail *(Chapter 2: Trip 11)*
Vogel State Park: Coosa Backcountry Trail *(Chapter 2: Trip 15)*
Smithgall Woods: Laurel Ridge Trail *(Chapter 3: Trip 13)*
Black Rock Mountain State Park: James E. Edmonds Backcountry Trail *(Chapter 3: Trip 26)*
Warwoman Dell & Becky Branch Falls Trail *(Chapter 3: Trip 27)*
Stone Mountain Park: Walk-Up Trail *(Chapter 5: Trip 11)*
Panola Mountain State Park: Microwatershed, Rock Outcrop, & Fitness Trails *(Chapter 5: Trip 13)*
Panola Mountain State Park: Panola Mountain Guided Hike *(Chapter 5: Trip 14)*
Reynolds Nature Preserve *(Chapter 5: Trip 15)*
Piedmont National Wildlife Refuge: Red-Cockaded Woodpecker Trail *(Chapter 7: Trip 6)*

Wildlife

Cohutta Wilderness: Hemp Top Trail *(Chapter 1: Trip 3)*
Cohutta Wilderness: Jacks River Trail *(Chapter 1: Trip 5)*
Pocket Recreation Area *(Chapter 1: Trip 12)*
Arrowhead Wildlife Interpretive Trail *(Chapter 1: Trip 14)*
Red Top Mountain State Park: Homestead Loop, Sweetgum, & White Tail Trails *(Chapter 2: Trip 8)*
Len Foote Hike Inn Trail *(Chapter 2: Trip 11)*
Vogel State Park: Coosa Backcountry Trail *(Chapter 2: Trip 15)*
Wagon Train Trail *(Chapter 3: Trip 9)*
Smithgall Woods: Ash Creek Trail & Wetland Loop *(Chapter 3: Trip 14)*
Chicopee Woods: West Lake & East Lake Trails *(Chapter 3: Trip 17)*
Moccasin Creek State Park: Non-Game Interpretive Trail *(Chapter 3: Trip 23)*
F. D. Roosevelt State Park: Wolfden Loop, White Candle, & Beaver Pond Trails *(Chapter 4: Trip 7)*
F. D. Roosevelt State Park: Dowdell Loop Trail *(Chapter 4: Trip 8)*

Chattahoochee River National Recreation Area: East Palisades Trail *(Chapter 5: Trip 1)*
Chattahoochee River National Recreation Area: West Palisades Trail *(Chapter 5: Trip 2)*
Chattahoochee River National Recreation Area: Cochran Shoals *(Chapter 5: Trip 4)*
Reynolds Nature Preserve *(Chapter 5: Trip 15)*
Fort Yargo State Park: Bird Berry Trail & Trails West of the Lake *(Chapter 6: Trip 2)*
Charlie Elliott Wildlife Center Loop *(Chapter 6: Trip 4)*
Hard Labor Creek State Park: Beaver Pond & Brantley Trails *(Chapter 6: Trip 5)*
Sprewell Bluff State Park: West Trails *(Chapter 7: Trip 1)*
Oconee National Forest: Ocmulgee River Trail *(Chapter 7: Trip 5)*
Piedmont National Wildlife Refuge: Red-Cockaded Woodpecker Trail *(Chapter 7: Trip 6)*

Appendix 2
Recommended Books & Maps

Books

Bartram, William, *Travels of William Bartram.* New York, N.Y.: Cosimo, 2007.

Baumgartner, Richard A., and Larry M. Strayer. *Kennesaw Mountain, June 1864: Bitter Standoff at the Gibraltar of Georgia.* Huntington, W.V.: Blue Acorn Press, 2000.

Beaton, Giff. *Birding Georgia.* Helena, Mo.: Falcon, 2000.

Brown, Claud L., and Katherine L. Kirkman. *Trees of Georgia and Adjacent States.* Portland, Ore.: Timber Press, 1990.

Brown, Fred. *The Riverkeeper's Guide to the Chattahoochee River.* Birmingham, Ala.: Menasha Ridge Press, 1997.

Cozzens, Peter. *This Terrible Sound: The Battle of Chickamauga.* Champaign, Ill.: University of Illinois Press, 1996.

Hally, David J. *Ocmulgee Archaeology, 1936–1986.* Athens, Ga.: University of Georgia Press, 1994.

Homan, Tim. *Hiking the Benton MacKaye Trail: A Guide to the Benton MacKaye Trail from Georgia's Springer Mountain to Tennessee's Ocoee River.* Atlanta: Peachtree Publishers, 2004. Homan provides detailed descriptions of each section of the Benton MacKaye Trail and describes various plant species.

———. *Hiking Trails of the Cohutta & Big Frog Wilderness.* Atlanta: Peachtree Publishers, 2000. Includes deep detail on flora and fauna of the Cohutta Wilderness.

Ketelle, Richard H., Don O'Neal, and Lisa Williams. *Appalachian Trail Guide to North Carolina–Georgia: Books and Maps.* Harpers Ferry, W. Va.: Appalachian Trail Conservancy, 2008. An essential companion if you choose to hike multiple sections of the Appalachian Trail, this book provides descriptions of features at specific mileage points and includes helpful comments on water sources and shelters.

Molloy, Johnny. *Long Trails of the Southeast.* Birmingham, Ala.: Menasha Ridge Press, 2002.

National Audubon Society. *National Audubon Society Field Guide to Trees: Eastern Region.* New York: Alfred A. Knopf, 2000.

Nourse, Hugh, and Carol Nourse. *Wildflowers of Georgia.* Athens, Ga.: University of Georgia Press, 2000.

Tekiela, Stan. *Birds of Georgia Field Guide.* Cambridge, Minn.: Adventure Publications, 2002.

Maps

The Appalachian Trail Official Map: Springer Mountain to Bly Gap, Georgia. Harpers Ferry, W. Va.: Appalachian Trail Conservancy, 2008.

Chattahoochee National Forest. Gainesville, Ga.: U.S. Department of Agriculture Forest Service, 2007.

Cohutta and Big Frog Wilderness Georgia-Tennessee map. U.S. Department of Agriculture Forest Service, 1996.

Trails of the Chattahoochee-Oconee National Forests. Gainesville, Ga.: U.S. Department of Agriculture Forest Service, 1998.

Appendix 3
Agencies & Information Sources

State & Federal Agencies

Georgia Department of Natural Resources
www.georgiawildlife.com

Charlie Elliott Wildlife Center
543 Elliott Trail
Mansfield, GA 30055
(770) 784-3059

Commissioners Office
2 Martin Luther King, Jr. Drive, S.E.,
Ste. 1252, East Tower
Atlanta, GA 30334
(404) 656-3500

Wildlife Resources Division
2592 Floyd Springs Rd.
Armuchee, GA 30165
(706) 295-6777

Georgia State Parks
www.gastateparks.org
(800) 864-7275

Amicalola Falls State Park
418 Amicalola Falls Lodge Rd.
Dawsonville, GA 30534
(706) 878-3087

Black Rock Mountain State Park
3085 Black Rock Mtn. Pkwy.
Mountain City, GA 30562
(706) 746-2141

Cloudland Canyon State Park
122 Cloudland Canyon Park
Rising Fawn, GA 30738
(706) 657-4050

F. D. Roosevelt State Park
2970 GA Highway 190
Pine Mountain, GA 31822
(706) 663-4858

Fort Mountain State Park
181 Fort Mountain Park Rd.
Chatsworth, GA 30705
(706) 422-1932

Fort Yargo State Park
210 S. Broad St.
Winder, GA 30680
(770) 867-3489

Georgia State Parks Headquarters
2 Martin Luther King, Jr. Dr.,
Ste. 1352 East
Atlanta, GA 30334
(404) 656-2770

Hard Labor Creek State Park
Knox Chapel Rd.
Rutledge, GA 30663
(706) 557-3001

Moccasin Creek State Park
3655 Highway 197
Clarkesville, GA 30523
(706) 947-3194

New Echota Historic Site
12 Chatsworth Hwy. NE
Calhoun, GA 30701
(706) 624-1321

Panola Mountain State Park
2600 GA Hwy. 155 SW
Stockbridge, GA 30281
(770) 389-7801

Pickett's Mill Battlefield Historic Site
4432 Mt. Tabor Church Rd.
Dallas, GA 30157
(770) 443-7850

Red Top Mountain State Park and Lodge
50 Lodge Rd. SE
Cartersville, GA 30121
Visitors Center: (770) 975-4226
Reservations: (800) 864-7275

Smithgall Woods Conservation Area and Lodge
61 Tsalaki Trail
Helen, GA 30545
(706) 878-3087

Sprewell Bluff State Park
740 Sprewell Bluff Rd.
Thomaston, GA 30286
(706) 646-6026

Sweetwater Creek State Park
1750 Mt. Vernon Rd.
Lithia Springs, GA 30122
(770) 732-5871

Tallulah Gorge State Park
338 Jane Hurt Yarn Rd.
Tallulah Falls, GA 30573
(706) 754-7970

Unicoi State Park
1788 Highway 356 Rd.
Helen, GA 30545
(706) 878-2201

Victoria Bryant State Park
1105 Bryant Park Rd.
Royston, GA 30662
(706) 245-6270

Vogel State Park
7485 Vogel State Park Rd.
Blairsville, GA 30512
(706) 745-2628

Watson Mill Bridge State Park
650 Watson Mill Rd.
Comer, GA 30629
(706) 783-3336

National Park Service
www.nps.gov

Chattahoochee River National Recreation Area
1978 Island Ford Pkwy.
Atlanta, GA 30350
(678) 538-1200

Chickamauga Battlefield
P.O. Box 2128
Fort Oglethorpe, GA 30742
(706) 866-9241

Kennesaw Mountain National Battlefield Park
900 Kennesaw Mountain Dr.
Kennesaw, GA 30152
(770) 427-4686

Ocmulgee National Monument
1207 Emery Hwy.
Macon, GA 31217
(478) 752-8257

U.S. Army Corps of Engineers
www.usace.army.mil

Carters Lake
P.O. Box 96
Oakman, GA 30732
(706) 334-2248

U.S. Forest Service
www.fs.fed.us

Blue Ridge District
1881 Hwy. 515
Blairsville, GA 30512
(706) 695-6736

Chattahoochee-Oconee National Forests
1755 Cleveland Hwy.
Gainesville, GA 30501
(770) 297-3000

Chattooga River District
809 Hwy. 441 S.
Clayton, GA 30525
(706) 782-3320

Conasauga District
3941 Hwy. 76
Chatsworth, GA 30512
(706) 695-6736

Oconee District
1199 Madison Rd.
Eatonton, GA 31024
(706) 485-3180

Other Parks, Preserves, & Private Facilities

Brasstown Valley Resort
6321 U.S. Hwy. 76
Young Harris, GA 30582
(706) 379-9900
www.brasstownvalley.com

Elachee Nature Science Center
2125 Elachee Dr.
Gainesville, GA 30504
(770) 535-1976
www.elachee.org

Gwinnett County Parks & Recreation
75 Langley Dr.
Lawrenceville, GA 30045
(770) 822-8840
www.gwinettcounty.com

Len Foote Hike Inn
240 Amicalola Falls State Park Rd.
Dawsonville, GA 30534
(800) 581-8032
www.hike-inn.com

Sandy Creek Park
400 Holman Rd.
Athens, GA 30601
(706) 613-3631
www.sandycreekpark.com

Stone Mountain Park
U.S. Hwy. 78 E., Exit 8
Stone Mountain, GA 30087
(770) 498-5690
www.stonemountainpark.com

William H. Reynolds Memorial Nature Preserve
5665 Reynolds Rd.
Morrow, GA 30260
(770) 603-4188
http://web.co.clayton.ga.us/reynolds/about.htm

Appendix 4
Conservation Organizations & Trail Groups

Appalachian Trail Conservancy
799 Washington St.
Harpers Ferry, WV 25425
(304) 535-6331
www.appalachiantrail.org

Atlanta Audubon Society
Box 29189
Atlanta, GA 30359
(770) 913-0511
www.atlantaaudubon.org

Benton MacKaye Trail Association
P.O. Box 53271
Atlanta, GA 30355
www.bmta.org

Georgia Appalachian Trail Club
P.O. Box 654
Atlanta, GA 30301
(404) 634-6495
www.georgia-atclub.org

Georgia Botanical Society
2718 Stillwater Lake Ln.
Marietta, GA 30066
(770) 827-5186
www.gabotsoc.org

Georgia Wildlife Federation
11600 Hazelbrand Rd.
Covington, GA 30014
(770) 787-7887
www.gwf.org

Pine Mountain Trail Association
P.O. Box 5
Columbus, GA 31902
www.pinemountaintrail.org

Sierra Club
Georgia Chapter Office
1401 Peachtree St. NE, Ste. 345
Atlanta, GA 30309
(404) 607-1262, ext. 221
http://georgia.sierraclub.org

Index

C

M

N

S

T

U

About the Author

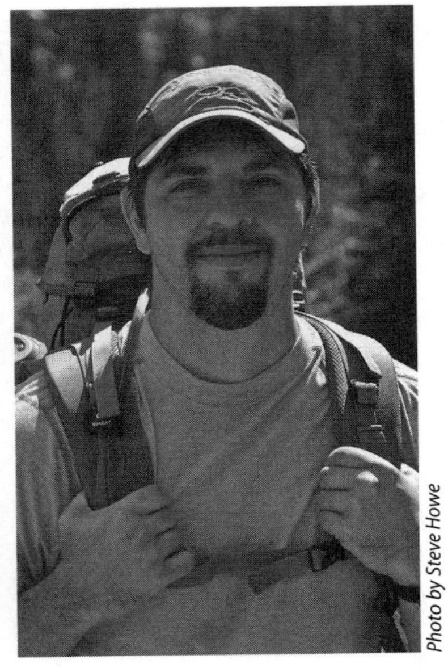

Photo by Steve Howe

Marcus Woolf has written for outdoor publications, such as *Outside* and *Backpacker* magazines, for more than a decade. He is senior editor for *GearTrends*, the leading trade publication for the outdoor recreation industry. While doing the legwork for this book, he survived a nose-to-nose encounter with a bear at 2 AM and a charge from a particularly mean opossum. Woolf is based in the Southeast where he continues his never-ending search for the perfect river rope swing.